OSCE CASES WITH MARK SCHEMES

OSCE CASES WITH MARK SCHEMES

Authors

Dr. Susan Shelmerdine, MBBS (Dist), BSc (hons), MRCS Eng
Specialty Registrar in Clinical Radiology, St. George's Hospital, London

Dr. Tamara North, MBBS
Senior House Officer, Obstetrics and Gynaecology, Royal Surrey County Hospital, Guildford

Mr. Jeremy Lynch, MBChB, MRCS Eng
Core Surgical Trainee, Queen Victoria Hospital, East Grinstead

Miss Aneesha Verma, MBBS (Dist), BSc (hons), MRCS Eng
Core Surgical Trainee, St. Mary's Hospital, London

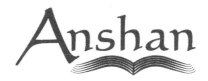

OSCE Cases with Mark Schemes

Published by:

Anshan Ltd
11a Little Mount Sion
Tunbridge Wells
Kent. TN1 1YS

Tel: +44 (0) 1892 557767
Fax: +44 (0) 1892 530358

e-mail: info@anshan.co.uk
website: www.anshan.co.uk

© 2012 Anshan Ltd

ISBN: 978 1 848290 631

All rights reserved. No part of this publication may be reproduced, stored in a retrieval system, or transmitted in any form or by any means, electronic, mechanical, photocopying, recording or otherwise, without the prior written permission of the publisher.

The use of registered names, trademarks, etc, in this publication does not imply, even in the absence of a specific statement that such names are exempt from the relevant laws and regulations and therefore for general use.

While every effort has been made to ensure the accuracy of the information contained within this publication, the publisher can give no guarantee for information about drug dosage and application thereof contained in this book. In every individual case the respective user must check current indications and accuracy by consulting other pharmaceutical literature and following the guidelines laid down by the manufacturers of specific products and the relevant authorities in the country in which they are practicing.

British Library Cataloguing in Publication Data

Copy Editor: Catherine Lain

Cover Design: Susan Shelmerdine

Cover Image: Susan Shelmerdine

Typeset by: Kerrypress Ltd, Luton, Bedfordshire

Printed and bound by: The Lavenham Press, Lavenham, Suffolk

CONTENTS

SECTION 1 – COMMUNICATION SKILLS

Co-written by Dr. S. Shelmerdine, Dr. T. North, Miss A. Verma & Mr. J. Lynch

- Cardiac and Respiratory Stations
- Gastroenterology Stations
- Neurology Stations
- Rheumatology Stations
- Endocrinology Stations
- General Surgery and Urology Stations
- Ear, Nose and Throat Stations
- Ophthalmology Stations

Written by Miss A. Verma

- Depression
- Bipolar Disorder
- Schizophrenia
- Eating Disorder
- Deliberate Self Harm

Written by Dr. S. Shelmerdine & Mr. J. Lynch

- Failure to Thrive
- Developmental Delay
- Abdominal Pain
- Jaundice
- Seizures
- Rash
- Cough

SECTION 2 – CLINICAL SKILLS

ABOUT THE AUTHORS

Dr. SUSAN CHENG SHELMERDINE, MBBS (Dist), BSc (hons), MRCS Eng
Specialty Registrar in Clinical Radiology, St. George's Hospital, London

Susan Shelmerdine graduated from St George's Hospital Medical School where she achieved first class honours in her intercalated BSc degree in Medical Imaging and qualified with distinction in her MBBS. She completed her MRCS during her foundation training and has an active interest in undergraduate education having taught on several courses at the Royal Society of Medicine, Imperial College London and St. George's University. She is currently completing a Postgraduate Certificate in Medical Education and is also an OSCE examiner at St. George's, University of London.

Dr. TAMARA GEORGIA NORTH, MBBS
Senior House Officer, Obstetrics and Gynaecology, Royal Surrey County Hospital, Guildford

Tamara North studied at St George's Hospital Medical School and developed the idea for this current book with Susan Shelmerdine during their undergraduate training. She is currently working in the field of obstetrics and gynaecology with a particular interest in obstetric care. Tamara completed her MRCOG Part 1 during her foundation training and participates actively in teaching undergraduate medical students.

Mr. JEREMY OLIVER LYNCH, MBChB, MRCS Eng
Core Surgical Trainee, Queen Victoria Hospital, East Grinstead

Jeremy Lynch qualified from Bristol University and has had a keen interest in undergraduate education since his medical school days. He is the creator of the popular medical student revision website www.passmed.co.uk and is an OSCE examiner at St. George's, University of London and at Brighton and Sussex Medical School. He has worked in a broad range of surgical specialties and published research in well-respected journals. Jeremy's interests lie in a career in vascular surgery.

Miss ANEESHA RATAN VERMA, MBBS (Dist), BSc (hons), MRCS Eng
Core Surgical Trainee, St. Mary's Hospital, London

Aneesha Verma graduated with a distinction from Imperial College London in 2008. Her intercalated BSc was in Neuroscience and she attained her MRCS in 2010. She tutors for OSCE and PACES medical examinations and has helped set up and deliver a 20-week revision lecture programme for undergraduate students. Aneesha has taught during conferences at the Royal Society of Medicine and the Royal College of Surgeons of England. She has completed formal teaching courses and was a faculty member for the Training and Assessment in Practice course. Aneesha has enjoyed gaining experience in a broad range of specialties including cardiothoracic, vascular, colorectal, breast, orthopaedic, upper gastrointestinal and plastic surgery.

ACKNOWLEDGEMENTS

The authors would like to acknowledge their parents, friends and families for their support and encouragement throughout the writing of this book.

INTRODUCTION

It's nearing the examination and you still feel you know nothing ...

Don't worry, you're not alone! This is an almost universal feeling every medical student goes through at some point in their training – even the most famous professor you can think of was once in your position. The trick is to revise wisely. You may even surprise yourself by your knowledge.

That is where this book comes in. There are countless revision books on the market instructing you on what you need to do and how you should be performing various examinations, but once you have a grasp on that, what next? No other book on the market offers candidates a way of revising and putting into practice what they have learnt. In addition, we have noticed that many medical students are good at knowing what they should be doing but somehow don't always translate this into successful examination results. Our book is unique in providing you with a peek at the type of answers examiners are looking for and providing you with numerous practice stations to test your skills.

We created this book not as a primary instructional tool but as a revision aid for anyone who feels they have a good grasp of basic concepts and is ready to take the next step in fine-tuning their knowledge. This book accurately reflects the examination experience. The best time to use this book is in the weeks running up to the examination after having read through a good general medical textbook.

Some of our top tips on performing well at the examination include the following:
1) Summarise, signpost and check your patient's understanding – this can gain you easy marks, prevent you looking like you don't know what to say, give you time to think of your next question and also remind the examiner of the questions you have already asked in case they didn't hear you the first time!
2) Dress like a doctor – after all, the OSCE is trying to assess whether you act like one! For women this means no low-cut or backless tops. Wear instead clothes which cover your shoulders, skirts at least knee length or longer, hair tied back in either a ponytail or bun. Remove any facial piercings. For men this means an ironed shirt, clean shaven or well-trimmed facial hair and polished shoes. Although you don't get marks awarded for your dress sense, examiners are all human and making a good impression can mean the difference between being offered the benefit of the doubt or not if you make a minor mistake.
3) Do your research – certain universities have 'favourite' stations or topics that seem to be repeated in some form or another every year. Make sure you ask your seniors what they remember being examined on. We're not saying that they will definitely come up, but if they do – you're going to wish you knew beforehand!
4) Practice! Practice! Practice! For clinical examinations it is crucial to practice examining, speaking out loud and getting friends and family to watch and critique you. Take every opportunity you are offered for extra bedside teaching by doctors and ensure you ask clinicians for their feedback on your performance too. You will be examined by several examiners all with slightly different opinions on what they think is good practice, so get as many opinions on your performance as possible to see what the general consensus is on your technique and bedside manner.

Good luck! We hope you find this revision aid useful and welcome any comments for future improvements.

S. Shelmerdine, T. North, J. Lynch, A. Verma

HOW TO USE THIS BOOK

The book is best used for group study in the weeks running up to your OSCE. Each chapter within this book (with the exception of the data interpretation and part of the clinical skills sections) is divided into three broad divisions:

- Scenarios

  This section contains the candidate instructions along with the recommended time allowance in which to complete the task.

- Simulated patient briefings

  This section includes directions and instructions for the 'actor' or 'patient'.

- Mark schemes

  This section contains the list of tasks which the candidate is expected to complete within the station. The examiner is expected to tick which action the candidate has performed within the time limit and also provide some feedback on how well the candidate performed the tasks. In some cases the tasks are allocated a mark of either 0, 1 or 2, whereas others are marked out of 0 or 1. Guidance on what students need to achieve in order to score the higher marks is given within the mark scheme.

  The last check boxes at the bottom of the mark schemes ask for a 'global rating' ranging from 0 to 5. This is not supposed to reflect how many points the candidate has scored but a global impression that the examiner has of the candidate. In real life this ranking helps to determine the pass mark for the station. This is done by constructing a graph with the 'global rating' of all candidates for the station in question lying on the x axis plotted against their station score on the y axis. The average score at which most 'borderline' candidates achieve will then determine the pass mark for the station. As this will obviously alter depending on the year group, the pass mark per station is not necessarily fixed and therefore a 'pass score' per station is not provided in this book. However, we recommend that students using this book aim to achieve a score for each station above 75% to be confident that they will achieve either a 'clear pass' or 'very good' score in their real examinations.

This book has been designed to be used ideally by three students working in a study group, with one person playing the candidate, one person acting as examiner and another pretending to be the patient. However, it is also possible to use this book in pairs (with one person playing both patient and examiner) or in groups larger than three (with perhaps two examiners who provide feedback or another person pretending to be a concerned relative).

Please note that the patient names used in this book are all fictional and do not refer to any real people or actual patients. Any co-incidental correlation of such names with real patients is entirely unintentional.

ABBREVIATIONS

A&E	Accident and Emergency
ABG	Arterial Blood Gas
ABPI	Ankle Brachial Pulse Index
ADLs	Activities of Daily Living (e.g. washing clothes, shopping, cleaning the house etc.)
ADH	Anti-diuretic Hormone
AFP	Alfa-fetoprotein
ANA	Antinuclear Antibody
AST	Aspartate Transaminase
AXR	Abdominal X-ray
BCG	Bacillus Calmette-Guérin
bd	twice a day
BE	Base Excess
B-HcG	Beta-human Chorionic Gonadotrophin
BPH	Benign Prostatic Hypertrophy
bpm	beats/breaths per minute
Ca	Calcium
CABG	Coronary Artery Bypass Graft
CEA	Carcinoembryonic Antigen
CIN	Cervical Intraepithelial Neoplasia
Cl	Chloride
CLO	Campylobacter-Like Organism (used in the phrase 'CLO test' to look for Helicobacter Pylori when investigating a patient with gastric/duodenal ulcers)
CNS	Central Nervous System
CO2	Carbon Dioxide
COPD	Chronic Obstructive Pulmonary Disease
CRP	C-reactive Protein
CSF	Cerebrospinal Fluid
CT	Computed Tomography
CT KUB	Computed Tomography of Kidneys, Ureters and Bladder
CVA	Cerebrovascular Accident
CXR	Chest X-ray
DEXA	Dual Energy X-ray Absorptiometry
DKA	Diabetic Ketoacidosis
DMARD	Disease Modifying Anti-Rheumatic Drugs
DNAR	Do Not Attempt Resuscitation
DVT	Deep Vein Thrombosis
ECG	Electrocardiogram
ECHO	Echocardiogram
EDH	Extradural Haemorrhage
EEG	Electroencephalogram
ERCP	Endoscopic Retrograde Cholangio-Pancreatoduodenoscopy
ERPC	Evacuation of Retained Products of Conception
ESR	Erythrocyte Sedimentation Rate
ETOH	Alcohol
ETT	Exercise Tolerance Test
FBC	Full Blood Count
FBS	Foetal Blood Sampling
FNA	Fine Needle Aspiration

GCS	Glasgow Coma Score
GDM	Gestational Diabetes Mellitus
GP	General Practitioner
GTN	Glycerine Trinitrate
Hb	Haemoglobin
HbA1C	Glycated Haemoglobin
HCO3	Bicarbonate
HIV	Human Immunodeficiency Virus
HLA-B27	Human Leukocyte Antigen – B27
HONK	Hyperosmolar Hyperglycaemic Non-Ketotic Acidosis
ICB	Intracerebral Bleed
IMB	Intermenstrual Bleeding
inh	Inhaler
INR	International Normalised Ratio
ISMN	Isosorbide Mononitrate
IUGR	Intra-Uterine Growth Retardation
IV	Intravenous
IVF	In Vitro Fertilisation
IVU	Intravenous Urogram
JVP	Jugular Venous Pulse/Pressure
K	Potassium
KCI	Potassium Chloride
KUB	Kidney, Ureters, Bladder (an abbreviation used in conjunction when talking about a computed tomography or X-ray imaging scan to describe the renal system being examined)
LDH	Lactate Dehydrogenase
LFT	Liver Function Tests
LLETZ	Large Loop Excision of the Transformation Zone
MAU/AMU	Medical Assessment Unit/Acute Medical Unit
MC&S	Microscopy, Culture & Sensitivity
MDI	Metered Dose Inhaler
MHA	Mental Health Act
MI	Myocardial Infarct
MRCP	Magnetic Resonance Cholangiopancreatography
MRI	Magnetic Resonance Imaging
Na	Sodium
NG	Nasogastric
NKDA	No Known Drug Allergies
NSAIDs	Non-Steroidal Anti-Inflammatory Drugs
O2	Oxygen
OA	Osteoarthritis
OCP	Oral Contraceptive Pill
od	once a day
OGD	Oesophogastroduodenoscopy
on	once a night
PA	Posterior-Anterior
PaCO2/PCO2	Partial Pressure of Carbon Dioxide
PaO2/PO2	Partial Pressure of Oxygen
PAPP-A	Pregnancy Associated Plasma Protein A
PC	Presenting Complaint
PCA	Patient Controlled Analgesia
PCB	Post-coital Bleeding

PCR	Polymerase Chain Reaction
PE	Pulmonary Embolism
PEFR	Peak Expiratory Flow Rate
PMB	Post Menopausal Bleeding
po	per oral
PR	Per Rectum
prn	as required
PSA	Prostate Specific Antigen
PV	Per Vaginal
qds	four times a day
RA	Rheumatoid Arthritis
SAH	Subarachnoid Haemorrhage
sc	Subcutaneous
SDH	Subdural Haemorrhage
SIADH	Syndrome of Inappropriate ADH
sl	Sublingual
SOB	Shortness of Breath
SPD	Symphysis Pubis Dysfunction
TB	Tuberculosis
tds	three times daily
TIA	Transient Ischaemic Attack
ToP	Termination of Pregnancy
TURP	Transurethral Resection of the Prostate
U&E	Urea and Electrolytes
V/Q	Ventilation-Perfusion
VTE	Venous Thromboembolism

SECTION 1 – COMMUNICATION SKILLS

CHAPTER 1: GENERAL MEDICAL AND SURGICAL HISTORIES

Co-written by Dr. S. Shelmerdine, Dr. T. North, Miss A. Verma & Mr. J. Lynch

- Cardiac and Respiratory Stations
- Gastroenterology Stations
- Neurology Stations
- Rheumatology Stations
- Endocrinology Stations
- General Surgery and Urology Stations
- Ear, Nose and Throat Stations
- Ophthalmology Stations

THE STATIONS

CARDIAC AND RESPIRATORY STATIONS

STATION 1
Time allowed: 10 minutes

You are a junior doctor working in a general practice.

Mr Nassir Trujillo is a middle-aged man who has come into your clinic today complaining of chest pain. He looks rather worried and he has asked for an urgent appointment.

Please take a focussed history from him and formulate a management plan.

STATION 2
Time allowed: 10 minutes

You are a junior doctor working in the Accident and Emergency department.

Miss Martha Albertson has come into the department complaining of chest pain and looks out of breath. She has been brought in by her boyfriend who is keen for her to be seen as soon as possible.

Please take a focussed history from her and formulate a management plan.

STATION 3
Time allowed: 10 minutes

You are a junior doctor working in general practice.

Mr Trevor Jakab, a young man, has come into the surgery today with his mother complaining of chest pains.

Please take a focussed history from him and suggest a differential diagnosis.

The examiner will stop you at 7 minutes to ask you a few questions.

STATION 4
Time allowed: 10 minutes

You are a junior doctor working in the Accident and Emergency department.

Mrs Nadine Bieber is a middle-aged lady who has come into the department with her daughter complaining of feeling nauseated, dizzy and generally 'not right'.

Please take a focussed history from her and suggest a differential diagnosis.

The examiner will stop you at 7 minutes to ask you a few questions.

STATION 5
Time allowed: 10 minutes

You are a junior doctor working in the Accident and Emergency department.

Mr Gopala Kaur, a middle-aged man, has attended the department complaining of feeling unwell, is short of breath and coughing up blood. He looks drawn out and tired but says he needs to be investigated straight away.

Please take a focussed history from him and formulate a differential diagnosis.

STATION 6

Time allowed: 10 minutes

You are a junior doctor working in the Accident and Emergency department.

Mrs Thulani Patel, an elderly lady, has just been brought into the department by ambulance from her nursing home with difficulty breathing.

Please take a focussed history from her and formulate a differential diagnosis.

The examiner will stop you at 7 minutes to ask you a few questions.

STATION 7

Time allowed: 10 minutes

You are a junior doctor working on the general medical ward.

Mr Cyrano Stoppelheim, an elderly man, has been admitted to your ward with weight loss and shortness of breath.

Please take a history from Mr Stoppelheim and formulate a differential diagnosis.

After 7 minutes the examiner will stop you to ask you some questions.

STATION 8

Time allowed: 10 minutes

You are a junior doctor working in general practice.

Mrs Rosie Birchling has come to see you in clinic because she is concerned that she is getting more 'puffy' these days.

Please take a history from Mrs Birchling regarding her symptoms.

After 7 minutes the examiner will ask you for your differential diagnoses.

GASTROENTEROLOGY STATIONS

STATION 9

Time allowed: 10 minutes

You are a junior doctor working in the Accident and Emergency department.

Mr Young is an elderly gentleman who complains of feeling bloated and says he has been vomiting.

Please take a focussed history from him and formulate a management plan.

The examiner will stop you at 7 minutes to ask you a few questions.

STATION 10

Time allowed: 10 minutes

You are a junior doctor working in the Accident and Emergency department.

Mrs Johnson is brought in by ambulance still wearing her pyjamas after having vomiting a large amount. She is unkempt, looks unwell and is very anxious.

Please take a focussed history from her and formulate an emergency management plan.

The examiner will stop you at 7 minutes to ask you a few questions.

STATION 11
Time allowed: 10 minutes

You are a junior doctor working in the Accident and Emergency department.

Mr Hodge has come to the department with his friends after a night out. His friends are laughing and prodding him. They jokingly poke him and say 'Come on, dude, stop pretending! We've brought you to hospital now!' The patient looks very tired, annoyed and worse for wear.

Please take a focussed history from him and formulate a management plan.

The examiner will stop you at 7 minutes to ask you a few questions.

STATION 12
Time allowed: 10 minutes

You are a junior doctor and your consultant asks you to see the following patient in his outpatient clinic.

Mr Lewis is an elderly chap with a history of difficulty swallowing who has been referred by her General Practitioner.

Please take a focussed history from him and formulate a management plan.

The examiner will stop you at 7 minutes to ask you a few questions.

STATION 13
Time allowed: 10 minutes

You are a junior doctor in an outpatient clinic.

Mr Joles is a middle-aged gentleman who presents with a history of passing blood through his back passage. He appears rather shaken and alarmed.

Please take a focussed history from him and formulate a management plan.

The examiner will stop you at 7 minutes to ask you a few questions.

STATION 14
Time allowed: 10 minutes

You are a junior doctor working in general practice.

Mr Butcher has come to see you as he has been passing blood from his back passage. You notice that he is looking rather pale.

Please take a focussed history from him and formulate a diagnosis and management plan.

After 7 minutes the examiner will stop you to ask questions.

STATION 15
Time allowed: 10 minutes

You are a junior doctor working in the Accident and Emergency department.

Miss Sharma is a young lady who has come to hospital complaining of abdominal pain. You notice that she is stooped over and is holding onto her abdomen as she walks. Her eyes look wet as if she has been in tears recently.

Please take a history from her and formulate a diagnosis and management plan.

After 7 minutes the examiner will stop you to ask questions.

STATION 16
Time allowed: 10 minutes

You are a junior doctor working in general practice.

Mrs Poole is a rather rotund young lady who has come to see you today complaining of abdominal pain and really wants something sorted as she is upset that she hasn't been able to eat as much as usual.

Please take a history from her and formulate an appropriate management plan.

After 7 minutes the examiner will ask you some questions.

STATION 17
Time allowed: 10 minutes

You are a junior doctor working in the Accident and Emergency department.

Mrs Mumford has come to the hospital today with abdominal pain. She is accompanied by her husband who looks very concerned and tells you that his wife needs urgent help.

Please take a history and formulate a diagnosis and management plan.

After 7 minutes the examiner will ask you some questions.

STATION 18
Time allowed: 10 minutes

You are a junior doctor working in general practice.

Mr James O'Leary is a young man who has come to see you in clinic today with his mum as he has been having diarrhoea. He looks rather embarrassed to have her in the room with him.

Please take a history from the patient and formulate a differential diagnosis and management plan.

After 7 minutes the examiner will stop you to ask you some questions.

STATION 19
Time allowed: 10 minutes

You are a junior doctor working in the Accident and Emergency department.

Miss Casey Lee has come into hospital as she has been having diarrhoea. You notice that her tank top and jeans look rather loose on her delicate frame.

Please take a history from the patient and formulate a differential diagnosis and management plan.

After 7 minutes the examiner will stop you to ask you some questions.

NEUROLOGY STATIONS

STATION 20
Time allowed: 10 minutes

You are a junior doctor working in a general practice.

Miss Blanchard is a young lady who has come into your surgery looking tired and wearing dark sunglasses. She is holding her head in her hands and is complaining of a headache.

Please take a focussed history from her and formulate a management plan.

STATION 21
Time allowed: 10 minutes

You are a junior doctor working in the Accident and Emergency department.

Miss Vamos has come into the department and is complaining of feeling generally run down and unwell. She has been brought in by her friends as she is too weak to walk into the department herself.

Please take a focussed history from her and formulate an emergency management plan.

The examiner will stop you at 7 minutes to ask you a few questions.

STATION 22
Time allowed: 10 minutes

You are a junior doctor working in the Accident and Emergency department.

Mrs Hodgkiss is a middle-aged lady who has come into the department with her husband complaining of a bad headache.

Please take a focussed history from her and formulate a management plan.

The examiner will stop you at 7 minutes to ask you a few questions.

STATION 23
Time allowed: 10 minutes

You are a junior doctor working in the Medical Assessment Unit (MAU).

Mrs Mabellie, an elderly woman, has just been admitted to your ward with headaches.

Please take a focussed history from her and suggest a differential diagnosis.

The examiner will stop you at 7 minutes to ask you a few questions.

STATION 24
Time allowed: 10 minutes

You are a junior doctor working in the Accident and Emergency department.

Miss Parkins has just been brought into the department by ambulance looking rather pale and clammy.

Please take a focussed history from her and formulate a differential diagnosis.

STATION 25
Time allowed: 10 minutes

You are a junior doctor working in the Accident and Emergency department.

Mr Gordon has been brought into the department by his friends after collapsing whilst playing football in the park. He is currently alert but quite drowsy.

Please take a focussed history from him and formulate a differential diagnosis and management plan.

After 7 minutes the examiner will stop you to ask questions.

STATION 26
Time allowed: 10 minutes

You are a junior doctor working on the general medical ward.

Mrs Lafayette has been admitted to your ward with bruising and complaining of being 'off legs'. She is an elderly woman and looks a little confused and bewildered at being in hospital. Her daughter has accompanied her.

Please take a history from Mrs Lafayette's daughter regarding her mother's admittance to hospital.

After 7 minutes the examiner will stop you to ask for your differential diagnoses.

STATION 27
Time allowed: 10 minutes

You are a junior doctor working in general practice.

Mr Warding has come to see you in clinic because his wife has been complaining that he has been getting a lot more forgetful.

Please take a history from Mr Warding regarding his symptoms and paying attention to his concerns.

After 7 minutes the examiner will ask you for your differential diagnoses.

STATION 28
Time allowed: 10 minutes

You are a junior doctor working in general practice.

Mrs Lacey is an elderly lady who has come to visit you in clinic accompanied by her carer. Her carer is concerned that she has been getting more confused lately.

Please take a history from the carer and formulate a differential diagnosis and management plan.

After 7 minutes the examiner will ask you for your differential diagnoses.

STATION 29
Time allowed: 10 minutes

You are a junior doctor working in the Accident and Emergency department.

Mr Kettering is a middle-aged man who has been brought into the hospital by his wife after waking up and complaining of left-sided weakness.

Please take a history from the patient and formulate a differential diagnosis and immediate management plan.

After 7 minutes the examiner will stop you to ask you some questions.

STATION 30
Time allowed: 10 minutes

You are a junior doctor working in general practice.

Mr Scott has come to see you today because he has not been feeling himself for the last week or so. He has told the receptionist that he is complaining of 'strange sensations' and feeling 'different somehow'.

Please take a history from Mr Scott and formulate a differential diagnosis.

After 7 minutes the examiner will stop you to ask you a few questions.

STATION 31

Time allowed: 7 minutes

You are a junior doctor working in the Accident and Emergency department.

Mr Timothy McAfee stopped drinking two days ago and presents today feeling very unwell. He tells you he feels rotten and wants your help desperately.

Please take a complete medical history from Mr McAfee in the allocated time.

RHEUMATOLOGY STATIONS

STATION 32

Time allowed: 10 minutes

You are a junior doctor working in general practice.

Mrs Goring complains of painful joints in her hands. You notice that she is wrapped up under many layers of clothing.

Please take a focussed history from her and formulate a management plan.

The examiner will stop you at 7 minutes to ask you a few questions.

STATION 33

Time allowed: 10 minutes

You are a junior doctor working in general practice.

Mrs Bets complains of painful joints. As she walks into your clinic's office you notice she is limping.

Please take a focussed history from her and formulate a management plan.

The examiner will stop you at 7 minutes to ask you a few questions.

STATION 34

Time allowed: 10 minutes

You are a junior doctor working in the Accident and Emergency department.

Mr Bowman is complaining of painful joints. He has his right wrist bandaged up and is holding it rather gingerly, whilst taking care that no one walks into him.

Please take a focussed history from him and formulate a management plan.

The examiner will stop you at 7 minutes to ask you a few questions.

STATION 35

Time allowed: 10 minutes

You are a junior doctor working in general practice.

Mrs Larson is complaining of painful hands. She is looking rather impatient in the waiting room and really wants you to help her.

Please take a focussed history from her and formulate a management plan.

The examiner will stop you at 7 minutes to ask you a few questions.

STATION 36
Time allowed: 10 minutes

You are a junior doctor working in general practice.

Mr Henry is a young gentleman who has come in to see you complaining of lower back pains.

Please take a focussed history from him and formulate a management plan.

The examiner will stop you at 7 minutes to ask you a few questions.

ENDOCRINOLOGY STATIONS

STATION 37
Time allowed: 10 minutes

You are a junior doctor working in general practice.

Mrs Ahern has attended your clinic because of feeling generally fatigued and is complaining of weight loss.

Please take a history from her and formulate a differential diagnosis.

After 7 minutes the examiner will stop you to ask you a few questions.

STATION 38
Time allowed: 10 minutes

You are a junior doctor working in general practice.

Miss Evergreen has come to see you today because she has been feeling 'just not with it' recently. She has told the nurse that she just can't seem to find the energy anymore to go about her daily tasks and wants to find out if there is a medical cause for this.

Please take a history from Miss Evergreen and formulate a differential diagnosis.

After 7 minutes the examiner will stop you to ask you a few questions.

GENERAL SURGERY AND UROLOGY STATIONS

STATION 39
Time allowed: 10 minutes

You are a junior doctor working in general surgery.

Mr Arthur Monty attends the urology clinic complaining of haematuria.

Please take a history from this patient and formulate a differential diagnosis.

After 7 minutes the examiner will stop you to ask you a few questions.

STATION 40
Time allowed: 7 minutes

You are a junior doctor working in the urology clinic.

Mr Albert Clower is a new patient who has come to you today with a lump in his left scrotum. He is rather embarrassed about this and would prefer to see a male doctor but will 'settle' for a female doctor if there isn't anyone else around.

Please take a complete medical history from Mr Clower regarding this new lump.

After 7 minutes the examiner will stop you to ask you a few questions.

STATION 41
Time allowed: 7 minutes

You are a junior doctor working in the urology clinic.

Mr Harold Mariano is a very prim elderly patient who has come to see you complaining of poor urinary stream. He has come with his wife but would like her to not be present during your consultation as he is a little shy of talking about such 'vulgar' matters.

Please take a complete medical history from Mr Mariano regarding his urinary complaints.

After 7 minutes the examiner will stop you to ask you a few questions.

STATION 42
Time allowed: 10 minutes

You are a junior doctor working in general practice.

Mrs Melinda Jasper is a new patient who has come to you today with a breast lump. She would like to be seen by a female doctor and will only speak to a male doctor if he promises not to examine her.

Please take a history from this patient and formulate a differential diagnosis.

After 7 minutes the examiner will stop you to ask you a few questions.

STATION 43
Time allowed: 7 minutes

You are a junior doctor working in general practice.

Miss Louise Easterling has presented today with 'stuff' coming out of her right breast.

Please take a complete medical history from Miss Easterling in the allocated time.

After 7 minutes the examiner will stop you to ask you a few questions.

STATION 44
Time allowed: 10 minutes

You are a junior doctor working in Accident and Emergency.

Mr Roger Palmer, an elderly gentleman, has attended your department today complaining of a lump in his groin. You notice he is wearing rather baggy trousers.

Please take a history from this patient and formulate a differential diagnosis.

After 7 minutes the examiner will stop you to ask you a few questions.

EAR, NOSE AND THROAT STATIONS

STATION 45
Time allowed: 10 minutes

You are a junior doctor working in a busy ENT clinic.

Mrs Gertrude Mclaurin is a patient who has come to see you today. She looks flustered and says that she has been suffering from almost daily nosebleeds.

Please take a history from this patient and formulate a differential diagnosis.

After 7 minutes the examiner will stop you to ask you a few questions.

STATION 46
Time allowed: 10 minutes

You are a junior doctor working in general practice.

Mrs Judith Shumaker is a patient who has been having trouble with her hearing recently. You have to call her name three times before she perks up and hears you. As she walks over to you she says 'Speak up now won't you?!'

Please take a history from this patient and formulate a differential diagnosis.

After 7 minutes the examiner will stop you to ask you a few questions.

STATION 47
Time allowed: 10 minutes

You are a junior doctor working in general practice.

Mrs Rhonda Smyth is a middle-aged lady who has come to you today to discuss her dizzy spells. She looks rather fed up and keeps holding her head in her hands.

Please take a history from this patient and formulate a differential diagnosis.

After 7 minutes the examiner will stop you to ask you a few questions.

OPTHALMOLOGY STATIONS

STATION 48
Time allowed: 10 minutes

You are a junior doctor working in general practice.

Mr Donner, a rather large gentleman, has come into the surgery today to speak to you about problems with his vision.

Please take a history from him and formulate a differential diagnosis.

After 7 minutes the examiner will stop you to ask you a few questions.

STATION 49
Time allowed: 10 minutes

You are a junior doctor working in general practice.

Mr Raphael Lakeside is a young gentleman who attends clinic with red and itchy eyes.

Please take a history from this patient and formulate a differential diagnosis.

After 7 minutes the examiner will stop you to ask you a few questions.

STATION 50
Time allowed: 10 minutes

You are a junior doctor working in general practice.

Miss Jemima Rolando is a young lady who attends clinic with red and itchy eyes. She appears to be rather distressed.

Please take a history from this patient and formulate a differential diagnosis.

After 7 minutes the examiner will stop you to ask you a few questions.

STATION 51
Time allowed: 10 minutes

You are a junior doctor working in general practice.

Mr James Smythson is a young gentleman who attends clinic with red and itchy eyes and appears rather impatient to talk to you.

Please take a history from this patient and formulate a differential diagnosis.

After 7 minutes the examiner will stop you to ask you a few questions.

STATION 52
Time allowed: 10 minutes

You are a junior doctor working in general practice.

Miss Sarah Young attends clinic complaining with problems with her sight.

Please take a history from this patient and formulate a differential diagnosis.

After 7 minutes the examiner will stop you to ask you a few questions.

SIMULATED PATIENT BRIEFINGS

STATION 1

Name: Mr Nassir Trujillo

Age: 53 years old

Job: Retired shopkeeper

PC:

You are known to have angina, diagnosed about five years ago, which you think is relatively well controlled. You usually get central chest pain and heaviness after running for a bus or after a big meal. When this happens you take a few puffs of your GTN spray and the pain subsides.

However, for the first time last week you experienced the same chest pain whilst watching television. This was the first time it has ever happened at rest. The pain was central, tight and did not radiate anywhere. You felt clammy and sweaty at the time but did not vomit or faint. You deny palpitations or shortness of breath. The severity of the pain was probably 7 out of 10. The intense pain only lasted for three minutes and gradually subsided over the next 20 minutes. You tried to use your GTN spray but it did not help. You decided to ignore the episode at the time because you felt better afterwards and did not want to cause a fuss.

Nevertheless you experienced a similar episode today whilst reading a magazine in the park about one hour ago. The pain, severity and characteristics were identical to the event last week. The event lasted a bit longer this time, for about seven minutes and you are still in pain now although it is starting to ease off. Nothing makes the pain better or worse. Again your GTN spray did not help.

You have not been abroad anywhere, have not had any infective symptoms and do not suffer from orthopnoea or paroxysmal nocturnal dyspnoea. You deny any recent hospital admissions.

Past Medical History:

Angina, hypertension, hypercholesterolaemia.

You have never had any heart attacks or heart surgery.

You do not know what the doctor is talking about if they mention the words 'coronary angiogram'.

Your angina has been solely managed by your GP and you have never had any referrals to cardiology.

Drug History:

You do not have any allergies.

GTN spray, 2 puffs, sublingual, prn

Simvastatin 20mg po on

Aspirin 75mg po od

Bisoprolol 1.25mg po od

Lisinopril 5mg po od

Social History:

You have smoked 20 cigarettes a day for the last 30 years and only drink alcohol in social settings.

You lead a very sedentary lifestyle and spend your days either visiting friends, doing the crossword and Sudoku puzzles, reading the newspaper or pottering around the house.

You do not do any exercise but you say that it is good for your health to not do this because 'you don't want to bring on the angina'.

You love fatty, fried food and have a very sweet tooth.

Family History:

Your father died of a heart attack aged 54 years old and your brother has recently had to undergo a cardiac bypass operation for 'blocked arteries'.

Ideas/Concerns/Expectations:

You are very worried that you are having a heart attack. You think that because you ignored the first event this means the damage is much worse and there is probably no hope for you now.

Diagnosis:

Acute coronary syndrome – unstable (crescendo) angina

Differentials:

Myocardial infarct

Management:

The management of unstable (crescendo) angina should be treated as a medical emergency.

Immediate investigations include:

Blood tests (FBC, U&E, LFTs, glucose, serial troponins)

ECG to look for ST segment changes

Chest X-ray

Referral for coronary angiogram +/- angioplasty if necessary.

Immediate medical management should include:

Oxygen (high flow)

Analgesia (e.g. morphine with an antiemetic)

Aspirin 300mg po stat

Clopidogrel 300mg po stat (important to still give this medication even if the patient is known to be going for a coronary angiogram +/- percutaneous coronary intervention).

Consider a glycoprotein 2b/3a inhibitor (e.g. tirofiban) in patients who are high/intermediate risk.

And offer unfractionated heparin to patients if coronary angiography will be within 24 hours (if it will be in over 24 hour's time then fondaparinux is acceptable).

STATION 2

Name: Mrs Martha Albertson

Age: 30 years old

Job: Fashion designer

PC:

For the last 10 hours you have been experiencing an odd sort of right-sided chest pain. It is sharp and constant in nature but worse on breathing in. You have taken paracetamol to make it go away but this doesn't completely help. The severity of the pain is about 7 out of 10. You do not think the pain is getting worse but it is certainly not improving at all. Although you are not short of breath, you do find it hard to breathe in deeply because of the pain. You have not had any haemoptysis or sputum production. You are not feverish or clammy or sweaty and deny any rigors. No one close to you has had similar symptoms. You have never had this sort of feeling before and don't know what it is.

You were married one month ago and have recently been away for three weeks on your honeymoon to Tahiti in the French Polynesian islands. The flight was about 10 hours long and you only arrived back to England yesterday.

Only if questioned you reveal to the doctor that you think in the last 24 hours your right calf is also a little tender and perhaps slightly swollen. You didn't think to mention it because you normally wear quite high heels and thought that perhaps your feet were just a little tired from walking in them.

Past Medical History:

You are generally fit and well.

Bilateral breast augmentation operation done privately about four years ago.

Regular botox injections to the upper lip and sides of the eyes.

No one in your family has ever had a stroke, heart attack, pulmonary embolism or any blood disorders.

Drug History:

You are allergic to penicillin. It causes you to have a severe rash and a tight throat but you have never had to be admitted to hospital for this and do not carry an EpiPen with you.

Microgynon 30 oral contraceptive pill

Paracetamol 1g po qds prn

Social History:

You are a fashion designer and have quite a hectic life travelling the world and visiting fashion shows. You like to experience fashion in different cultures and want to bring that 'international feel' to your designs.

You gave up smoking three months ago as you want to try for a family soon and think this is a good idea, and you only drink at social occasions. When you used to smoke you only had 5 cigarettes a day for 10 years.

You do not take any recreational drugs.

Ideas/Concerns/Expectations:

You and your husband would really like to try for a family. Although you are on the OCP currently, you would really like to stop it in the next few months and try for a child. You would like to know if you need any medication and if it would be dangerous to try for a baby whilst on this medicine.

Diagnosis:

Pulmonary embolism

Differentials:

Lower respiratory tract infection pneumonia pneumothorax, aortic dissection

Management:

After a full history, examination and clinical observations the initial investigations should include:

Blood tests (FBC, U&E, LFT, CRP, d-dimer, serial troponins if history unclear)

Chest X-ray

ECG (the classical sign of S1Q3T3 is actually quite rare – you are more likely to find just a sinus tachycardia in patients with a pulmonary embolism, or the ECG may just be normal)

ABG (to check PaO2 levels and saturations – on air if possible)

CT pulmonary angiogram (CTPA) to identify location of pulmonary embolism or V/Q perfusion study*

* If the patient is pregnant and also complains of calf swelling it is wise to obtain a Duplex Scan of her leg to determine whether there is a deep venous thrombosis present instead of using ionising radiation. This is because the treatment option for a DVT is the same as for a PE and therefore ordering a CTPA for sole identification of a PE is inconsequential.

Management would include anticoagulation:

Oxygen (high flow)

Analgesia (morphine if severe)

Low molecular weight heparin injections subcutaneously (e.g. dalteparin) initially until INR in range with warfarin or if there are contraindications to starting warfarin (e.g. pregnancy)

Warfarin (loading dose of 5mg until INR in range of 2.0–3.0 for at least three months and in some cases a period of 6 months is warranted)

TEDS (thromboembolic deterrent stockings)

Advice on the future prevention of thromboembolic disease i.e. hydration, exercise, stop smoking, cessation of the contraceptive pill etc.

IVC filters are controversial but in some instances such as recurrent thrombotic events, they may be considered. Discuss these cases with an interventional radiologist and haematologist.

STATION 3

Name: Mr Trevor Jakab

Age: 19 years old

Job: Economics student

PC:

You have been feeling very 'fluey' recently and just 'not right'. For the last week you have had high temperatures, a cough, sore throat and general muscle ache. Many students in your halls of residence have similar symptoms and you think you all passed the 'flu' around to each other. You visited your GP last week at the start of your symptoms and he told you it was most likely viral and to stay hydrated in bed at home and have plenty of sleep.

You followed his advice and things were getting a bit better until the last day or so when you noticed that you developed some chest pains and spiked another high temperature. The pains are central and stabbing in nature, and get worse on breathing inwards. You do feel a little short of breath but no more so than you have felt in the last week. You do not have any rigors, sweating or vomiting associated with this chest pain. You think the pain is slightly better when you sit up and forwards and for this reason you have tried to sleep in this position all night and are now very tired! The pain is constant, does not radiate and is about a 6 out of 10 in severity. You describe it as a dull ache. It does get slightly worse if you press on your chest wall.

You have never had any chest or heart problems in your life and have never had any previous cardiac investigations. You certainly have never had any symptoms like this.

Past Medical History:

You are fit and well.

Drug History:

You do not take any regular medications and do not have any allergies.

Paracetamol 1g po qds prn (since the flu started)

Social History:

You live in the university halls of residence.

You like to go out drinking but only socially and do not smoke.

You have been living at home with your parents since the flu and your mother has been looking after you throughout this event.

Family History:

None significant.

Ideas/Concerns/Expectations:

You are worried that you are having a heart attack and very upset that something like this can happen to you at such a young age when you don't even have a family history of it. You think this is all totally unfair.

Diagnosis:

Pericarditis

Differentials:

Gastroenteritis, costochondritis, pericardial effusion

Management:

Infection with a virus is the most common cause of pericarditis. The infective culprit is classically Coxsackie B virus but can include mumps, influenza or echoviruses.

Blood test: FBC, U&E, LFTs, CRP.

Other: Chest X-ray, ECG, ECHO.

Management is usually conservative with NSAIDs such as ibuprofen and most patients have an uneventful recovery within a few weeks without any long-term cardiac damage.

STATION 4

Name: Mrs Nadine Bieber

Age: 56 years old

Job: Unemployed

PC:

You were out and about in town this afternoon with your daughter shopping for clothes to wear to your best friend's birthday party this weekend when you suddenly came over all 'funny'. You say that almost out of the blue you felt sweaty and clammy and knew you needed to sit down. When you found a bench in the shop to sit on you felt very nauseated and dizzy like everything was spinning. Your daughter says you looked very pale and that she noticed you panting to catch your breath. The whole episode lasted about five minutes and afterwards you just felt very sleepy and drained. You did not have any chest pains during the episode and deny being sick although you desperately thought you were going to be.

You have not had any similar episodes before. You deny palpitations, neurological symptoms or any shortness of breath. At the moment all you want to do is lie down and have a nap. Your daughter was very worried and thought coming to the hospital first would be a better idea than continuing to go shopping or sleeping at home.

In the last month you have been feeling fine and did not suffer from any colds, flues or coughs. You have not had any contact with anyone suffering from infections and have not travelled abroad. You have not lost weight or had any change in your appetite or bowel habits. You do not suffer from orthopnoea and sleep with one pillow at night. You never wake up in the middle of the night and you are a deep sleeper.

Past Medical History:

Type 2 diabetes (Your diabetes is poorly controlled and your last HbA1c a month ago was 11%. Your BMs are always erratic and so you don't really bother checking them as you don't really understand what do to about them. You do not admit this to the doctor unless specifically asked.)

Hypertension

Hypercholesterolaemia

Laser therapy to retinas several times for diabetic retinopathy

Gout

You deny ever having any cardiac investigations or a previous heart attack.

Drug History:

NKDA

Metformin 500mg po bd

Doxazosin 2mg po od

Pravastatin 40mg po od

Allopurinol 300mg po od

Social History:

You have smoked 20 cigarettes a day for the last 10 years. You drink about three glasses of wine a week, mostly during the weekends at mealtimes with your friends and family. You do not take any recreational drugs.

You are divorced and live in your own small one bed roomed apartment. You have one daughter who is 30 years old and works in a bakery. You do not do work and spend most of your days either visiting your daughter or meeting up with your friends.

Family History:

Your father died at the age of 58 years old after a sudden severe brain haemorrhage.

Your mother and aunt both suffered with type 2 diabetes when they were in their fifties.

Ideas/Concerns/Expectations:

You think that this funny episode was all due to a 'mini-stroke' and you worry that it may only be a matter of time before you experience a full-blown stroke and die in the same way your father did!

Diagnosis:

Silent myocardial infarct

Differentials:

Vasovagal syncope, panic attack, viral flu, angina

Management:

Immediate investigations include:

Blood tests (FBC, U&E, LFTs, glucose, lipids, clotting screen, serial troponins)

ECG to look for ST segment changes

Chest X-ray

Referral for coronary angiogram +/- angioplasty if necessary (in some centres thrombolysis may be an alternative consideration).

Immediate medical management should include:

Oxygen (high flow)

Analgesia (e.g. 5–10mg morphine with an antiemetic)

Aspirin 300mg po stat

GTN sublingual

Heparin subcutaneous injections (e.g. enoxaparin 1mg/kg every 12 hours subcutaneous injections after an initial loading dose of 30mg bolus administered intravenously).

STATION 5

Name: Mr Gopala Kaur

Age: 41 years old

Job: Restaurant manager

PC:

For the last week you have been suffering with increasing shortness of breath, rigors, fevers and a very bad cough. The shortness of breath is constant and gets worse when you exert yourself, even just doing chores around the house, so you have taken a few days off work to try to recover. Nevertheless instead of getting better you actually think your symptoms are worse and have come to see if the doctor can prescribe you something for them. In the last three days you have also noticed that you are having night sweats, have lost your appetite completely and on two occasions coughed up a small amount of fresh blood (approximately a teaspoonful each time). You don't think you have lost a significant amount of weight but feel that you look rather pale and drained when you see your reflection in the mirror. You are very anxious and have never had any similar episodes before.

You have not been vomiting or suffering with any chest pains or change in bowel habits. You deny any cardiac related symptoms.

If questioned you mention that you and your family recently returned from a lovely summer holiday visiting your family in southern India. Whilst you were there you also did a lot of sight-seeing and visited many small rural villages and ate a lot of exotic food as you wanted to show your sons what life was like on the other side of the world (it was their first ever visit to India). You can't remember being close to anyone who was very ill but are not entirely sure.

Past Medical History:

You are normally very active and keep fit and well.

You were born in the UK but do not remember if you were given the BCG vaccine as a child. You do not have a scar on your arm.

Drug History:

You do not have any drug allergies.

Social History:

You have smoked 10 cigarettes per day for the last 15 years but do not drink alcohol or take recreational drugs.

You enjoy sports especially cricket.

You have two sons (aged 12 and 15) and a wife and you all live together in a semi-detached house in the suburbs.

You enjoy your job and don't think you have been particularly stressed at all lately as you have just been on a lovely summer holiday with the family! You were born and bred in England all your life but your grandparents and cousins live in southern India.

Family History:

Father died of a heart attack aged 48 years old. Mother is a type 2 diabetic and is still alive.

No one in your household is suffering from any infective symptoms.

Ideas/Concerns/Expectations:

You are the only member of your immediate family who has a job and you have a rather busy restaurant to run. You are concerned that feeling ill will mean that you need time off work and you are just not sure how to manage this without any other source of income coming in.

You feel very guilty about your smoking habit and you are also very anxious that the doctor will tell you that you may have lung cancer.

Diagnosis:

Tuberculosis

Differentials:

Atypical pneumonia, emphysema, lung cancer

Management:

Initial investigations would include:

Routine blood tests: FBC, U&E, LFTs, CRP

Sending 3 sputum samples for acid fast bacilli (ideally with one being an early morning sample)

Blood cultures, urine for MC&S and also early morning urine to test for acid fast bacilli

Other: ABG, ECG, CXR

CT chest

Management would include:

Referral to respiratory team

A standard first-line drug management of the condition would include the 'RIPE' treatment: i.e. rifampicin, isoniazid, pyrazinamide and ethambutol daily for four months followed by isoniazid and rifampicin three times a week for four months.

STATION 6

Name: Mrs Thulani Patel

Age: 72 years old

Job: Nursing home resident

PC:

You have come into hospital today with your nursing home staff as they are getting rather worried about you. In the past six days you have started to feel increasingly short of breath and it seems to be getting a lot worse. If asked, you deny any wheezing or associated chest tightness. The shortness of breath is constant, happens at rest and is exacerbated by any activity that you do. This is having an effect on your daily routine as you now prefer to stay in bed and not get up because you don't want to tire yourself out.

You also have a bad cough and have been bringing up some green thick sputum in the last three days. You find it difficult to quantify the exact amount of sputum but say that there is a lot and it happens almost every time you cough. There is no blood with the sputum. You feel shivery and think you may have a fever although the nursing home staff has not taken your temperature. You do not suffer from any cardiac related symptoms and deny any chest pain.

For the last week you have been getting more and more muddled and confused. Although you do admit you are rather forgetful sometimes, you find that you are now worse and cannot remember what you were talking about even in the middle of a sentence! In addition you can't remember if you've eaten or had your meals yet and so have been avoiding eating as you don't feel hungry thinking that you must have already had dinner.

You deny any weight loss, change in bowel habits or urinary symptoms.

Past Medical History:

3 x TIAs several years ago – no residual neurological weakness

Mild asthma – only on 'reliever' inhalers and rarely need to use these

Mild Alzheimer's disease

Depression

Right total hip replacement 10 years ago

Drug History:

You are allergic to peanuts and get swollen lips and a tight throat. The staff in the nursing home carry an EpiPen just in case you come into contact with any nuts.

Aspirin 75mg po od

Salbutamol inhaler, prn, 2 puffs

Citalopram 20mg po od

Paracetamol 1g po qds prn

Social History:

You live in a nursing home and have full-time 24 hour carers in the home.

You mobilise independently with a Zimmer frame although you find the initial standing up part is very difficult.

You can feed yourself but need help cleaning and dressing.

You do not smoke and never have. You used to drink a glass of wine every night when you were younger but find that alcohol at your age tends to make you more forgetful and sleepy so you avoid it. You do not have any close family left after your husband died eight years ago so your only friends are those that live in the nursing home with you.

Ideas/Concerns/Expectations:

You wonder if your 'time is up' and whether the doctors are going to be able to really cure you or are just being nice to you so you won't get too upset about not reaching your 73rd birthday.

Diagnosis:

Community acquired pneumonia

Differentials:

Exacerbation of asthma, pleural effusion

Management:

Routine blood tests: FBC, U&E, LFTs, CRP

Sputum sample for MC&S

Blood cultures, urine MC&S

Other: ABG, ECG, CXR, supplementary oxygen

Admission to hospital under general medical or respiratory team in light of frail and elderly stature.

Maintain hydration and monitor urine output.

Commence antibiotic regime in accordance with local hospital anti-microbial guidelines.

STATION 7

Name: Mr Cyrano Stoppelheim

Age: 69 years old

Job: Retired information technology specialist

PC:

For the past three months you have noticed yourself becoming increasingly short of breath. You used to be quite fit for your age and loved to go jogging in the evenings around the local park (for about 5 km). However, now you find yourself out of breath when you haven't even completed one lap around the park (after about 2 km). When you stop to catch your breath you also find it takes you a bit longer to get back to normal again. The shortness of breath never happens at rest and you have no problems sleeping or lying down flat.

You find it strange that even though you are doing less exercise now than you used to, you have actually lost more weight. You can't say how much but your clothes are fitting more loosely on you and your friends have been commenting on how gaunt you now look. You deny any chest pain but do have a bit of backache which only came on in the last four months in your lower back. It is constant and worse on palpation and all movements.

You have not had any flu-like symptoms, no infections, no fevers and you deny any change in bowel habits. You were not going to come to the GP but it has been going on a while now and even your mother has started to notice that you are 'not right'.

Only if questioned you mention that last week you had one episode of haemoptysis. This was an isolated case and you noticed when you coughed you had a bit of blood in your handkerchief. It was fresh bright red in colour without any clots. You can't really estimate the amount but you didn't think it was significant and thought perhaps it was because you had coughed very hard.

Past Medical History:

COPD – you have a chronic non-productive cough and tend to get a few chest infections in the winter months. You go to your GP for the flu jab every year to try to prevent this but it never seems to work! You are on inhalers which you use very rarely, mainly when you have a chest infection so you don't get any uncomfortable chest tightness.

Hypercholesterolaemia

Hypertension

Drug History:

You are not allergic to any medications.

Salbutamol inhalers, 2 puffs, prn

Simvastatin 20mg po on

Doxazosin 3mg po od

Paracetamol 1g po qds prn for the backache

Family History:

Your mother has had three strokes in the last four years since the age of 83 years old.

Your father died at the age of 69 years old from lung cancer.

You have two brothers who are both fit and well.

Social History:

You live with your mother and are her sole carer. She is dependent on you for most of her care including washing, feeding and shopping since her strokes.

You are not married and do not have any children.

You have smoked all your life, roughly 25 cigarettes a day for the last 55 years since the age of 14.

You enjoy a beer now and again with your mates down the pub but don't consider yourself a heavy drinker.

You do not take any recreational drugs.

Ideas/Concerns/Expectations:

You are worried that there is something serious going on and wonder how you will cope with caring for your mother if you need to be admitted to hospital.

Diagnosis:

Lung cancer

Differentials:

Bronchiectasis, infective exacerbation of COPD, congestive cardiac failure, pneumonia

Management:

Routine blood tests: FBC, U&E, LFTs, CRP, clotting screen, blood cultures

Other: Chest X-ray, ABG, ECG, urine dip and MC&S

CT chest, abdomen +/- pelvis for cancer staging

Bronchoscopy or CT guided biopsy of lung lesion depending on site

Referral to MDT meeting for discussion and referral to respiratory and oncology teams.

STATION 8

Name: Mrs Rosie Birchling

Age: 72 years old

Job: Retired bookkeeper

PC:

For the last month or so you feel that you have been getting rather 'puffy' especially at the end of the day. Specifically you think that both of your legs and calves are swollen and you are not sure why this is. It isn't just any kind of swelling though as there is no redness to the skin, no pain in your legs and when you try to massage your legs to get the swelling down you notice that there is a lasting impression in the skin in the areas you have been pressing! Very peculiar! You think the swelling is worse when you are on your feet during the day or have been out for a long walk in the park and better when you sit and watch television with your feet up for at least an hour or so.

There is no swelling to your face, arms or lower back. The calf swelling only extends to just below your knees. You deny any trauma to your ankles and have not had any recent fractures or surgery to your legs. The last time you were on a long-haul flight was over 20 years ago.

You are usually short of breath anyway and can manage walking about 20 m until you feel you need a little rest. In the last two weeks this is slightly worse and you can only manage about 15 m. You do not have any chest pain or palpitations. You sleep with three pillows at night (which is normal for you and has not changed for a long time) and you deny waking up suddenly in the middle of the night with shortness of breath. You find you are very short of breath if you are made to lie flat.

Past Medical History:

Gallstones

Hypertension

Cardiac failure – first diagnosed three years ago. You had a recent ECHO three months ago and the doctor told you that your left side of the heart wasn't pumping as well as it should.

DVTs and PEs diagnosed 5 years ago – used to be on warfarin, but now stopped.

Osteoarthritis in both hips – bilateral total hip replacements performed over 10 years ago.

Drug History:

NKDA

Furosemide 40mg po bd (if questioned you do not have any side effects to this drug apart from needing to go to the toilet more frequently)

Lisinopril 5mg po od

Bisoprolol 2.5mg po od

Social History:

You have never smoked in your life.

You enjoy the occasional glass of wine but only on special occasions.

You like going for little walks in the park even though you need to rest quite regularly.

You live with your daughter in a little country cottage and she helps to care and cook for you.

You are able to walk independently and climb stairs but prefer to use a stick 'just in case'.

You can feed and dress yourself and do not need help washing.

Your husband died over 20 years ago from lung cancer.

Ideas/Concerns/Expectations:

You wonder if all of this puffiness can be related to your heart condition and want to know if there is any medication you can take to make it go away.

Diagnosis:

Congestive cardiac failure

Differentials:

Pulmonary oedema, exacerbation of COPD, silent myocardial infarct triggering worsening of heart failure

Management:

Initial investigations may include:

Routine blood tests: FBC, U&E, LFTs, CRP, NT-pro-BNP, glucose, serial troponins

Other: Chest X-ray, repeat ECHO, ECG, ABG

The management of this patient will take into account the following:

Monitoring of urine output and daily fluid intake/weights

Increasing the dose of the patient's diuretic.

If the patient developed acute pulmonary oedema and was in severe shortness of breath, high flow oxygen, intravenous morphine, a nitrate infusion and also high dose diuretics would be initiated.

STATION 9

Name: Mr Chris Young

Age: 76 years old

Job: Retired accountant

PC:

You have had an awful crampy pain in the centre of your stomach for the last two days. Initially you thought it was just a bit of 'trapped wind' but the pain has been gradually worsening and is now generalised across the whole of your abdomen. There isn't one single area where you can pinpoint it being the worst. You felt nauseous overnight so didn't get much sleep and this morning you started vomiting a large amount of greenish, foul tasting liquid. There is no food in the vomitus as you haven't been eating very much and neither is there any blood. Since this morning you have vomited at least six times but now that there is nothing left to vomit up you have started retching.

Your bowel habits are normally pretty regular but for the last day or so you have not opened your bowels. You are still passing gas. You do not have any urinary symptoms or pain elsewhere. You have not noticed any 'lumps' in your groin or otherwise. Although you have had poor appetite in the last two days, you actually think your tummy is looking much bigger than usual and had been feeling really rather bloated until you started vomiting today.

You have not lost any weight recently and you do not have a fever either. You have not had any bleeding from your back passage. There is no pain anywhere else except in your stomach and you desperately want the doctor to give you some painkillers as soon as possible!

Past Medical History:

Appendicectomy aged 10 years old

Laparascopic cholecystectomy aged 55 years old

Hypertension

Drug History:

No known drug allergies

Ramipril 5mg po od

Social History:

You have smoked 20 cigarettes a day for the last 20 years and enjoy three pints of beer a week, usually on weekends.

You live in a small flat with your wife and pet dog, Buster.

You deny visiting any dodgy restaurants lately and do not know anyone who has the same pain as you at the moment.

Family History:

Your father and older brother both had colon cancer when they were in their sixties and they required big operations to remove the tumours.

Ideas/Concerns/Expectations:

You are worried that this might be cancer and you keep asking the doctor whether they think it is cancer. You really want to avoid an operation as much as possible.

Diagnosis:

Small bowel obstruction

Differentials:

Small bowel obstruction tends to cause the symptoms of vomiting and 'bloatedness' early on and constipation is one of the later signs, compared with large bowel obstruction where this is the opposite case. The main differentials for small bowel obstruction include adhesions or hernia. In rare cases, the cause for obstruction could be secondary to a tumour, which could be an adenocarcinoma, a lymphoma or a gastro-intestinal stromal tumour.

Management:

Full clinical examination including per rectal examination and routine observations and blood tests: FBC, U&Es, LFTs, CRP, group and save and possibly tumour markers – CEA.

ABG to check for lactate, base excess which if raised, can signify bowel ischaemia.

Obtain an abdominal X-ray and erect chest X-ray to look for obstructed bowel loops and perforation.

Admit the patient and keep them nil by mouth.

Insert an NG tube and catheter and ensure hourly fluid monitoring with 4 hourly aspiration of the NG tube.

Start IV fluids and give antiemetics (cyclizine, metaclopromide) and analgesia – NSAIDs (ibuprofen, diclofenac), paracetamol.

The patient will require a CT scan given the differential of a tumour causing the obstruction.

STATION 10

Name: Mrs Stefanie Johnson

Age: 58 years old

Job: Unemployed

PC:

You woke up late this morning at about 11am (as usual) and felt rather unwell in yourself. As you got up to go to the toilet you suddenly felt the urge to vomit and then noticed a large amount of fresh blood in toilet bowl. You don't know exactly quite how much you vomited up but you know it was definitely more than two cupfuls. After the event you felt extremely faint and dizzy and couldn't stand up properly without needing to lie down again on the toilet floor. This made you extremely anxious and you dialled 999 for an ambulance to bring you to hospital straight away, hence the reason you are still in your pyjamas.

You have not and did not experience any chest pains or abdominal pains during or before the episode. You have vomited up blood before, the last episode being two weeks ago after having a lot to drink, but it was not as much as this morning and you certainly did not feel faint. You deny any recent weight loss or change in bowel habits but say that your stools are a little darker than usual. You do not have any urinary symptoms, fevers, night sweats and deny any bone or muscle pains. You generally have a bad diet and do not eat healthily anyway but you do not think your appetite has changed. Your last food intake was at 2pm yesterday.

Past Medical History:

Hepatitis B and C

Alcoholic liver disease

Dilated cardiomyopathy (You had chest pains on an off for the last year and a medical doctor arranged an ECHO scan for you. They told you your heart was very large and dilated and said they wanted to follow you up but you got scared and have never gone back to see them.)

Drug History:

You don't take any medications and do not have any allergies. You think you are supposed to be on some vitamin B tablets as your GP had brought this up before but you aren't the 'medicine taking type' and so don't worry yourself about these things!

Social History:

You live alone in a council flat and complain that it is always messy as you are too busy to clear up. However, you are currently unemployed and have not held down a steady job for the past 20 years. You are estranged from your ex-husband and two children who you are no longer in touch with and you do not know where they live.

You have smoked 30 cigarettes a day for the last 40 years and drink 1–2 bottles of vodka a day. You have been a heavy drinker most of your life but have been drinking this amount for at least five years. You did try to give up drinking two years ago but it 'didn't work out' and you were tired of 'going in and out of rehab all the time'. You don't believe it helps and you believe you feel better on alcohol, so why make yourself unhappy?

You do not use drugs anymore though you used to inject intravenous drugs including heroin until five years ago. You stopped using drugs when you were diagnosed with hepatitis B and C.

Ideas/Concerns/Expectations:

You hate coming to hospital and want to go home. You just got scared at the amount of blood you saw but if the doctor suggests running some tests you say you now feel fine and really only came into hospital to hear that from someone else. You don't want to stay in overnight.

Diagnosis:

Variceal bleed

Differentials:

Mallory-Weiss tear, upper GI cancer

Management:

Infectious risk – double glove, wear an apron and eye protection when taking blood etc.

Immediate treatment: x2 large bore intravenous access, take blood tests: FBC, U&E, LFT, CRP, coagulation profile, group and save and crossmatch 4 units of blood.

Start intravenous fluids and resuscitate the patient.

Call on call gastroenterologist regarding patient – they will require an emergency upper GI endoscopy.

STATION 11

Name: Mr James Hodge

Age: 22 years old

Job: Medical student

PC:

You are captain of the men's rugby team at university and have been out all night celebrating your team's success at a recent tournament. You admit you have had a lot to drink but have been paying dearly for it by vomiting and retching up everything you have drunk all night. You vomited twice in the nightclub and then three times on the way home at 4am. You then vomited about six times overnight and you noticed there were steaks of bright red blood in your vomit of the last few occasions. In addition to this you have got a mild dull ache in your upper abdomen which does not radiate anywhere and feels like acid reflux.

There is no blood in your stools, you do not have urinary symptoms and you deny any recent weight loss. Up until last night you have been well in yourself without any recent illnesses.

Your flatmates (who are also in the rugby club) have continued drinking all night and have brought you into hospital because they thought you were messing around when you told them you were bleeding into your vomit. They thought if they brought you to see a doctor you would deny the whole thing and they could have a good laugh about it. They are all very rowdy and still quite drunk.

Past Medical History:

Fit and well.

Drug History:

No regular medications.

No known drug allergies.

Social History:

You are in your fourth year of medical school and are captain of the rugby team.

You do not smoke or take any recreational drugs.

You drink at your rugby club social circle every Wednesday evenings and can drink anywhere up to 5 pints of beer. This evening you can't remember how much you drank as you mixed your drinks and had some cocktails, shots, beer and vodka with mixers. You really would not be able to say exactly how many units or even glasses. You lost count after 6 drinks.

Family History:

None significant.

Ideas/Concerns/Expectations:

You were not worried until you saw the blood. Now you are feeling quite anxious and very hung-over. It really doesn't help that your flatmates are poking you and jeering. You would like the doctor to tell them to go away so you can get some rest.

Diagnosis:

Mallory-Weiss tear

Differentials:

Gastritis, variceal bleed, reflux disease

Management:

Blood tests: FBC, U&E, LFT, CRP, coagulation profile & group and save.

Chest X-ray to look for mediastinal air.

Give IV antiemetics and proton pump inhibitors (omeprazole).

Contact the gastroenterologist as the patient will require an emergency upper GI endoscopy.

STATION 12

Name: Mr Henry Lewis

Age: 72 years old

Job: Retired lawyer

PC:

You have been finding it difficult to swallow for the past two months which has been progressively getting worse, so you went to see your GP a few weeks ago. Initially you were able to eat all foods but then two months ago you noticed that at times you had a feeling of the food getting stuck in your upper throat and this would make you cough.

About five weeks ago you noticed that you had to swallow smaller mouthfuls than normal, and in the last week you have found that you can only swallow very soft food such as banana or yoghurt. You have not noticed any neck swellings and you deny any aspiration of your foods. You have not had any recent chest infections and deny shortness of breath. You think you have lost weight though you are not sure how much – but you have noticed you need to do up your belt tighter and your shirts are loose around the collar. You do not suffer from any reflux symptoms and you do not have any abdominal pain. You have not had any vomiting though sometimes you feel nauseous after eating. You have not had any blood loss from the back passage and have not had any change in your bowel habit.

Past Medical History:

Hypercholesterolaemia

Drug History:

You do not have any known drug allergies.

Simvastatin 20mg po od

Social History:

You live at home with your wife who is also a retired lawyer.

You smoke a pipe (once a day) and occasionally drink alcohol.

You enjoy your retired life and keep busy playing golf and going on short breaks around Europe with your wife.

Family History:

None significant.

Ideas/Concerns/Expectations:

You are worried about what the problem could be and want to know if there are any vitamins you should take given that you cannot eat as much as you used to.

Diagnosis:

Oesophageal cancer

Differentials:

Achalasia, peptic stricture, scleroderma

Management:

Blood test: FBC, U&E, LFTs, CRP.

Refer patient for urgent two week rule referral for upper GI endoscopy.

A barium/gastrograffin swallow may also reveal a stricture in the oesophagus and confirm your diagnosis.

A CT scan of the chest, abdomen and pelvis may not reveal the primary tumour but can be useful for staging any metastatic spread of disease.

Urgent referral to the upper gastrointestinal MDT meeting and specialist is vital.

STATION 13

Name: Mr Helmut Joles

Age: 43 years old

Job: Investment banker

PC:

You are a bit concerned that for the last few months you have been passing small amounts of blood from your back passage. The blood is bright red and you usually notice it on the toilet paper or streaked on the stool. It appears separate to the stool and not mixed with it. Your stools are usually light brown and never black. You have not had any change in your bowel habits but you are usually a little constipated and do have to strain to pass your stools. You open your bowels every day. You have not lost any weight nor had any episodes of vomiting.

You often work late and eat out or get takeaways, which is the lifestyle you have become accustomed to. You do not have any abdominal pain or reflux symptoms.

Past Medical History:

Hypertension

Drug History:

You do not have any drug allergies.

Ramipril 5mg po od

Social History:

You have smoked 15 cigarettes a day for the last 20 years and are currently cutting down.

You drink socially most nights and indulge in the occasional line of cocaine but nothing regular and no intravenous recreational drugs.

You live in your own apartment and have a girlfriend who you have not told about this.

Ideas/Concerns/Expectations:

You are quite embarrassed and feel awkward answering questions about your bowel habits.

Diagnosis:

Haemorrhoids

Differentials:

Colon cancer, inflammatory bowel disease

Management:

Full clinical examination including per rectal examination.

Send routine blood tests: FBS, U/E, LFT, CRP, clotting screen.

Patient will require proctoscopy and rigid sigmoidoscopy in an outpatient clinic.

Then he should be referred for a colonoscopy to rule out any proximal lesion.

STATION 14

Name: Mr Peter Butcher

Age: 81 years old

Job: Retired gardener

PC:

For the last few months you have noticed blood in your stools. It is not there all the time and tends to only occur occasionally. It appears to be unpredictable. When the blood is present, however, you notice it is dark red and mixed with the stool although sometimes your stools are very dark brown, almost black looking and smell awful! You have ignored this for a while but your wife has made you come today as she is very worried and wants you to get checked out.

You have not had any abdominal pains, fevers, vomiting or night sweats but you do think that your bowel habit is not what it used to be. Before you were very frequent and passed stools daily which were medium brown in colour, well-formed and did not smell as strongly as your stools do now. In the last year though you have been feeling rather constipated (despite no change in what you have been eating) and when you do go to open your bowels you are not always sure if you have completed the motion. Sometimes you think there is still something there to pass.

You think you have also lost quite a bit of weight. An embarrassing situation happened last week where you were talking to your wife about some flowers you had recently planted and whilst gesturing, your wedding ring flew off your finger across the room! You always used to find the ring rather tight and restricting (a bit like your marriage) but recently it has felt rather loose. You feel that the weight loss is because your appetite has decreased a little (although the types of food you eat have not changed) and you think that it is probably normal for your appetite to decrease as you get older.

Past Medical History:

None – you have been fit and well all your life and have never been admitted to hospital for anything.

Drug History:

None and no allergies.

Multivitamin pills once a day

Social History:

You do not smoke and only very occasionally drink alcohol.

You live alone with your wife and both of you manage independently with no home help.

You pride yourself with your generally high level of health and fitness and put it all down to years of gardening and being active outdoors.

You continue to jog for 30 minutes every morning and enjoy a round of golf every weekend with some of your friends at the golf club.

Family History:

None.

Ideas/Concerns/Expectations:

You are not keen on coming to the doctors and say that you think everything is fine. You only came as your wife made you and you can no longer stand her constant nagging around the house. You have been fit and healthy all your life and although you know your symptoms are not 'normal' you feel actually quite well and not at all ill in yourself.

Diagnosis:

Colorectal cancer

Differentials:

Colorectal polyps, constipation

Management:

Routine blood tests: FBC, U&E, LFTs, CRP, possibly tumour markers e.g. CEA, AFP.

Referral for a two week wait for colonoscopy and also to the colorectal surgical outpatient clinic.

If colorectal cancer is strongly suspected then a staging CT chest, abdomen and pelvis may also be requested including a MRI of the rectum for local staging if rectal cancer is diagnosed on colonoscopy. The fact that the patient is suffering from symptoms of tenesmus tends to indicate a rather low-lying tumour. The majority of colorectal cancers are situated within the sigmoid colon or rectum.

STATION 15

Name: Miss Natasha Sharma

Age: 19 years old

Job: Studying engineering at university

PC:

You have been feeling generally unwell since yesterday morning while you were at your lectures in university. You developed central abdominal pain after you had your lunch (a ham and cheese sandwich) yesterday and this pain has gradually worsened. When you went to bed in the evening you noticed that you felt hot and sweaty but thought it was because the weather was rather stuffy. You only started to get rather concerned when you awoke the next morning feeling even worse, having had very little sleep and you were completely off your breakfast. You did not attend university today and had a bout of vomiting at about 11am. There was no blood in the vomit but you were concerned that you were really rather ill. You tried to get an appointment at your GP but none of the doctors were available and so you decided to come to hospital.

The pain has become worse today and now is more in your lower right abdomen. You do not have any urinary symptoms and have not opened your bowels since yesterday. Apart from not yet opening your bowels today you have not noticed any change in bowel habits recently. You deny any preceding coryzal symptoms and have not been in contact with anyone that you know with similar symptoms. You are not sure if you could be pregnant or not as you are currently on the oral contraceptive pill and run them back to back to avoid periods so can't remember your last period date. You also say that although you are on the pill you aren't particularly good at remembering to take them all the time, so if you were pregnant it would be a shock but wouldn't totally surprise you either. You do not have any vaginal discharge or any bleeding that you have noticed on your knickers.

You ate out the night before last at a new Thai restaurant in the town and you think your symptoms are related as you don't usually eat spicy foods and your diet is really quite westernised.

Past Medical History:

Asthma

Drug History:

Salbutamol inh 2 puffs prn

Microgynon 30 (oral contraceptive pill)

Social History:

You live in University Halls and your mother is on her way to the hospital to come see you as you are worried about being in hospitals on your own.

You smoke 5 cigarettes a day and drink occasionally.

You are sexually active and have not had any previous STIs. Your last full STI check was about five months ago and was clear. You have been seeing a new boyfriend for the last six months and you also made sure he was tested and clear before you started sleeping together.

Ideas/Concerns/Expectations:

You are hoping it was just something you ate. You are very scared of needles so you do not want anyone to take blood. You really don't like the idea of having an operation and if the doctor suggests this you ask if there is any chance you can have antibiotics to settle the symptoms down instead.

Diagnosis:

Appendicitis

Differentials:

Ectopic pregnancy, ovarian torsion, ovarian cyst, gastroenteritis

Management:

Full clinical examination including per rectal examination.

Routine blood tests: FBC, U&E, LFTs, CRP, BHCG, amylase, blood cultures, clotting and group and save.

Urine dipstick (will show septic pyuria) including B-hCG.

Admit patient – nil by mouth, IV fluids, analgesia.

Imaging:

Arrange an urgent abdominal and transvaginal ultrasound to rule out gynaecological pathology.

If the ultrasound does not visualise the appendix and shows no gynaecological pathology, the patient will still require a diagnostic laparoscopy +/- laparoscopic or open appendicectomy.

In some hospitals an out-of-hours ultrasound scan may not be possible to request and occasionally these patients may have a CT Abdomen and Pelvis performed (although not if pregnancy is a possibility and the patient is of childbearing age). If the patient is clinically septic with raised inflammatory markers and there is a strong clinical suspicion of appendicitis then it is prudent to proceed to appendicectomy rather than to wait for imaging to be performed.

A suspicion of a perforated appendix may be confirmed by an erect chest X-ray and visualisation of free air under the diaphragm, although a normal erect film will not exclude this diagnosis.

STATION 16

Name: Mrs Sally Poole

Age: 49 years old

Job: Secretary

PC:

You developed abdominal pain this morning on your way to work. The pain was so bad that you decided not to go to work and you instead called your GP to book an emergency appointment. The pain started at approximately 7am as you were getting on the bus. You had awoken that morning feeling fine and had cereal and milk for breakfast as usual. You report the pain was in the right upper part of your abdomen and it was a constant pain. You felt nauseous but have not vomited.

When you arrived at the surgery you felt rather silly as the pain had resolved on its own on your way there. The whole episode lasted about one hour but as you were at the surgery you decided to see the GP anyway to find out if there was a cause for this pain. You have had a few of these episodes over the last few months and are starting to feel worried because you were hoping you could ignore them and they would just go away.

The pain normally comes on after you have eaten and you don't think it is related to anything in particular that you do eat although you admit your diet is rather rubbish and you like deep fried fatty foods or anything that looks sugary. Whenever the pain comes on you are nauseous with it but you have not had any vomiting episodes. You do not have any urinary symptoms or weight loss, though you do feel you need to lose weight. You have not had any change in bowel habit or any blood loss per rectum.

Past Medical History:

Diabetes type 2 – well controlled on oral hypoglycaemics. No severe diabetes-related complications.

Hypertension

Gastro-oesophageal reflux disease

Drug History:

No drug allergies.

Metformin 500mg po BD

Amlodipine 5mg po OD

Omeprazole 40mg po OD

Social History:

You do not smoke and you occasionally drink alcohol.

You live with your husband and two teenage sons.

Ideas/Concerns/Expectations:

You are worried as your company is down-sizing and you have had four days off work sick in the last two months with the same abdominal pain, but as it only lasts an hour or so you were hoping it was nothing serious and would just go away.

Diagnosis:

Biliary colic – gallstones

Differentials:

Acute cholecystitis, gastritis

Management:

Routine blood tests: FBC, U&E, LFTs, CRP.

Referral for an ultrasound and to general surgical outpatient clinic to discuss the option of a cholecystectomy.

STATION 17

Name: Mrs Lucy Mumford

Age: 62 years old

Job: Home-maker

PC:

You are suffering from terrible pains in the right upper part of your abdomen which radiates round your body to affect also the right side of your back. The pain started two days ago and wasn't that bad so you put off seeing the doctors but ever since this afternoon, about four hours ago, it has been progressively getting worse. It is a constant sharp pain and it doesn't seem to get better or worse with any movements, neither does it come on worse when eating or drinking. You feel unwell and nauseous and just vomited once whilst waiting to be seen in A&E. If the doctor asks you, the vomitus only contained a sandwich and some cereal you had earlier on in the day but no blood.

You are feeling hot and shivery and the triage nurse mentioned to you that you had a temperature when she was taking your observations. You deny any recent night sweats and until two days ago your appetite was normal (since all this has been building up you have been a little off your food). You do not have any urinary symptoms and you have not had any change in your bowel habit. You have lost some weight but you have been trying to with exercise and it has only been about 4lbs over the last four months. You have not had any blood loss per rectum. You also deny thinking that your skin is turning yellow.

You have had pain in the right upper part of your abdomen before on and off over the last few years, but it usually only lasts a short while before going away so you have never seen a doctor about it or had any scans to find out what it is. You have never felt this unwell with the pain though and you certainly have never vomited or had fevers with it, which is why you came to hospital today.

Past Medical History:

High cholesterol

Drug History:

NKDA

Simvastatin 20mg po od

Social History:

You live with your husband and cat. You have three children who are all grown up and live abroad. Your husband has just retired and you are both currently planning a trip to visit your sister in Australia for Christmas.

You do not smoke or drink alcohol regularly. Your normal diet is not the healthiest and you do admit to particularly enjoying red wine and French cheeses as well as the odd fast food indulgence.

You have never been a very active person in your life and you really have only started doing some exercise now as a group of your friends and yourself are planning to do a sponsored fun run for charity in two month's time.

Ideas/Concerns/Expectations:

You are worried this might interfere with your Christmas holidays and that it will prevent you from taking part in the charity fun run with your friends.

Diagnosis:

Acute cholecystitis

Differentials:

Ascending cholangitis, pyelonephritis, biliary colic

Management:

Full clinical examination.

Routine blood tests: FBC, U&E, LFTs, CRP, clotting and group and save.

Full septic screen: Urine dip and MSU for microbiology, cultures and sensitivities, blood cultures, CXR.

Admit the patient, keep them nil by mouth and start on intravenous antibiotics such as cefuroxime and metronidazole (although the exact regime will depend on your local hospital antimicrobial guidelines).

Arrange an abdominal ultrasound to look for gallstones as the cause for the acute cholecystitis and to rule out any suspicious liver lesions. If there is a gallstone in the common bile duct causing dilatation the patient will require an ERCP.

STATION 18

Name: Mr James O'Leary

Age: 18 years old

Job: In school

PC:

You have come to the GP practice with your mother as you have been having diarrhoea for the past few weeks. You are very embarrassed talking about this but your mother has said you have to see the doctor so she has brought you in today.

It started while you were on holiday with your friends in Ibiza three weeks ago to celebrate your graduation from school. You were in Ibiza for one week and the diarrhoea started two days before your return to the UK. You were passing stool up to six times a day for the first few days but now are passing stool three times a day. There is bright red blood mixed with the stool as well as thick clear mucus. You also notice you frequently get crampy lower abdominal pain often before you pass stool. You have to go to the toilet immediately if you feel you need to pass stool and only if the doctor directly questions you do you report that you have been incontinent on two occasions – once in Ibiza and once last week. You have not been out much since returning from Ibiza as you are worried that you might suddenly need the toilet and have an accident.

This initially scared you but you really didn't want to cause a fuss with all your friends around so you didn't seek help abroad. You hadn't eaten anything different to the rest of your mates so you just thought that perhaps all the alcohol you were drinking was 'taking its toll on your body' and this episode would pass when you got back to the UK, but it didn't. You have not felt nauseous, feverish or been vomiting at all. You have not lost any weight and your appetite is not greatly changed. You have not had any mouth ulcers or problems with your eyes and deny any skin lesions on any part of your body.

Past Medical History:

You have had lower back pain for the past six months which you assume is due to a football-related injury though you cannot recall any injury specifically – you play football for your school. You are seeing a physiotherapist for this. The pain is worse in the mornings and usually goes away by lunch time and when you are up and about moving a little more. A hot water bottle or heat pack on the back also tends to make the pain much less although paracetamol doesn't do anything.

Drug History:

No drug allergies.

You occasionally take some ibuprofen when the back pain is bad.

Social History:

You do not smoke and only drink when you are with your friends. Although you only drink in moderation usually, whilst in Ibiza you did drink much larger quantities of alcohol than usual. You can't recall how much but you are pretty sure it was over the recommended limit. (You find this very difficult to admit with your mother in the room, so if asked about alcohol you will try to avoid telling the doctor the amount you drank in Ibiza unless questioned directly.)

You do not take any other recreational drugs. You live at home with your parents but will be moving away to university in a few months to study law.

Family History:

Your grandfather died of colon cancer at the age of 87 years old.

Ideas/Concerns/Expectations:

You are worried about how this is affecting your life and want some medication to make the symptoms go away. You really do not want to be stuck indoors or have this hold you back from making new friends at university during Freshers' Week.

Diagnosis:

Ulcerative colitis

Differentials:

Crohn's disease, infectious colitis

Management:

Routine blood tests: FBC, U&E, LFTs, CRP, blood cultures.

Stool microscopy and culture to rule out an infective cause.

Urine microscopy, sensitivities and cultures with dipstick test to rule out concomitant urinary tract infection.

Referral to gastroenterology outpatient clinic as well as for sigmoidoscopy/colonoscopy and biopsy for histological diagnosis.

STATION 19

Name: Miss Casey Lee

Age: 21 years old

Job: Waitress

PC:

You have been suffering with ongoing diarrhoea for the last three days and you are now starting to feel extremely fragile, fatigued and weak. The very first episode a few days ago woke you up in the early hours of the morning with crampy abdominal pains. At that time you felt you desperately needed the toilet and the subsequent stool that you passed was slightly loose, light brown in colour but did not contain any blood. You then went to work but had to leave early as you were feeling unwell and had opened your bowels six times that day. Each time the stools you passed were progressively looser.

You became slowly to feel more and more nauseated and vomited that day on your way home from work on the bus and a further four times that evening. Since this time you have not returned to work and you feel as though things are getting worse and not better. There is never any blood in your vomitus, only food that you had eaten during the day.

You have opened your bowels about eight times per day for the last two days passing very small amounts of very watery and offensive-smelling stool. You have noticed that there was a slight amount of bright red blood on the toilet paper (never in the toilet bowl or mixed with your stools) when you opened your bowels the last few times and you have found it quite sore when opening your bowels. You presume this is because you have been going to the toilet a lot and the repeated use of the toilet paper on your skin has made it very sore and sensitive.

You have not been eating anything except a piece of toast now and again and you have been drinking water and Ribena. You have lost about 2kg in weight over the last three days. You deny any previous similar episodes. It does not hurt you to pass urine and you do not think you go to urinate any more frequently than usual. Your periods are regular, the last one being only two weeks ago and you are currently not in a relationship and deny pregnancy. You have not had any recent foreign travel nor have you eaten anything new or unusual that you can recall.

Past Medical History:

Pyelonephritis (3 years ago)

Appendicectomy as a teenager

Drug History:

NKDA

Nil regular medications.

Social History:

You smoke 5 cigarettes a day and drink a glass of wine most evenings after your shift at work.

You do not take any other recreational drugs.

You live with a flatmate in rented accommodation.

Family History:

None.

Ideas/Concerns/Expectations:

You are feeling very weak and tired and want some medication to stop the diarrhoea.

Diagnosis:

Gastroenetritis, infective colitis (e.g. giardia, shigella, salmonella)

Differentials:

Inflammatory bowel disease

Management:

Routine observations including pulse, blood pressure, temperature.

Full clinical examination including per rectal examination.

Routine blood tests: FBC, U&E, LFTs, CRP, blood cultures.

Urine dip stick (and microscopy, sensitivity and cultures) and B-hCG.

Stool microscopy and culture to check for an infective cause.

Patient will likely require admission at least overnight for IV fluid rehydration given that she is feeling so weak and tired.

STATION 20

Name: Miss Sarah Blanchard

Age: 35 years old

Job: Accountant

PC:

This morning when you woke up you felt an intense pain in the whole of the left half of your head. It doesn't radiate into your neck or cause any neck stiffness. You would describe the pain as throbbing and an intense ache. You didn't have any alcohol to drink last night and don't recall banging your head on anything. It's been five hours since it started now and doesn't seem to be settling.

You have found that bright lights hurt your eyes and you are generally weak and very tired. You had to call in sick to work today because of the pain and decided to come to see your GP because you have vomited twice this morning and that worried you.

Past Medical History:

You have had about five similar episodes like this before but the last time it happened was over 10 years ago and you're not sure if this is related. You are generally fit and well.

Drug History:

You don't take any medications and do not have any allergies.

You took two 500mg tablets of paracetamol this morning and it didn't touch your pain.

Social History:

You don't smoke and only drink alcohol in social settings.

You have not travelled anywhere recently or eaten any strange foods.

At the moment you are undergoing a stressful period at work with many deadlines to meet. In addition you split up with your boyfriend last week and are finding it hard to cope without him.

Family History:

Your sister has been diagnosed in the past by her GP with migraines.

Ideas/Concerns/Expectations:

You think that perhaps you are coming down with flu and should take some antibiotics.

Diagnosis:

Migraines

Differentials:

Tension headache, cluster headache

Management:

No specific test to confirm diagnosis.

Full clinical examination and routine observations and blood tests: FBC, U&Es, LFTs, CRP.

Medication may include antiemetics (cyclizine, metaclopromide) and analgesia – NSAIDs (ibuprofen, diclofenac), paracetamol, aspirin.

Certain cases may be appropriate for 'triptan' medication e.g. sumatriptan to prevent future attacks.

Avoid codeine phosphate or any triggers which appear to cause the migraines (in some patients this may include red wine and cheese).

STATION 21

Name: Miss Judy Vamos

Age: 18 years old

Job: Student

PC:

For the last 1–2 days you have been suffering with flu-like symptoms – in particular feeling hot and cold, having generalised muscle weakness and nausea. In the early hours of this morning you vomited three times and in the last two hours you have started to feel a generalised crampy headache all over your head. It feels like it radiates into your neck and it is getting increasingly more difficult to move your neck. You also find bright lights irritate your eyes and you've been spending the whole morning in bed with the covers over your head.

You currently feel very irritable and drowsy and keep falling asleep as the junior doctor tries to take your history. You do not have any skin rashes but one of your friends took your temperature at home and said it was very high at 41^{0}C.

Past Medical History:

You are generally fit and well.

Drug History:

You don't take any medications and do not have any allergies. You haven't taken any medicines or painkillers today.

Social History:

You are a Spanish language student at university and love it.

You live with five flatmates in your student flat and share a communal kitchen and bathroom.

You have not been abroad recently or eaten any strange foods.

You do not know of any infectious contacts that may have passed on any illnesses to you.

You smoke and drink alcohol in small amounts and only in social settings.

Ideas/Concerns/Expectations:

You feel silly for coming to hospital and were made to come by your flatmates who you think are overreacting. You have your term examinations soon and don't want to be kept in hospital. You keep begging the doctor to let you go home and start to get really irritable if they tell you that you need to be admitted.

Diagnosis:

Meningitis

Differentials:

Encephalitis, subarachnoid haemorrhage, brain abscess

Management:

Immediate treatment: cefotaxime 2mg IM injection, intravenous fluids, supportive management and monitoring.

Treat any seizures according to local protocols.

Blood tests: FBC, U&E, LFT, CRP, blood cultures, glucose, coagulation profile.

Other tests: Lumbar puncture, septic screen – to include MSU, sputum cultures and above blood tests.

Radiological tests: CT head, CXR.

STATION 22

Name: Mrs Elizabeth Hodgkiss

Age: 56 years old

Job: Librarian

PC:

You woke up this morning with the worst headache you have ever suffered from in your life. It is predominately around the back of your head but you think it spreads a bit down the back of your neck and you find yourself having difficulty moving your neck. You have felt really drowsy and just 'not right'. You tried to go to work but couldn't quite keep your balance walking. That was when you decided you needed to come to hospital. You vomited twice in the car on the way in and each time you vomited the headache was much worse. You deny any visual disturbance or photophobia. You are not feverish and have not had any episodes of seizures. You have no focal neurology but feel confused. You do not normally suffer from headaches. You deny any head trauma. You have not taken any medication or painkillers today. You have been feeling otherwise well until today.

Past Medical History:

Atrial fibrillation

Drug History:

Warfarin – 5mg od po (Your most recent INR taken two weeks ago was 3.)

Social History:

You do not drink or smoke or take any recreational drugs.

You live at home with your husband and have two children who are grown up.

You have not travelled abroad recently nor have you had any change in your diet.

Family History:

None significant.

Ideas/Concerns/Expectations:

You are very worried that you may be suffering from a brain tumour because you don't usually suffer from headaches and can't understand why you are getting confused and vomiting.

Diagnosis:

Subarachnoid haemorrhage

Differentials:

Meningitis, encephalitis, migraine

Management:

CT head +/- CT angiogram if SAH diagnosed on scan.

Lumbar puncture to look for xanthochromia if CT head is negative (performed no sooner than 12 hours from onset of headache).

All patients should be started on calcium channel antagonist (nifedipine), seizure activity controlled and supportive management started (e.g. monitoring, intravenous fluid administration).

Referral to neurosurgical unit for either surgical clipping or endovascular embolisation of bleeding point.

STATION 23

Name: Mrs Jolanda Mabellie

Age: 72 years old

Job: Retired secretary

PC:

You have been suffering from headaches on both sides of your head which came on about a week ago and are not going away. They are sharp and severe in nature but do not really radiate anywhere. They are most painful on the sides of your head just between your eyes and ears. It is tender when you touch your head and you have also found it painful to comb your hair in these areas. When you eat food you also notice pain in your jaw on chewing. Although you don't feel like you have flu, you have been feeling sweaty at night and a little feverish. You have not had any visual disturbance or pain in your eyes. You don't have any neurology and you have never had a severe headache in your life. You have tried to take some paracetamol for your headache but this has not helped.

You do not have any muscle pain or any weight loss. You have still been able to perform most of your daily activities.

Past Medical History:

You suffer from high blood pressure and high cholesterol.

Drug History:

Lisinopril 5mg po od

Simvastatin 20mg od

Social History:

You live at home with your daughter and her family who help to care for you although you can do most of your daily activities on your own.

You don't smoke or drink any alcohol.

Family History:

None significant.

Ideas/Concerns/Expectations:

You are worried that there is no cure for this headache and you will have to put up with it forever!

Diagnosis:

Temporal arteritis

Differentials:

Polymyalgia rheumatica, tension headache

Management:

Blood test: FBC (anaemia), U&E, LFTs, CRP, ESR (raised).

Other: temporal artery biopsy, colour duplex scan of temporal artery blood flow.

Medication: High dose steroids (prednisolone) with osteoporosis protective cover (vitamin D and calcium supplements). Low dose aspirin (75mg) with proton pump inhibitor cover (omeprazole) has been shown to reduce the likelihood of vision loss and strokes in patients with temporal arteriritis.

Referral for ophthalmology review if sight in danger or patient develops amorisis fugax.

STATION 24

Name: Miss Hannah Parkins

Age: 21 years old

Job: Student

PC:

You were out in the shopping centre this afternoon with a group of friends today when you suddenly came over all giddy and weak. All you remember is feeling very hot before blacking out. When you awoke you noticed a lot of people surrounding you and asking if you were OK. You felt weak and tired when you awoke but not in any pain and you currently feel back to normal. You did not wet yourself or bite your tongue. Your friends said that you were unrousable for about 1–2 minutes and that you were shaking a little bit when you collapsed. They told you that your hands and legs but not your body were gently shaking for about 20 seconds and that you didn't hurt yourself or bang your head when you fell. They said you looked very pale and clammy during this episode. You deny any chest pain or palpitations.

You have not had similar episodes in the past and you have been feeling well in yourself recently. You have been stressed and not sleeping properly lately because of your studies and missed having breakfast this morning.

Past Medical History:

No history of epilepsy or previous collapses.

Drug History:

None. No allergies.

Social History:

You have smoked 5 cigarettes a day for the last three years.

You drink only on the weekends with your friends and usually have 2–3 small glasses of wine each time you go out.

Ideas/Concerns/Expectations:

You think that you have just had a simple faint because you were hot and missed breakfast but your friends and family were concerned and asked you to see a doctor to be sure.

Diagnosis:

Vasovagal collapse

Differentials:

Simple syncope, epilepsy less likely

Management:

Avoidance of triggers, maintain hydration.

Rule out underlying cause for syncope by performing full cardiovascular and neurological examination, routine blood tests (FBC, U&E, LFTs, CRP), CXR, ECG and routine clinical observations (BP measurement, pulse, respiratory rate, temperature).

(In some instances graded compression stockings and reducing doses of antihypertensive medications may be beneficial – not in this clinical scenario though.)

STATION 25

Name: Mr Peter Gordon

Age: 34 years old

Job: Marketing manager

PC:

You were playing football in the park with a few friends this afternoon at about 4pm when you remember feeling a strange nauseating sensation and numbness around your mouth. You don't remember much after this but awoke to find yourself on the grass with all your friends staring at you and looking worried. You felt all your muscles were really sore and that your tongue was bleeding and painful. You did not lose continence. You do not think you hit your head and you haven't seen any bruising on your body. However, you did feel very drowsy and tired and still feel like this now. Your friends tell you that during the time you were on the floor you were unconscious and shaking your arms and legs rhythmically and violently. They saw you first go stiff, fall down then shake. The whole episode lasted for three minutes and they were all very worried. You have not had any recent infections, have not travelled abroad, changed your diet or had any weight loss or change in appetite. You generally feel well within yourself.

Past Medical History:

You have suffered with epilepsy for the last 10 years and it is generally very well controlled. Your last seizure was over five years ago and you stopped taking epileptic medication about three years ago because you felt that things were going OK and you were not fitting without them – until now.

You had been regularly seeing your neurologist with your last appointment three years ago but have not had a check up since then. You had a CT scan of your head when you were first diagnosed and there was nothing abnormal discovered on the scan. An EEG was also performed but nothing unusual was found on that either. You are generally a fit and healthy person and maintain a healthy diet with lots of exercise.

Drug History:

None and no drug allergies.

Social History:

You have smoked 10 cigarettes per day for the last 15 years.

You drink alcohol within moderation. You usually only have one glass of wine three times a week and the odd beer on the weekend if out with friends.

You do not take any illicit drugs.

You are single and live alone in your own flat in London and work in the city in quite a stressful job where you are regularly having important meetings and needing to give presentations.

Family History:

Your brother and father both suffered with epilepsy. They are currently on medication for this but you don't know what type.

Ideas/Concerns/Expectations:

You are very disappointed this has happened. You understand that epilepsy can occur without a cause and that one may not be found in this case. You are reluctant to go back on medication after you had been doing so well for the last three years off it. This is really upsetting you, however if persuaded, you would take some pills as you don't want to risk having a fit in the middle of an important business meeting.

Diagnosis:

Tonic-clonic epilepsy

Differentials:

Simple syncope, vasovagal event, derangement of metabolites e.g. hypoglycaemia, intracranial event (e.g. space occupying lesion), infection (e.g. meningitis)

Management:

Routine blood tests: FBC, U&E, LFTs, CRP

Other: CT Head, ECG, CXR

Referral to neurologists for discussion regarding restarting antiepileptic medication.

STATION 26

Patient's Name: Mrs Liesl Lafayette

Daughter's Name: Miss Sandra Lafayette

Age: 85 years old

Job: Retired (used to be a housewife)

PC:

Your mother currently lives with you and your husband at home and you help to care for her. This afternoon whilst washing up in the kitchen you heard a loud 'bang' from the living room. You rushed in to find your mother lying on the floor after having fallen from standing height. She had a big bruise on the front of her forehead and it looked as if she had hit her head on the coffee table. She did not lose consciousness and apart from a headache where she was bruised denied having any chest pain, headache or palpitations prior to the fall. She did not look pale or sweaty or clammy.

You helped her up and sat her in a chair after the fall but realised that over the last two hours she has been getting acutely more confused and sleepy. It is almost as if she is drifting in and out of consciousness. She is still rousable but looks irritated and when you ask her simple questions such as 'Do you know where you are?' she replies only with muttering and incomprehensible sounds. She is normally very alert and orientated. She does not suffer from dementia or have any previous history of strokes or heart attacks. She has had previous falls but has not been harmed by them and never needed admitting to hospital. You have examined her and you don't think she hurt any other part of her body from the fall. She does not complain of pain anywhere else in her body.

Past Medical History:

Atrial fibrillation

Hypercholesterolaemia

Hypertension

Had had several DVTs in the past prior to treatment on warfarin 10 years ago.

Drug History:

Warfarin 3mg od po – INR last checked two weeks ago was 3. Target range is between 2 and 3.

Simvastatin 20mg od po

Digoxin 1.25mg od po

Amlodipine 5mg od po

Social History:

You live with your mother and your husband in a bungalow. There are no pets in the house.

Your mother is normally able to walk around the house with the aid of a walking stick although she has become more unsteady in her old age. She is normally not confused and able to hold a normal conversation. She requires help cooking, cleaning, washing and dressing but can feed herself and is continent.

Your mother has never smoked and no longer drinks alcohol. She used to enjoy an after dinner glass of sherry.

Ideas/Concerns/Expectations:

You are concerned about your mother's new confusion and head injury from her fall. You wonder if the fall was severe enough to cause her any brain damage or concussion.

Diagnosis:

Mechanical fall with subdural haematoma

Differentials:

Other forms of intracranial haemorrhage such as extradural or subarachnoid haemorrhage (although the top diagnosis of subdural haematoma is most likely in this age group), fall secondary to poor lighting/poor gait/poor eyesight, acute cerebrovascular accident (CVA) which are less likely.

Management:

Routine blood tests: FBC, U&E, LFTs, CRP and check INR levels.

CT Head +/- referral to neurosurgery for burr hole decompression.

Other: ECG, CXR, cardiac enzymes.

Occupational health assessment at home.

Physiotherapy assessment.

STATION 27

Name: Mr Harold Warding

Age: 72 years old

Job: Retired salesman

PC:

Over the last six months your wife has been complaining that you are getting more and more forgetful about things. For example, last week your house was broken into and your wife's jewellery stolen because you forgot to close the front door, which is out of character for you. A few days ago you left the stove on when you went to walk your dog and only realised when you came home – fortunately no damage occurred. You keep misplacing things and not realising where you last put them, then find them in odd places like your wallet in the fridge. You do not have a headache and do not have any neurology of note. Although you think your memory is fading, you would not say that you have had any change in your personality. You do not suffer from any mental health problems; you deny any depression and have not had any recent head trauma.

Past Medical History:

Diabetes type 2 – well controlled on oral hypoglycaemics. No severe diabetes related complications.

Hypertension

Benign prostatic hypertrophy

Gastro-oesophageal reflux disease

Drug History:

NKDA

Omeprazole 20mg po od

Amlodipine 5mg po od

Metformin 500mg po od

Social History:

You have smoked all your life. On average you have had 15 cigarettes a day for the last 50 years. You do not drink any alcohol.

You are independent of all activities of daily living.

You live with your wife in a small cottage in the nearby village. You have one dog and like taking long country walks.

Since you have starting being forgetful you feel that your relationship with your wife has become rather strained and she is starting to get rather irritated by you. You had a big argument when the house was burgled last week and your wife was very upset her things were stolen. You feel helpless because you can't remember doing these things and certainly didn't mean to leave the door open on purpose!

Ideas/Concerns/Expectations:

You wonder if you have had a mini-stroke to cause this confusion and also worry about having a brain tumour. You want to know if the doctor will send you for a brain scan to check that there is nothing serious going on. You would like to know if there is any medication that you can take to improve your memory.

Diagnosis:

Dementia (Alzheimer's)

Differentials:

Vascular dementia, Lewy Body Dementia

Management:

Routine blood tests: FBC, U&E, LFTs, CRP.

Confusion screen: CT head, vitamin B12 and folate levels, syphilis screen, glucose, TFTs, MSU.

Mini Mental State Examination, MMSE.

Old age psychiatry referral for diagnosis under DSM-IV criteria.

Medication may include NMDA antagonists (memantine) or acetylcholinesterase inhibitors (donepezil, rivastigmine).

STATION 28

Carer's name: Jessie Smith

Patient's Name: Mrs Isabelle Lacey

Age: 84 years old

PC:

For the last five days you have noticed a member of your care home, Isabelle Lacey, has become rather confused and muddled for no apparent reason. She is normally a very chatty member of the home and enjoys her afternoon tea by the fireplace with the other care home residents. She is very good at card games and loves the newspaper Sudoku. Recently, however, she has been filling out all the puzzles wrongly in the paper and other care home residents are struggling to make sense of her conversations.

She has not demonstrated any fevers, rigors or complained of any tummy pains. Some of the staff have noticed that she has been incontinent more times than usual and that when cleaning her underwear there is a strange smell. They have not noticed any blood on the underwear. She has not had any recent change in her medication or diet or been in contact with any other residents with illnesses. She has no neurology and no one has noticed any skin rashes. She has not lost any weight but her appetite is slightly decreased.

Past Medical History:

High blood pressure

Increased cholesterol

Myocardial infarct about 10 years ago

Drug History:

NKDA

Aspirin 75mg po od

Simvastatin 20mg po od

Bisoprolol 2.5mg po od

Lisinopril 5mg po od

Social History:

Mrs Lacey lives in a care home with 20 other residents.

Her family visit three times a week.

She is unsteady on her feet and mobilises with a Zimmer frame. She requires help going to the toilet, washing, dressing, doing laundry and cleaning. She is able to feed herself. She is occasionally incontinent of urine so wears pads for this which need to be changed by the staff at the home.

Ideas/Concerns/Expectations:

The care home staff think Mrs Lacey may be having flu or just suffering a bit of 'old age confusion'. They also wonder if she has had a mini-stroke perhaps.

Diagnosis:

Urinary tract infection

Differentials:

Other source of infection such as gastroenteritis or respiratory tract infection although less likely.

Dementia, transient ischaemic attack (TIA), cerebrovascular accident (CVA), small vessel ischaemia

Management:

Routine blood tests: FBC, U&E, LFTs, CRP.

Routine observations: Temperature, pulse, blood pressure, oxygen saturation and respiratory rate.

Full septic screen: MSU for microbiology, cultures and sensitivities, blood cultures, CXR.

Imaging: Renal ultrasound scan to identify any renal damage/abscess/scarring, CT head for confusion.

Antibiotics: Oral antibiotics such as trimethoprim, nitrofurantoin or co-amoxiclav (although be careful in the elderly to risk causing pseudomembranous colitis).

Advice: Maintain hydration, nurse in a well lit and familiar surroundings to avoid agitation.

STATION 29

Name: Mr Kevin Kettering

Age: 58 years old

Job: Gardener

PC:

This morning whilst you were getting out of bed you noticed your left leg and arm were extremely weak. In fact you almost fell to the floor because you could not hold your own weight but managed to fall back into bed without hurting yourself. You thought you just slept funny and that once the blood supply returned it would be all right, but this lasted for 30 minutes. During the episode you felt that the left side of your body was numb and you were not able to move properly. You did not feel any pain or tingling. You did not have any speech disturbance. You are systemically well without any recent foreign travel, flu-like symptoms or fevers. This has never happened to you before.

Your wife was fast asleep during this time and you didn't want to wake her as you thought the whole episode would just pass. After 30 minutes the symptoms gradually resolved. You are now much stronger although a slight numb feeling still persists in the left arm and leg. You have come into hospital now to get a proper check up because you are worried you are having a stroke.

Past Medical History:

Diabetes type 2 – diagnosed 10 years ago. It is relatively well controlled without any serious complications from diabetes apart from a raised blood pressure. No foot ulcers, renal damage or retina damage. Your latest HbA1c was 8%.

High blood pressure – diagnosed six years ago and started on medication. It is within the normal limits.

Drug History:

NKDA

Metformin 500mg po od

Amlodipine 5mg po od

Social History:

You have smoked 20 cigarettes a day for the last 20 years.

You only drink a glass of wine on the weekends with meals.

You are currently fully independent of ADLs. You enjoy long walks in the countryside and work as a gardener, spending all your time outdoors. On weekends you enjoy playing golf with your friends and consider yourself an active member of the country golf club. You live with your wife in a bungalow and have no children.

Family History:

Mother died of a heart attack aged 52 years old.

Father had a stroke aged 60 years old.

Ideas/Concerns/Expectations:

You are worried about having a stroke because you saw your father go through years of loss of his independence and having carers help with daily activities of living. You don't know how you would cope if this happened to you.

Diagnosis:

Cerebrovascular accident (CVA), transient ischaemic attack (TIA)

Differentials:

Space occupying lesion (brain tumour, abscess) – less likely

Management:

CT head +/- MRI head

Routine blood tests: FBC, U&E, LFTs, CRP.

Other blood tests: fasting glucose, cholesterol, homocysteine levels.

Other investigations: ECG, ECHO, Carotid Doppler tests, CXR, BP measurements.

Referral to stroke unit for treatment and rehabilitation.

Treatment depends on the type of stroke (i.e. whether haemorrhagic or thrombotic or other).

If thrombotic (majority of cases), and not suitable for thrombolysis, medication includes high dose (300mg) aspirin for at least the initial two weeks followed by lower dose aspirin long-term with proton pump inhibitor cover (PPI). Risk factor modification and treatment of possible causes for the event are addressed (e.g. rate control or rhythm control for atrial fibrillation, treatment of high blood pressure, carotid endarterectomy etc.).

STATION 30

Name: Mr Adam Scott

Age: 50 years old

Job: Stock broker

PC:

For the last four months or so you have not been feeling quite yourself. You feel that you are forgetting lots of bits of information that you are normally quite sharp on such as what the stocks and shares are doing in your line of work. In addition, for the last two months you notice a strange sort of ringing in your left ear that doesn't seem to go away. Over the past week you have started to feel rather 'butter fingered'. When you are texting the messages don't make sense because you keep missing the letters you want to type and last week when you were at a business meeting you spilt a big cup of water even though you were certain you were holding the cup tightly. This has never happened to you before and you are very worried.

Although you have sensation in your right arm and leg they feel muted. You occasionally have a sensation of tingling down that side of your body but it doesn't normally last very long – only about a few minutes. You do not have a headache. You are systemically well with no other symptoms. No recent travel abroad.

Past Medical History:

Nil of note.

Drug History:

NKDA

Social History:

Smoked 20 cigarettes a day for the last 30 years.

Drinks a glass of wine every night.

Lives in his own four bedroom house with two young children and his wife.

Busy stressful job as a stock broker. Business is not going very well.

Family History:

Your great grandfather suffered with a brain tumour but you don't know what happened to him.

Ideas/Concerns/Expectations:

You worry that you may have a brain tumour and want to rule this out. You demand that the doctors order you a MRI or CT scan to check this out urgently. You have two young children and a wife to support at home and worry that if you get ill then you can no longer do this.

Diagnosis:

Space occupying lesion (brain tumour)

Differentials:

Cerebrovascular accident (CVA)

Management:

Routine blood tests: FBC, U&E, LFT, CRP.

Full neurological examination.

Radiological investigations: CT head +/- MRI head.

Referral to neurosurgeons and discussion at neurology MDT.

STATION 31

Name: Timothy McAfee

Age: 45 years old

Job: Unemployed train driver

PC: Tremor

You are a heavy alcohol user and two days ago after a prolonged alcohol binge decided to stop drinking alcohol – you have not had a drink since. Today you woke up feeling very unwell. You feel nauseous and cannot stop shaking. You have had 'the shakes' before, and usually a shot of whisky has settled it (you put it down to nerves). You had a fever throughout the night, and didn't sleep very much. This morning you suffered an attack of severe anxiety, such that you thought you were going to die. You were very short of breath and at that point called an ambulance (although this attack only lasted 10–20 minutes in total). You keep having a feeling that something is crawling over your hands and feet, although nothing is there. You have the vague feeling that someone is causing this sensation to annoy you, although you cannot pinpoint who is persecuting you in this way. You do not have any respiratory/gastrointestinal/urinary symptoms.

You normally drink about half a bottle of vodka a day, beginning in the mornings, and have done so at this level for over a year. You are known for being able to drink the most in your local pub! You don't really have any interest in other types of alcohol. You have tried to stop drinking twice before, but after a couple of weeks you started again at similar levels.

You have had a very low mood recently as you lost your job and partner recently. You have not considered suicide, and mainly the vodka lets you forget about your problems.

Past Medical History:

Various broken bones and lacerations over the last few years.

No inpatient admissions.

Drug History:

Nil. No allergies.

Social History:

Your partner left you three months ago due to arguments about drinking. She took your two year old son with her, and you have only seen him a couple of times since.

You recently lost your job as a train driver, as one of your colleagues saw you sipping from a hip flask at work.

Family History:

Your father also drank excessively, but he died of lung cancer when you were young.

Your mother has dementia and lives in a nursing home.

Ideas/Concerns/Expectations:

You know that alcohol has a detrimental effect on your life, but don't seem to be able to cope without it. You would like try on this occasion, but this whole episode has given you quite a shock.

Diagnosis:

Delirium tremens

Management:

Patients with delirium tremens have a high mortality rate if untreated.

Bloods: FBC to exclude co-existing infection, U&Es may be deranged, and LFTs (and clotting) may be raised. Amylase should be taken to exclude pancreatitis. Glucose levels may be low.

CXR may be helpful to exclude (often co-existing) pneumonia.

ECG may reveal arrhythmias.

CT head if seizures have occurred.

Benzodiazepines (e.g. a reducing regime of chlordiazepozide) are important to prevent autonomic over activity and seizures.

Intramuscular/intravenous thiamine (to prevent Wernicke-Korsakoff syndrome) and oral vitamin B complex.

Intensive care may be needed in severe cases.

STATION 32

Name: Mrs Lorraine Goring

Age: 53 years old

Job: Cleaner

PC:

For the last 6–8 months or so you have been noticing increasing amount of pain and swelling in the joints of your hands. You have also noticed that they are getting rather stiffer and less mobile as time goes on. You find that the pain is often worse when you first wake up but once you start working (cleaning people's houses) the pain improves. This is starting to affect your life as it causes you to be late for work in the mornings because you find getting dressed, doing up buttons and packing your bag is really quite a challenge. Although you have tried to manage the pain yourself with paracetamol you find that this does not really work. The only thing that seems to make the pain better is if you keep your hands warm and so you have been trying to wear more layers of clothing, sometimes keeping gloves on and filling a hot water bottle up to take into your bed with you in the mornings before you get ready to get up and go to work.

Your joints are not red and the skin around your joints does not look infected or have any cuts or abrasions. You don't have pain in any other joints but have noticed some funny lumps on your elbows which are tender, firm and skin-coloured without any redness or hotness to them. You do not have any rashes. You have not had red eyes and have not noticed any dryness in your mouth or eyes. You have not had any diarrhoea and have not lost weight. You do not have any mouth or genital ulcers. You do not have any neurological symptoms.

Past Medical History:

Hypercholesterolaemia

Hypothyroidism

Drug History:

NKDA

You take simvastatin 20mg od.

Levothyroxine 100mcg po od

Social History:

You smoke 1–2 cigarettes a day and only occasionally drink alcohol.

You live alone in a one bedroom flat and your children are grown up.

You are divorced and have very little to do with your estranged ex-husband.

Family History:

Your mother died of a heart attack when she was aged 52 years old. Your grandparents had arthritis but you don't know any details about it.

Ideas/Concerns/Expectations:

You are worried that this will eventually affect your work and you will need to stop even though you are currently able to work. You never got a degree from university and have bills to pay. If you can't be a cleaner then you are not really sure what else there is for you to do or who will support you.

Diagnosis:

Rheumatoid arthritis

Differentials:

Osteoarthritis, crystal arthropathy

Management:

Send blood tests including: FBC, CRP, ESR, rheumatoid factor and anti-CCP antibodies.

Arrange X-rays of the hands.

Encourage regular exercise and the patient may require referral to physiotherapy and occupational therapy for aids/splints.

Manage cardiovascular and cerebrovascular disease risk factors as atherosclerosis is accelerated in rheumatoid arthritis.

Encourage smoking cessation as this increases symptoms of rheumatoid arthritis.

Referral to a rheumatologist for assessment – treatment will include DMARDS, steroids for flare ups, and NSAIDS for pain control.

STATION 33

Name: Mrs Julie Bets

Age: 63 years old

Job: Retired clothes shop owner

PC:

You attend your GP practice today with a rather painful limp. For the last few months you have noticed increasing pain in your left hip and right knee which is usually worse at the end of the day, particularly if you have been on your feet a lot or have been cooking for your grandchildren at home.

None of your joints are red or swollen although the knee pain is worse when you touch your knee. It is rather difficult to be specific about which areas are tender to touch as you feel the whole knee can be 'achy' at the end of the day and it really doesn't matter where you touch it. In addition your granddaughter (who is only 8 years old) says that when she tries to 'massage' your knee she can hear crackling in it as she moves it. You wonder if you have bits of bone in your joint but can't think how they got in there!

You deny any recent falls, injury or trauma to the affected areas. None of your other joints are affected and you have not noticed any swellings or lumps anywhere else in your body. You do not have any rashes. You have not had red eyes and have not noticed any dryness in your mouth or eyes. You have not had any diarrhoea and have not lost weight. You do not have any mouth or genital ulcers. You do not have any neurological symptoms.

Past Medical History:

None.

Drug History:

NKDA

Paracetamol 1g po prn

Ibuprofen 400mg po prn

Social History:

You do not smoke or drink.

You have one son who is always at work and very busy. His wife is also very career-orientated so you are usually left with your two granddaughters to look after when they come home from school. You enjoy playing with them but find it hard to keep up with their antics as your joint pain gets worse with excessive movements.

You used to do a lot of exercise as a youngster and ran three marathons in your day. You never had any sporting injuries but do feel that you have 'overused' your joints a bit and are paying the price now. Many of your friends have recently had joint replacement surgeries and you know they have not had great results so would like to put this off for as long as possible!

Ideas/Concerns/Expectations:

You did not want to bother the doctor but the pain is getting the better of you so you wanted to check what is wrong.

Diagnosis:

Osteoarthritis

Differentials:

Rheumatoid arthritis, crystal arthropathy

Management:

Arrange X-rays of hands and knee.

Encourage regular exercise.

Prescribe regular analgesics such as paracetamol/codeine/NSAIDS.

Reduce weight, is BMI >28.

Intra-articular steroid injections may temporarily alleviate severe symptoms.

Joint replacement is indicated for severe osteoarthritis.

STATION 34

Name: Mr Stuart Bowman

Age: 70 years old

Job: Retired accountant

PC:

You have come to see the GP today with your right wrist wrapped loosely in some bandaging. You have found that for the last week it has been painful, red, hot and swollen and whatever you do it just doesn't seem to get better. You find that wrapping it in bandages makes other people aware that you have pain in your wrist and stops them banging into you as the joint is very tender to touch. You report that two months ago your right ankle was swollen and painful but this went away by itself after a week and you took regular paracetamol for this.

The left wrist is fine and now your right ankle has also completely settled. You deny any other joint pain in your body and you have not had any fevers, night sweats or rigors. There are no bruising, skin abrasions or cuts over the right wrist and you have not had any recent trauma or surgery to the area.

Elsewhere in your body you deny any rashes and do not have red or itchy eyes. You deny mouth dryness and cannot recall any change in bowel habits or weight loss. You do not have any mouth or genital ulcers.

Although the joint is acutely swollen and tender you can still easily move your fingers and deny any neurological symptoms in the right hand. There is no obvious deformity (apart from the swelling) of your hands or right wrist.

Past Medical History:

Hypertension

Anxiety

Drug History:

No drug allergies.

Bendroflumethiazide 2.5mg od po

Fluoxetine 20mg po od

Paracetamol 1g po qds prn

Social History:

You do not smoke and usually drink only at the weekends, but admit it is really just a small amount.

You live with your wife and do not have any pets or children.

Your neighbours are very friendly and have been helping you do your shopping since you've been having this bad joint pain.

Normally you are really quite independent and still drive and do household chores on your own.

Family History:

None significant.

Ideas/Concerns/Expectations:

You are in quite a lot of pain and you came to hospital to get stronger painkillers.

Diagnosis:

Pseudogout

Differentials:

Gout, septic arthritis

Management:

Blood tests: FBC, U&E (including phosphate and magnesium), TFTs, CRP.

X-ray of affected joint.

Light microscopy of joint fluid.

Give analgesia – NSAIDS.

If not controlled with analgesia can try steroids or hydroxychloroquine.

STATION 35

Name: Mrs Nancy Larson

Age: 42 years old

Job: Teacher

PC:

For the last five months you have been noticing increasing pain particularly the joints of your hands and your feet. The pain appears to be worse first thing in the morning when you also get stiffness in the fingers but does gradually ease off during the rest of the day. You find this really rather annoying as you are a teacher and need to mark a lot of student papers and do typed student reports for the end of year assessments. None of your joints are red or hot but they do occasionally feel rather swollen. Again this is only usually first thing in the morning. You take ibuprofen for the pain and swelling, which seems to help a little bit.

In the rest of your body you deny swelling or pain in any other joints although you think as you get older you are getting some back stiffness like all your other friends your age. However, you have noticed that your eyes and mouth are getting rather dry for some reason and that your face is looking a little tight. You are delighted by this as you think it makes your wrinkles less obvious. You have not had red eyes, diarrhoea and have not lost weight although you will admit that in the last four months you have not been eating as much as you used to due to food getting stuck in your throat making you feel a little uncomfortable. You do not have any mouth or genital ulcers and deny neurological symptoms.

Past Medical History:

None significant.

Drug History:

You are allergic to morphine. When asked what sort of allergies you get you say it makes you constipated and you feel nauseated on it. You had to be given it once when you fractured your arm as a teenager falling off your horse.

Ibuprofen 400mg po od prn

Social History:

You do not smoke or drink.

You live at home with your husband and you have a very busy job. You were recently promoted to being Head of the English department at the high school where you work and you therefore have lots of reading, marking and meetings to attend.

Family History:

None significant.

Ideas/Concerns/Expectations:

You are not very worried but wanted to come and get checked out as you think with your new job responsibilities this pain and stiffness will only get worse and you need it to be sorted quickly!

Diagnosis:

Sjogren's syndrome

Differentials:

Rheumatoid arthritis

Management:

Blood test: FBC, CRP, rheumatoid factor, ANA, Anti-Ro and Anti-La antibodies.

Parotid gland biopsy would show focal lymphocytic aggregation.

Schirmer's test to test for dryness of the eyes and decreased lacrimal tear production.

Rose bengal staining and slit lamp examination may reveal keratitis in the eyes.

If severe disease – immunosuppressants such as steroids may be used.

STATION 36

Name: Mr Lawrence Henry

Age: 21 years old

Job: Engineering student

PC:

You have been having pretty severe pains in your hips and your lower back for the last two months. They initially started in the lower back but have gradually spread to include the back of your pelvis and both hips. You find it now increasingly hard to bend over and touch your toes like you used to and think that the pain is worse at night although the stiffness in the joints can be quite bad in the mornings too. As the day goes on this stiffness improves and you also find that the more exercise you do, the more it eases off. Your joints are not red, hot or tender. You have not noticed any swelling or pain in any other joints. You don't have any deformity of the fingers in your hands and you find that at university you are still able to do your assignments, type and handle the tools you use with no trouble.

You deny any rashes and have not had any eye problems such as redness but find your mouth and eyes do get rather dry sometimes. You have not had any diarrhoea and have not lost weight. You do not have any mouth or genital ulcers. There is no history of any trauma, surgery or sporting injury to your lower back or hips. You do not have any neurological symptoms.

Past Medical History:

Hay fever

Drug History:

No drug allergies. None regular.

Social History:

You smoke and drink occasionally but not enough to quantify a regular amount. If you had to estimate you would probably say about 20 cigarettes in a whole month and maybe three glasses of wine a week.

Family History:

None significant.

Ideas/Concerns/Expectations:

You are concerned that you are have arthritis but think you are too young to have this.

Diagnosis:

Ankylosing spondylitis

Differentials:

Osteoarthritis, secondary to trauma

Management:

Blood test: FBC, CRP, ESR, HLA-B27.

Lumbar X-ray – can be normal in early disease. MRI is more sensitive.

Exercise regimen.

NSAIDS, TNF alpha blockers.

Local steroid injections for temporary relief.

STATION 37

Name: Mrs Ursula Ahern

Age: 68 years old

Job: Retired accountant

PC:

For the last three months you have been feeling very fatigued and lacking in energy. You are normally not like this and enjoy going out and exercising as well as taking an active role in the care of your grandchildren. You are not sure of the reason for this. You deny travel abroad, eating anything strange or feeling flu-like or feverish. You have been sleeping well, in fact more so than you normally do but still feel tired. You have not had any change in your appetite but noticed that in the last two months you have lost 7kg without trying and think you look rather pale in the mirror.

Although you do not experience any pain or change in bowel habit, you have noticed a bit of blood in your stools now and again. It is usually mixed with the stools and dark. You have no pain passing stools. You have suffered from diverticulitis in the past where you did pass some blood in your stools but this was associated with left-sided abdominal pain which you don't have on this occasion. You have had colonoscopies in the past, the most recent one was over five years ago and it did not reveal anything suspicious.

Past Medical History:

Gallstones – you had your gallbladder removed 20 years ago laparascopically

Appendicitis as a teenager

Diverticulitis

Drug History:

NKDA. None.

Social History:

You have smoked 10 cigarettes a day for the last 40 years.

You do not drink alcohol except on social occasions.

You live with your husband and are both very active and can perform all activities of daily living. You have three sons and five grandchildren aged between 3 years old and 10 years old. You help take them to school and look after them when your children are busy at work.

Family History:

Your father was diagnosed with bowel cancer at the age of 79 years old.

Your mother died of breast cancer in her seventies.

Ideas/Concerns/Expectations:

You think all your symptoms are just down to getting a bit old and frail. You suspect the doctor will tell you not to worry and that the bleeding is just the diverticulitis.

Diagnosis:

Anaemia secondary to colorectal carcinoma

Differentials:

Diverticulitis/diverticular abscess

Management:

Routine blood tests: FBC, ferritin, U&E, LFTs, CRP and tumour markers e.g. CEA.

Colonoscopy +/- biopsy.

Staging CT thorax/abdomen/pelvis.

Referral to colorectal MDT.

Referral to general surgery team.

STATION 38

Name: Miss Rosie Evergreen

Age: 34 years old

Job: Personal Assistant, PA

PC:

Within the last two months you have been feeling very tired and lacking in energy. You also notice that you have been putting on a lot of weight very quickly without any increase in your appetite or diet. The amount of weight gained is roughly 10kg during the last month. You feel that your face is now very round and your waistline has increased so much that you are starting to see stretchmarks across your tummy.

You have also noticed that your skin is quite spotty and embarrassingly you think you have now developed an increase in the amount of your facial hair. Your periods are not irregular and appear to be normal. You do not notice any neurology or visual disturbances. You are rather depressed by all of this and feel very unattractive and ugly as a result.

Past Medical History:

Asthma (but not on steroids)

Diabetes type 2 – only diagnosed recently, within the last month by the GP.

Drug History:

NKDA

Salbutamol inhalers

Ipratropium bromide inhalers

Metformin 500mg po od

You do not take any steroids.

Social History:

You do not drink alcohol or smoke.

You attend aerobics classes twice a week for an hour and have also been going to the gym three times a week on top of this recently to try to lose weight but it hasn't helped.

You are sleeping well at night and can't understand why you are so tired. You are not going through a stressful time at work and everything is otherwise going well in your life.

Ideas/Concerns/Expectations:

You just want to get back to normal life and feel very upset about all this. You are not in a relationship and desperately want to get married soon and start a family but cannot see how any man would want to date you looking the way you do!

Diagnosis:

Cushing's syndrome

Differentials:

Hypothyroidism, chronic alcohol consumption, poorly controlled diabetes

Investigation:

Routine blood tests: FBC, U&E, LFTs, fasting glucose, HbA1c levels.

Blood tests for pituitary function such as thyroid hormones, prolactin, FSH, LH etc.

24 hour urinary cortisol levels.

Low dose dexamethasone suppression tests.

Midnight cortisol levels to look for loss of diurnal cortisol variation.

MRI of the pituitary gland.

Referral to endocrinologist for treatment.

STATION 39

Name: Mr Arthur Monty

Age: 75 years old

Job: Retired painter/builder/decorator

PC:

You have noticed that on three occasions in the past month your urine has looked red as if it was blood that you were passing. The first time was one month ago, the second time a week ago and the third time was yesterday. During the remainder of the time your urine is normal-coloured. The episodes were all painless. There was no connection you could make to anything different that has happened in your life or any diet you were on. You have not eaten beetroot in many years.

During the episodes of haematuria, the urine was red for the whole stream. You remember being very shocked to see it. You went to see the GP yesterday as you are really worried and you thought that perhaps the lack of pain was a good sign but the GP was also concerned and has sent you to the urology clinic in hospital today.

You do not have any pain on passing urine or any discharge from the penis. You do not have either abdominal pain or back pain. In the last year you have also noticed that whenever you go to urinate you have to wait a number of seconds before your urine starts to flow and it tends to dribble a bit more at the end, after you think you have finished. You pass urine about six times a day and now need to get up at night at least once to pass urine whereas you only previously passed urine about four times a day and never at night.

You have found yourself feeling rather tired and fatigued more than usual in the last six months and also think that you may have lost weight recently. You are not sure exactly how much but your clothes feel baggy now and your family have commented upon this as well.

Past Medical History:

None significant.

Drug History:

NKDA. Nil regular.

Social History:

You have smoked 20 a day for 30 years.

You drink a couple of pints of beer most evenings per week but no wine or spirits.

You have not worked with any dangerous chemicals (including aniline dyes) that you know of apart from the usual paints, cleaners etc.

You have never had any urine or sexual infections.

You don't travel outside the UK.

Family History:

Your parents are alive and well and there is no family history of any illness.

Ideas/Concerns/Expectations:

You are concerned that this is cancer and the fact that your GP arranged an urgent appointment makes you feel even more certain this is what is going on but no one wants to admit it. You are a matter of fact sort of patient and if it is something serious you would rather know sooner rather than later so that you can try to sort it out and get on top of it.

Diagnosis:

Cancer of the urinary tract (most often transitional cell carcinoma)

Differentials:

Infection: cystitis/urethritis, tuberculosis, schistosomiasis

Renal calculi

Tumour: bladder carcinoma, renal carcinoma, prostate cancer, urethral cancer

Trauma (unlikely in this instance)

Inflamation: glomerulonephritis, polyarteritis, Goodpasture's syndrome, Henoch-Schonlein purpura, IgA nephropathy

Coagulation disorders: anticoagulants, inherited clotting disorders

Toxins: NSAIDs

Foods: excessive beetroot

Not haematuria: porphyria, bilirubinuria

Management:

The patient's genitourinary system should be fully examined, and the prostate should be felt. The blood pressure should be taken.

The urine should be dipped to confirm the diagnosis of haematuria. Even if the sample is not currently red, it is likely to contain microscopic haematuria. The dipstick will also be useful to pick up infection and proteinuria. Cytology can be undertaken on the urine to help diagnose cancer.

The patient should have a FBC to exclude haematuria, clotting tests to exclude clotting disorders, and U&Es to exclude associated renal dysfunction. The patient should be admitted for a blood transfusion if the haemoglobin is low.

A flexible cystoscopy with biopsy in the first instance is essential to help diagnose bladder and urethral abnormalities. A pelvic CT or MRI scan can help stage the disease. Examination of the upper urinary system with bladder ultrasound and IVU may also be helpful.

Rigid cystoscopy under general anaesthesia and trans-urethral resection of bladder tumour (TURBT) allows cure if cancer is diagnosed. Intravesical chemotherapy (such as with BCG) and external beam radiotherapy reduce recurrence. Advising the patient to stop smoking also reduces the recurrence rate. In some advanced cases cystoprostatectomy is required to cure the disease.

STATION 40

Name: Albert Clower

Age: 37 years old

Job: Internet entrepreneur

PC: Left scrotal lump

Whilst in the shower a week ago you noticed that one of your testicles seemed bigger than the other. You weren't quite sure if they had always been like this, so you asked your girlfriend (a qualified nurse) to examine you. She was concerned and told you to go to the GP. The lump is not painful but you have noticed a kind of 'dragging' sensation. The overlying skin feels normal. You remember that a couple of weeks ago you were kicked in the groin whilst playing rugby, and are unsure if this is what started it. You think you might have put on a bit of weight recently, as your girlfriend has been making fun of your 'man-breasts'. You are not having any sexual problems. You have not experienced any abdominal pain or other gastrointestinal symptoms or urinary symptoms. You feel well in yourself.

Past Medical History:

As a child you had an operation to correct an undescended left testicle.

As a teenager you were treated for attention hyperactivity disorder (ADHD).

Drug History:

Nil. No allergies.

Social History:

You smoke socially (about 20 per week).

You indulge in binge drinking at weekends but would rather not tell the doctor exactly how much because you are embarrassed you will get told off!

You live with your girlfriend of two years and your relationship is going well.

Family History:

Your father suffered with type 1 diabetes and your mother had breast cancer.

Ideas/Concerns/Expectations:

You don't really think it is anything but want to avoid being pestered by your girlfriend and so will go along with whatever investigations are necessary.

Diagnosis:

Testicular tumour (seminoma)

Differential:

Other testicular tumour: lymphoma, non-germ cell testicular tumours

Hydrocele

Epididymal cyst

Infection: epididymo-orchitis, tuberculosis, syphilis, mumps

Torsion

Management:

Ultrasound scan to confirm diagnosis.

Staging scan by CT of the chest, abdomen and pelvis.

Tumour markers: Beta-human chorionic gonadotrophin (Beta-HCG) may be raised (Alpha-fetoprotein is not normally raised in seminomas, but may be raised for non-germ cell tumours).

Surgical management: orchidectomy via an inguinal approach (to avoid tumour seeding).

Radiotherapy and chemotherapy are indicated for certain stages of cancers.

Overall testicular tumours (seminomas) if found early have a very good prognosis. It is estimated that over 95% of testicular tumours in young men will be seminomas.

STATION 41

Name: Mr Harold Mariano

Age: 76 years old

Job: Retired bus driver

PC: Poor urinary stream

For six months you have had trouble emptying your bladder. You have to stand for ages over a toilet bowl until the water starts to come out, and then it only seems to come out slowly and with straining. Even at the end of the stream you still feel that there is a bit of dribbling at the end and you do not feel you have completely emptied your bladder. You frequently return within a few hours to have another go.

Overall you would say that you pass urine about 10 times a day. You get up 3–4 times a night to empty your bladder and your wife is getting rather annoyed at all the time you seem to be spending in the toilet. She wonders if you are trying to hide a secret from her or if you are trying to make secret telephone calls to another woman!

You have never suffered haematuria, loin pain, or dysuria. You occasionally suffer from constipation but you take laxatives to help things move along whenever you feel that is the case. There has not ever been a time when you couldn't pass any urine at all, and you have not suffered from urinary incontinence or urgency. You have not suffered back pain. You are not currently sexually active due to lack of sexual appetite rather than any issues with erectile dysfunction. You deny ever needing to go to hospital for catheterisation (only volunteer this information if asked).

Past Medical History:

Hypertension

COPD

Drug History:

No allergies.

Bendroflumethiazine 5mg OD

Salbutamol (PRN) and Seretide (2 puffs BD) inhalers

Social History:

You live with your wife, who suffered a hip fracture six months ago and has had poor mobility since then.

You are an ex-smoker (stopping five years ago) and used to smoke 10 cigarettes for 30 years.

You do not drink much alcohol but do however enjoy coffee and drink 4–5 cups a day.

You drive the school bus two days a week, but find that your urinary frequency interferes with this and are thinking of giving up this part-time job.

Family History:

Nil.

Ideas/Concerns/Expectations:

You are finding this annoyance is starting to interfere with your life and would like something done about it if possible.

You would also like to get your wife's suspicious thoughts put to rest!

Diagnosis:

Lower urinary tract symptoms due to benign prostatic hyperplasia

Differentials:

Prostate cancer

Bladder/urethral cancer

Urinary tract infection – chronic

Urinary tract stones

Detrusor muscle weakness

Chronic prostatitis

Polyuria, e.g. due to diabetes

Neurological: e.g. multiple sclerosis

Management:

Examination of the abdomen, genitalia and prostate.

Urine dipstick and cytology.

Bloods: FBC, CRP, U&Es (if renal dysfunction suspected), PSA.

Urinary frequency charting.

Flow-rate and post-void residual volume measurement.

Transrectal ultrasound scan of the prostate.

Advice regarding fluid and caffeine intake (can exacerbate symptoms).

Consider intermittent bladder catheterisation.

Drug treatment: alpha blockers (e.g. alfuzosin), 5-alpha reductase inhibitors (e.g. finasteride), late afternoon loop diuretic.

Surgery: transurethral resection of the prostate (TURP).

STATION 42

Name: Mrs Melinda Jasper

Age: 42 years old

Job: Financial planner

PC:

You discovered a breast lump a week ago in the shower, and it has taken this long to get a GP appointment (which you are rather unsatisfied with). The lump is in the upper, outer aspect of your breast and has not changed since you noticed it. It is painless, and is not associated with skin or nipple changes, or lumps under your armpits. You have never had any previous breast lumps or surgery to the breasts.

You had your menarche at age 12 and are not menopausal. You have one daughter, who you had when you were 32. You did not breastfeed her as it was too painful, although you did express into a bottle.

You are not on the oral contraceptive pill and never have been.

Past Medical History:

Anxiety and depressive disorder

Drug History:

No known drug allergies.

Citalopram 40mg od

Social History:

You are married and live in a semi-detached house in the suburbs with your husband and 10 year old daughter.

You are a social smoker (about 15 per week), and drink a glass of red every night.

You have never taken any recreational drugs.

You do not take anything over the counter or any homeopathic medication.

Family History:

Your mother suffered from breast cancer in her forties, and she had a mastectomy which was curative.

Ideas/Concerns/Expectations:

You are very worried that it might be cancer and would like this ruled out.

Diagnosis:

Breast cancer

Differentials:

Simple cyst

Papilloma

Fat necrosis

Fibroadenoma

Abscess

Lipoma or sebaceous cyst

Phyllodes tumour

Management:

The breast should be fully examined. The axilla should be examined for lymph nodes, and the abdomen and lungs for metastases.

The patient should be referred to the breast clinic in view of her family history. Mammography is useful to detect cancers. Ultrasound is useful in younger patients. Fine needle aspiration (FNA) or biopsy is often diagnostic. Blood tests are useful to detect anaemia and liver metastases. CXR (lung metastases), bone scans (bony metastases), and CTs are useful for staging. MRI and PET scans are occasionally required.

Depending on the stage of the tumour, lumpectomy, wide local excision, and mastectomy (with or without axillary node dissection) are used. Adjuvant hormonal therapy (tamoxifen, Anastrozole) is given if tumours are positive for hormonal receptors. Chemotherapy agents (such as doxorubicin) and radiotherapy can be given to reduce recurrence. Trastuzumab (Herceptin) can be given if the biopsy of the patient's cancer demonstrates HER2 receptors.

STATION 43

Name: Miss Louise Easterling

Age: 29 years old

Job: Nurse

PC: Right bloody nipple discharge

A week ago you noticed a bit of blood on your shirt around the right nipple but initially assumed that you must have cut yourself or wondered whether it was a bit of the patient's blood that you had taken earlier in the day (you work as a nurse). You have had on and off bloody discharge from the right nipple since then and are able to express it. It is watery bloodstained fluid. You find it difficult to quantify the amount as it seems to make a mess of your shirt and looks like it is probably more than it is. You do not suffer with any breast or nipple pain and deny having felt any lumps in your armpits or breast. Your left nipple does not seem to display the same symptoms.

You had your menarche at age 13, your periods are regular at every 29–31 days and you normally bleed for 3–5 days. You have never been pregnant and do not have any children. You have never breastfed.

Past Medical History:

Anxiety and depression

Drug History:

Citalopram 20mg od

You have used the OCP since you were 17 years old.

Social History:

You live with your boyfriend of two years, who has just been diagnosed with testicular cancer, and you are quite worried about him. You do not work smoke, and you drink socially (but not excessively).

You find your job a little stressful and you think that with all this talk about cancer going around you would be devastated if you had it, especially at such a young age.

Family History:

Your mother died of ovarian cancer at age 58.

Ideas/Concerns/Expectations:

With your medical background you know that there is a connection to breast cancer and this really worries you.

Diagnosis:

Intraductal papilloma

Duct ectasia

Differentials:

Breast cancer

Management:

The intention of investigation is to exclude breast cancer.

Examination of both breasts and axilla.

Examination of lungs and abdomen for metasteses.

Cytology of nipple discharge.

Mammography or ultrasound scan of the right breast.

Magnetic resonance galactography.

If papilloma is diagnosed then reassurance can be given. The papilloma can be excised to rule out with certainty that it is not a malignancy, or if it is troubling to the patient.

STATION 44

Name: Mr Roger Palmer

Age: 71 years old

Job: Retired engineer

PC:

You still enjoy carpentry and a couple of weeks ago whilst stooping to pick up a heavy piece of wood you suffered a sharp pain in your right groin and noticed a lump come out. It disappeared soon after but has reappeared twice since, and seems to come on when you are exerting yourself. The lump is present just inside your right groin crease. It is not painful and there have been no overlying skin changes. There have been no changes in the other groin. You feel well otherwise, and have not had any symptoms of constipation, vomiting or abdominal pain.

Past Medical History:

You have chronic obstructive airways disease and hypertension.

You have never had any other surgery in this or any other part of your body.

Drug History:

You do not have any drug allergies.

You are very bad at remembering your medications' names but know that you have two inhalers (blue, purple) and one 'fluid tablet' for your blood pressure.

Social History:

You are independent of all activities of daily living.

You do not consider yourself overweight but your wife is always pestering you to lose a few pounds.

You have smoked 15 cigarettes a day for the last 10 years and prior to this it was about 30 cigarettes a day for the last 50 years. You rarely drink alcohol.

Family History:

Nil of note.

Ideas/Concerns/Expectations:

You are not really bothered about the lump (in fact it was your wife who instructed you to come), but are happy to have whatever treatment is recommended for it.

Diagnosis:

Inguinal hernia

Differentials:

Femoral hernia

Infection: groin abscess, psoas abscess

Soft tissue: lipoma, sebaceous cyst, lymphadenopathy, haematoma

Vascular: femoral artery aneurysm, saphena varix

Cancer

Management:

The groin and abdomen should be fully examined. A per-rectal examination should be performed. If the lump is erythematous, irreducible, or tender the patient should be referred urgently to the surgical team for evaluation.

Inguinal hernias protrude above and medial to the pubic tubercle. They may contain bowel but most often simply have fat or omentum in them. Males are afflicted more commonly than females. They are more obvious on standing, and a positive cough impulse may be present. Although femoral hernias are often quoted as being more common in the female population (and this is true, women do get femoral hernias more often than men), overall a lump in the groin regardless of sex will be more likely to be an inguinal hernia.

The patient can be referred to the general surgery clinic if there is no evidence of obstruction or strangulation. The diagnosis is clinical, although ultrasound is occasionally useful. Inguinal hernias can be repaired using an open or laparoscopic approach (preferred in bilateral cases).

STATION 45

Name: Mrs Gertrude Mclaurin

Age: 83 years old

Job: Retired secretary

PC:

Up until two weeks ago you suffered from the occasional nosebleed but it has become much worse recently. Almost every day for the last 14 days you have suffered bleeds of various severity: usually ranging from 10 minutes to two hours. You attended A&E yesterday after a particularly heavy episode where they inserted a nasal pack until it settled down. The bleeding is only from the right nostril. You are not a frequent nose-picker or blower, and have not had any recent trauma to the nose. You do not feel pale, faint, tachycardic, and have no chest pain.

Past Medical History:

You had a hysterectomy many years ago and also had a DVT diagnosed four months ago.

Drug History:

No known drug allergies.

Warfarin (For the last four months due to a recent DVT your INR is titrated to between 2 and 3, however, your last check was three weeks ago and you are not sure what the latest INR is. Three weeks ago it was 3.2 and you were told to withhold a dose of warfarin by your doctor and then continue again as normal.)

Aspirin 75mg od (This has not been prescribed by a doctor; you just take it and buy it over the counter in the shops because you read somewhere that it prevents heart attacks.)

Social History:

You do not drink or smoke.

Family History:

Diabetes runs in the family (both your parents developed diabetes in later life).

No bleeding disorders or nasal problems.

Ideas/Concerns/Expectations:

The nosebleeds are becoming very disruptive to your life as you are afraid to leave the house to see your friends. You have a friend who had nasal cancer and are afraid this might be what you have too, although you will only admit this when you are asked what you think the cause of the bleeding is. You would like something done today if possible.

Diagnosis:

Epistaxis related to anticoagulant use

Differentials:

Trauma to the nose (such as nose picking)

Clotting or platelet disorders

Drugs: aspirin, warfarin

Vascular abnormalities: hereditary haemorrhagic telangiectasia

Irritants: nasal inhalant use (especially steroid-based ones), cocaine use

Malignancy of the nose

Management:

Acute epistaxis can occasionally be severe and require inpatient treatment. IV access should be secured and fluids given to correct dehydration/shock. Anaemia should be corrected if present and clotting abnormalities can be reversed. The nose can be packed and definitive surgical management delivered if necessary.

In the clinic setting risk factors should be excluded. In this case it should be ascertained whether the concomitant use of aspirin and warfarin is necessary. A full examination of the head and neck should be undertaken including nasal speculum, and rigid or flexible nasendoscopy to evaluate intra-nasal lesions. FBC and clotting should be undertaken if not already done. CT is occasionally indicated.

Silver nitrate cauterization is often successful. Advice can be given regarding decreasing risk factors and what to do to stop the bleeding successfully (lean forward and pinch the fleshy tip of the nose for 5–10 minutes).

STATION 46

Name: Mrs Judith Shumaker

Age: 68 years old

Job: Retired teacher

PC:

You are concerned because you think that your hearing is starting to fade. You have noticed recently that you have found it more difficult to understand your husband, and he is certainly getting fed up having to repeat himself! You have the TV set to the loudest level and yet you still cannot make out all the words spoken. Although these have only become problems recently you have a feeling that this may have been creeping up on you for a while. You were unsure if at first there was something stuck in your ear and so have been using cotton buds everyday to clean them out but there has been no improvement for the last month.

You don't think that your hearing is worse in any one ear. You have not experienced any pain, headaches, tinnitus, nausea, vertigo, aural discharge or facial weakness. You have never had any instrumentation or trauma to the ear.

Past Medical History:

Repeated UTIs – requiring two hospital admissions in the last year. During the admissions you were put on some strong antibiotics which you think started with a 'G' and ended in something like 'mycin'.

Hypertension

Osteoarthritis in knees and hips

Drug History:

No drug allergies.

Trimethoprim 200mg od po (long-term antibiotics to prevent recurrence of UTIs)

Furosemide 40mg bd po

Diclofenac 100mg po prn

Social History:

You do not drink or smoke.

You live at home with your husband who is also retired.

You both enjoy gardening and try to keep as fit as possible by having long walks in the countryside.

You are both independent of activities of daily living.

Family History:

You think that your mother also suffered from poor hearing in her old age.

Ideas/Concerns/Expectations:

As a teacher when you were younger you were famed for your strong, loud voice, and you consider it is possible you may have damaged your hearing by shouting! You would also quite like to get your hearing sorted out as you cannot afford a new louder television!

Diagnosis:

Cerumen (ear wax)

Differentials:
Conductive:

Foreign bodies

Exostosis

Infection: otitis media/externa

Tympanic membrane perforation

Growths: e.g. cysts or tumours

Cholesteatoma

Otosclerosis

Tympanosclerosis

Sensorineural:

Presbyacusis

Noise-induced hearing loss

Ototoxicity: e.g. aminoglycosides and salicylates

Autoimmune disease

Acoustic neuroma (usually unilateral)

Ménière's disease

Perilymphatic fistula

Management:

This patient may have more than one cause for her hearing loss. She has likely had Gentamicin exposure in hospital and loud noise exposure as a teacher. Cotton buds predispose to tympanic perforation, infection and foreign bodies (the tip can break off!). Luckily she has the most easily treatable disorder: ear wax.

Otoscopy confirms the diagnosis. Once it is removed in clinic via microsuction (under visualization using a microscope) the patient can undergo audiometry and tympanometry to exclude other diagnoses. Microsuction can be performed regularly in the ear clinic if necessary. Ear syringing is another treatment used but carries a higher risk of perforation. Olive oil ear drops are a harmless first-line treatment for the patient to take at home, and sodium bicarbonate drops may be used if this fails. Ear buds push wax further into the ear and should be avoided under all circumstances.

Treatment and management of the other causes depends on cause. Ultimately hearing aids may be necessary for non-reversible causes.

STATION 47

Name: Mrs Rhonda Smyth

Age: 52 years old

Job: Human resources manager

PC:

For the past couple of months you have had repeated episodes of severe dizziness (where the world is spinning around you). These are of sudden onset and last for just 30 seconds to one minute. You think they are provoked by certain head movements although you haven't been able to reproduce them. They are accompanied by slight nausea but not vomiting. You have not experienced any hearing loss, tinnitus, otalgia, photophobia, headaches, stiff necks. You haven't had any recent head injury.

Past Medical History:

You suffer from depression and also have had a right mastectomy and breast reconstruction for breast cancer 15 years ago. You did not have any metastatic disease and as far as you are aware the cancer is completely 'cured'.

Drug History:

Citalopram 20mg po od

Social History:

You do not smoke or drink any alcohol.

You live at home with your husband and two pet dogs. Things at home are difficult at the moment and you are not getting on well with your husband. He is always irritated that you are complaining about feeling dizzy and never in the mood to go out for dinner or watch a show in town.

Family History:

Your father died from a heart attack, and you can't recall any other diseases in the family.

Ideas/Concerns/Expectations:

These attacks of vertigo are contributing to your depression and putting a strain on your relationship with your husband, and you would like to know if your citalopram dose can be increased. You would really like to have something done about the vertigo but fear that no treatments exist.

Diagnosis:

Benign paroxysmal positional vertigo (BPPV)

Differentials:

Central:

Cerebrovascular disease (usually brainstem)

Migraine

Multiple sclerosis

Acoustic neuroma

Diplopia

Alcohol/drug toxicity

Peripheral:

Vestibular neuritis

Ménière's disease

Ototoxicity: e.g. gentamicin, salicylates

Infection: viral labyrinthitis, otitis media, Herpes zoster (Ramsay Hunt syndrome)

Management:

Otoscopy should be performed. A full neurological examination should be undertaken including inspection for nystagmus. Hallpike's manoeuvre is useful for diagnosing BPPV: a positive result is defined as vertigo and rotatory nystagmus towards the affected ear for several seconds.

Patients with vertigo should undergo audiometry to exclude cochlear dysfunction. Vestibular function can be evaluated using electronystagmography, calorimetry and brainstem-evoked responses. Neurological causes can be diagnoses on CT or MRI scans. Lumbar puncture can also be useful for diagnosing multiple sclerosis.

Explanation and reassurance is helpful for a patient suffering with BPPV, which is often self-limiting. Vestibular suppressants (such as prochlorperazine) can be useful for acute severe vertigo, but should not be used for prolonged periods. The Epley manoeuvre can be performed in clinic and has good efficacy in resolving vertigo. The patient can be instructed on exercises ('Brandt-Daroff' exercises) to be performed at home.

STATION 48

Name: Mr Kay Donner

Age: 45 years old

Job: Solicitor

PC:

Over the last month you have been rather irritated with yourself. You seem to keep bumping into things, only realising at the very last minute how close you are to them. In particular you can't seem to see things out of the corner of your eye as clearly – when you were trying to park your car the other day you banged your wing mirror and scratched the side of the car because you didn't realise how close it was to the car next door!

You also think that your appearance is changing. Over the last six months you've noticed that your skin is thick and greasy and a little spotty. Your hair is also rather dry even though you haven't changed shampoo. You don't think you look fatter than normal but somehow you don't fit into your trousers or shirts anymore. You deny any neurology but do occasionally suffer from generalised headaches, which never used to happen. You are systemically well and deny any travel abroad, change in medication or recent infections.

Past Medical History:

None.

Drug History:

NKDA.

None.

Social History:

You do not drink or smoke.

You work in the city and are not married.

Family History:

None.

Ideas/Concerns/Expectations:

You think all of this is strange and worry that it is all in your imagination. You wonder if you should really be seeing a doctor or a cosmetic surgeon instead to correct your strange new features!

Diagnosis:

Acromegaly caused by a macroadenoma of the pituitary gland

Differential Diagnosis:

Non-functioning macroadenoma of the pituitary gland.

Intracerebral tumour compressing on the optic chiasm or alternatively an intracerebral tumour with surrounding cerebral oedema which is causing a mass effect on the optic chiasm.

Management:

Full examination of the patient including cardiovascular and neurology assessment.

Investigation of any complications from acromegaly such as sight/visual assessment, blood pressure measurements, dental assessment, colonoscopy and blood glucose control.

Routine blood measurements: FBC, U&Es, LFTs and CRP.

Specific blood tests for acromegaly: oral glucose tolerance test to identify failure of suppression of growth hormone with elevated insulin-like growth factor levels. Isolated insulin-like growth factor – 1 (IGF-1) or binding protein 3 levels (IGFBP3). Other tests of pituitary function such as thyroid hormones, prolactin, gonadal hormones.

Radiological investigations: MRI pituitary gland, ECHO of the heart.

Referral to endocrinologist +/- neurosurgeon for treatment.

STATION 49

Name: Mr Raphael Lakeside

Age: 38 years old

Job: Used car salesman

PC:

At present both your eyes are red, teary and feel gritty. It all started two days ago when you noticed that your right eye was symptomatic. When you woke up this morning you noticed the symptoms had spread and are now in your left eye as well. You do not have any problems with your vision apart from the blurriness due to the tears and have never had any problems with or operations on your eyes in the past. You are short-sighted and wear contact lenses, which you keep in a container with both right and left lenses together in the same solution. You try your best to keep your hands and the lenses clean and always wash your hands before touching your contact lenses. You do not remember rubbing or scratching your eyes at any point and are otherwise fit and well. You have no systemic features (no headache/fever/dysuria/diarrhoea/vomiting/abdominal pain).

Past Medical History:

The only time you've been in hospital was for an appendicectomy at 15 years old.

Migraines.

You used to have asthma as a boy but you grew out of it and no longer use inhalers.

Drug History:

NKDA.

Pizitofen for migraine prophylaxis (dose unknown).

Social History:

You do not smoke, and drink about 14 pints of beer a week.

You and your wife use condoms as contraception and you have had no sexual contact with anybody else.

You are married with two children. Your eldest son has two hamsters. Your son Joseph has had a similar problem with his eyes a week ago and had to go and see the GP for some eye drops. (Only disclose if specifically asked about contacts.)

Family History:

Neither you, nor anybody in your family, suffer from hay fever, eczema or rheumatological diseases.

Ideas/Concerns/Expectations:

You are concerned because you don't feel like you can visit your clients with such red eyes. As a result you have had to take a couple of days off work, but unfortunately your salary depends on commission so you cannot afford to take any more time off.

Diagnosis:

Infective conjunctivitis

Differential Diagnosis:

Scleritis, corneal abrasion, allergic conjunctivitis

Management:

Examine patient's eyes for visual acuity, pupillary response and fundoscopy.

Obtain swabs from any purulent discharge to send to microbiology.

Medication may include chloramphenicol or fusidic acid eye drops.

Advice on prevention of spread such as avoiding contact lens wearing until episode clears up, using a new pair of lenses and maintaining them in different solutions for different eyes, washing hands, using separate towels to other family members.

Clean the eye from discharge by using cotton wool soaked in warm water.

STATION 50

Name: Miss Jemima Rolando

Age: 23 years old

Job: Actress

PC:

You've noticed that over the last three weeks that your eyes have become red and itchy. Some days it is worse than others and you have also had a runny nose. You have had no problems with your vision, pain in your eyes, and no other systemic symptoms or changes in your skin, hair or nails. You do not wear glasses or contact lenses.

Past Medical History:

Asthma (well controlled, no previous hospitalizations, last attack 5 years ago).

No previous surgical operations.

Drug History:

NKDA.

Beclomethasone inhaler (two puffs twice a day)

Salbutamol inhaler (prn)

Social History:

You are engaged to your boyfriend and are currently on the pill, but have had no other sexual contacts or noticed any abnormal vaginal discharge.

You have smoked 15 cigarettes a day since you were 15 years old and drink a couple of glasses of wine every evening. You have no pets at home, however, your mother had a cat when you were growing up and you remember being allergic to it and sneezing a lot around the house.

Family History:

Your mother suffers from bad eczema for which she has to take steroid cream (you have never met your father and don't know anything about him) but as far as you know nobody else is atopic in the family or suffers from rheumatological diseases.

Ideas/Concerns/Expectations:

You are concerned because you have an important audition in two day's time and do not think you can go if you continue to feel like this.

Diagnosis:

Seasonal allergic rhinitis and conjunctivitis

Differential Diagnosis:

Allergic rhinitis – non-seasonal related

Non-allergic rhinitis

Influenza viral infection

Management:

Medical treatments may include antihistamines such as loratadine, cetirizine, promethiazine.

Eye drops containing antihistamines are also sometimes beneficial.

Advise patients to avoid precipitating factors (if possible and known).

If the allergies do become a severe problem then allergen testing can be performed to determine which precipitating factors are responsible and low dose steroid medication may be prescribed.

STATION 51

Name: Mr James Smythson

Age: 19 years old

Job: Business studies university student

PC:

You've noticed your eyes have become particularly sore, red and itchy over the last week. You have also noticed joint pain on movement in both knees; but have never suffered from problems with your joints or eyes before and do not wear glasses. You haven't taken any painkillers but have tried rubbing Tiger Balm into your knees, which has eased the pain slightly. Your knees don't appear swollen, hot or tender to touch. You do not remember any trauma to your joints or banging them recently.

You have also noticed pain on passing urine for the last two days and do not feel as if you can pass urine as freely as before. (If questioned, you haven't passed urine for over 24 hours and are starting to suffer from supra-pubic pain.) You feel hot and clammy but have not had any vomiting, diarrhoea, headache or visual disturbances.

Past Medical History:

You broke you thumb playing rugby three years ago but apart from this have never had to go to hospital before. You are otherwise fit and well. You do not suffer from hay fever, asthma or eczema.

Drug History:

NKDA. Nil regular.

Social History:

You have smoked 20 cigarettes a day since you were 16 years old and drink over 30 pints a week, sometimes more if you are having a heavy weekend.

You had a one-night stand a few weekends ago with a girl you had never met before and did not use a condom.

You live at home with your parents.

You have two pet dogs.

Family History:

Your father suffers from rheumatoid arthritis and had to retire at 40 because he could no longer be a carpenter.

Ideas/Concerns/Expectations:

You know that your father has also had problems with his eyes in the past related to his arthritis and are concerned the same thing is happening to you because of your knee pain and eye complaints.

Diagnosis:

Reiter's syndrome (sexually acquired reactive arthritis)

Differentials:

Inflammatory bowel conditions e.g. ulcerative colitis although less likely

Investigations:

Blood tests including a full blood count, urea and electrolytes, blood cultures, HLA-typing.

Urethral swabs for a sexually transmitted infection screen with possible HIV counselling and testing.

Midstream urine sample of microbiology and dipstick testing.

Aspiration of the knee joint if an effusion is present for microbiology review.

Management:

Catheterise to relieve urinary retention from urethritis.

Prescription of NSAIDs for pain relief +/- PPI protection.

Treatment of any underlying sexually transmitted infection (e.g. doxycycline for chlamydia) and contact tracing of partner for treatment.

STATION 52

Name: Miss Sarah Young

Age: 25 years old

Job: Unemployed

PC:

You have noticed a gradual loss in your vision in both eyes over the last 8 months with the right slightly worse than the left. When you look into the distance everything is blurred and when driving you feel that you can no longer clearly make out the road signs or the number plate of the car in front of you. You do not have any redness or pain in your eye unless you have been straining your eyes by trying to read things in the distance for a long time. You do not have any neurology or headaches and there is no problem with your near vision or colour vision. You do not complain of floaters, halos, flashes of light or any heaviness within the eyes.

You have never worn glasses and can't remember the last time you had your eyes tested.

Past Medical History:

None significant.

Drug History:

NKDA. Nil regular.

Social History:

You have smoked 20 cigarettes a day for the last 10 years.

You drink about 3 pints of beer a week but do not take any illicit drugs.

You live in a council flat with your two children aged 5 and 3 years old and are unmarried and unemployed. There are no pets at home.

Family History:

Both your parents are in their fifties and wear glasses for reading.

Ideas/Concerns/Expectations:

You think you are going blind and concerned about what will happen to your children growing up with a blind single parent. You no longer speak to the father of your children and already struggle bringing them up on your own. You cannot imagine doing it blind!

Diagnosis:

Refractive error

Differentials:

Chronic open angle glaucoma

Diabetes related retinopathy

Optic nerve compression

Hereditary retinal dystrophies

Papilloedema

Management:

This patient gives a clear history of refractive error and there is no reason to suspect any of the other differentials at this stage. It can be easily confirmed with use of a pin-hole device to improve the acuity. The use of Snellen charts would diagnose the severity, and allow monitoring of the rate of deterioration.

A full neurological examination would help to exclude neurological causes. Inspection of the optic disc reveals papilloedema (pale, swollen optic disc), and checking visual fields and relative afferent pupillary defect can help to diagnose optic nerve lesions. Diabetes can cause refractive error due to hyperglycaemia changing the shape of the lens. It can be easily excluded by a BM in this instance. Tonometry and gonioscopy can diagnose glaucoma, and if present a referral to the ophthalmologist would be advised.

This patient should be referred to an optician for discussion of treatment options.

GENERAL MEDICAL AND SURGICAL HISTORIES

Candidate Number:	University:
Date:	Year of Study:

STATIONS 1, 2 & 3 – CHEST PAIN

	Appropriate introduction (1=full name and role), checks patient's name (1)	2	1	0
	Explains purpose of interview and checks consent (2=does well, 1=adequately, 0=poorly or not done)	2	1	0
	Starts with an open question and listens without interrupting (1=both)		1	0
	Presenting Complaint:			
	Establishes the site (1) of the pain including any radiation (1)	2	1	0
	Enquires after the onset (1) and duration of the pain (1)	2	1	0
	Enquires after the severity of the pain (1) and whether patient has taken any analgesia or medication already to alleviate the symptoms (1)	2	1	0
	Establishes the character of the pain (1) i.e. stabbing, heavy, sharp, pleuritic and asks about exacerbating/relieving factors (1) i.e. worse lying down, straining, movement, palpation etc.	2	1	0
	Asks about associated cardio-respiratory symptoms such as shortness of breath, palpitations, orthopnoea, paroxysmal nocturnal dyspnea, haemoptysis, sputum production, calf swelling/pain (2=any three symptoms, 1=any two symptoms)	2	1	0
	Asks about associated systemic symptoms such as nausea, fevers, weight loss, pain elsewhere, sweating, vomiting (2=any three symptoms, 1=any two symptoms)	2	1	0
	Asks about risk factors for venous thromboembolic events (VTE): recent surgery, long haul flights, past history of VTE, family history of clotting disorders, history of malignancy (2=any three risk factors, 1=any two risk factors)	2	1	0
	Asks about risk factors for heart disease: diabetes, high cholesterol, high blood pressure, family history of cardiac disease, previous heart disease, recent cardiac interventions etc. (2=any three risk factors, 1=any two risk factors)	2	1	0
	Enquires after previous similar episodes (and treatments for this)		1	0
	Explores patient's ideas and concerns regarding the presenting complaint	2	1	0
	Other relevant history:			
	Relevant past medical and surgical history (especially cardiac related)	2	1	0
	Medication history (1) including allergies and the nature of the allergy (1)	2	1	0
	Relevant family history (especially of heart disease and age of death of family members and/or of thrombotic events)		1	0
	Smoking, alcohol and drug use (2=all three, 1=any two factors)	2	1	0
	Relevant social history e.g. exercise, lifestyle, diet, housing circumstances, dependents, occupation etc.		1	0
	Appropriate closure (e.g. explains next step, thanks patient and summarises) (2=does well, 1=adequately, 0=poorly or not done)	2	1	0
	Communication Skills			
	Appropriate questioning style (mix of open and closed questions) (2=does well, 1=adequately, 0=poorly or not done)	2	1	0
	Invites questions (1). Listens actively (1).	2	1	0
	Organised approach to history-taking (e.g. systematic, summarises, signposts change in focus of question)	2	1	0
	Simulated patient score (2=very good, 1=satisfactory, 0=poor)	2	1	0
	Examiner to ask: 'What are your differential diagnoses?'			
	Candidate states an appropriate diagnosis (1) and offers a differential (1) (see patient scenarios for possible diagnoses)	2	1	0
	Examiner to ask: 'What investigations/management would you recommend?'			
	Candidate suggests appropriate investigations (1) followed by a sensible line of management (1) (see patient scenarios for possible management options)	2	1	0
	Total Score			

Global Rating	1 Clear Fail	2 Borderline	3 Clear Pass	4 Very Good	5 Outstanding

Candidate Number:	University:
Date:	Year of Study:

STATION 4 – NON-SPECIFIC SYMPTOMS

	Appropriate introduction (1=full name and role), checks patient's name (1)	2	1	0
	Explains purpose of interview and checks consent (2=does well, 1=adequately, 0=poorly or not done)	2	1	0
	Starts with an open question and listens without interrupting (1=both)		1	0
	Presenting Complaint:			
	Establishes circumstances around recent events (1) and if patient lost consciousness (1)	2	1	0
	Establishes onset (1) and duration (1)	2	1	0
	Enquires whether patient knew event was about to happen (i.e. any warning symptoms such as palpitations or feelings of impending doom) (1) and how patient felt after the event (i.e. confused, dizzy, tired etc.) (1)	2	1	0
	Asks about associated cardio-respiratory symptoms such as shortness of breath, palpitations, orthopnoea, paroxysmal nocturnal dyspnea, haemoptysis, sputum production, calf swelling/pain (2=any three symptoms, 1=any two symptoms)	2	1	0
	Asks about associated systemic symptoms such as nausea, fevers, weight loss, pain elsewhere, sweating, vomiting, change in bowel habits (2=any three symptoms, 1=any two symptoms)	2	1	0
	Asks about risk factors for venous thromboembolic events (VTE): recent surgery, long haul flights, past history of VTE/CVA, family history of clotting disorders, history of malignancy (2=any three risk factors, 1=any two risk factors)	2	1	0
	Asks about risk factors for heart disease: diabetes, high cholesterol, high blood pressure, family history of cardiac disease, previous heart disease, recent cardiac interventions etc. (2=any three risk factors, 1=any two risk factors)	2	1	0
	Enquires after previous similar episodes		1	0
	Explores patient's ideas and concerns regarding the presenting complaint	2	1	0
	Other relevant history:			
	Relevant past medical and surgical history (1) including specific details of diabetic control (1)	2	1	0
	Medication history (1) including allergies and the nature of the allergy (1)	2	1	0
	Relevant family history (especially of heart disease or neurological problems)		1	0
	Smoking, alcohol and drug use (2=all three, 1=any two factors)	2	1	0
	Relevant social history (e.g. exercise, lifestyle, diet, housing circumstances, dependents, occupation etc).		1	0
	Appropriate closure (e.g. explains next step, thanks patient and summarises) (2=does well, 1=adequately, 0=poorly or not done)	2	1	0
	Communication Skills			
	Appropriate questioning style (mix of open and closed questions) (2=does well, 1=adequately, 0=poorly or not done)	2	1	0
	Invites questions (1). Listens actively (1).	2	1	0
	Organised approach to history-taking (e.g. systematic, summarises, signposts change in focus of question)	2	1	0
	Simulated patient score (2=very good, 1=satisfactory, 0=poor)	2	1	0
	Examiner to ask: 'What are your differential diagnoses?'			
	Candidate states an appropriate diagnosis (1) and offers a differential (1) (see patient scenarios for possible diagnoses)	2	1	0
	Examiner to ask: 'What investigations/management would you recommend?'			
	Candidate suggests appropriate investigations (1) followed by a sensible line of management (1) (see patient scenarios for possible management options)	2	1	0
	Total Score			

Global Rating	1 Clear Fail	2 Borderline	3 Clear Pass	4 Very Good	5 Outstanding

Candidate Number:	University:
Date:	Year of Study:

STATION 5 – TUBERCULOSIS

	Appropriate introduction (1=full name and role), checks patient's name (1)	2	1	0
	Explains purpose of interview and checks consent (2=does well, 1=adequately, 0=poorly or not done)	2	1	0
	Presenting Complaint:			
	Obtains an overview of recent events		1	0
	Establishes onset (1) and duration (1) of the shortness of breath	2	1	0
	Enquires after the triggers for the shortness of breath		1	0
	Establishes onset of haemoptysis (1) and number of episodes (1)	2	1	0
	Enquires after volume of blood (1) and whether it is fresh or contains clots in it (1)	2	1	0
	Establishes whether patient was in pain during the haemoptysis (1) and has chest pain (1)	2	1	0
	Asks about the progression of the symptoms i.e. worsening or getting better		1	0
	Asks about associated systemic symptoms such as chest pain, nausea, fevers, weight loss, pain elsewhere, night sweats, vomiting (2=any three symptoms, 1=any two symptoms)	2	1	0
	Asks about associated cardio-respiratory symptoms such as shortness of breath, palpitations, orthopnoea, paroxysmal nocturnal dyspnea, haemoptysis, sputum production, calf swelling/pain (2=any three symptoms, 1=any two symptoms)	2	1	0
	Asks about risk factors for venous thromboembolic events (VTE): Recent surgery, past history of VTE, family history of clotting disorders, history of malignancy. (2=any three risk factors, 1=any two risk factors)	2	1	0
	Asks about risk factors for heart disease: diabetes, high cholesterol, high blood pressure, family history of cardiac disease, previous heart disease etc. (2=any three risk factors, 1=any two risk factors)	2	1	0
	Asks about recent travel to exotic countries (1) and any infectious contacts (1)	2	1	0
	Asks patient if they have ever been vaccinated against tuberculosis with the BCG vaccine		1	0
	Enquires after previous similar episodes (and treatments for this)		1	0
	Explores patient's ideas and concerns regarding the presenting complaint	2	1	0
	Other relevant history:			
	Relevant past medical and surgical history	2	1	0
	Medication history (1) including allergies and the nature of the allergy (1)	2	1	0
	Relevant family history		1	0
	Smoking, alcohol and drug use (2=all three, 1=any two factors)	2	1	0
	Relevant social history e.g. exercise, lifestyle, diet, housing circumstances, occupation etc.		1	0
	Appropriate closure (e.g. explains next step, thanks patient and summarises) (2=does well, 1=adequately, 0=poorly or not done)	2	1	0
	Communication Skills			
	Appropriate questioning style (mix of open and closed questions) (2=does well, 1=adequately, 0=poorly or not done)	2	1	0
	Invites questions (1). Listens actively (1).	2	1	0
	Organised approach to history-taking (e.g. systematic, summarises, signposts change in focus of question)	2	1	0
	Simulated patient score (2=very good, 1=satisfactory, 0=poor)	2	1	0
	Examiner to ask: 'What are your differential diagnoses?'			
	Candidate states an appropriate diagnosis (1) and offers a differential (1) (see patient scenarios for possible diagnoses)	2	1	0
	Examiner to ask: 'What investigations/management would you recommend?'			
	Candidate suggests appropriate investigations (1) followed by a sensible line of management (1) (see patient scenarios for possible management options)	2	1	0
	Total Score			

Global Rating	1 Clear Fail	2 Borderline	3 Clear Pass	4 Very Good	5 Outstanding

Candidate Number:		University:
Date:		Year of Study:

STATIONS 6 & 7 – SHORTNESS OF BREATH

		2	1	0
	Appropriate introduction (1=full name and role), checks patient's name (1)	2	1	0
	Explains purpose of interview and checks consent (2=does well, 1=adequately, 0=poorly or not done)	2	1	0
	Starts with an open question and listens without interrupting (1=both)		1	0
	Presenting Complaint:			
	Establishes onset (1) and duration (1) of the shortness of breath	2	1	0
	Enquires after the triggers for the shortness of breath i.e. at rest, on exertion, sleep related, positional (2=any three factors, 1=any two factors)	2	1	0
	Asks about the progression of the shortness of breath i.e. worsening (1) and over how long it has been worsening/improving (1)	2	1	0
	Enquires after the severity of shortness of breath (i.e. What is the patient able to do/not able to do anymore? What was their exercise tolerance before and now?)	2	1	0
	Enquires after factors which relieve the shortness of breath i.e. rest, inhalers (if patient has any), medication the patient takes, fresh air etc. (2=any two, 1=any one)	2	1	0
	Detailed history about associated cardio-respiratory symptoms such as chest pain, palpitations, orthopnoea, paroxysmal nocturnal dyspnea, haemoptysis, sputum (2=any three symptoms, 1=any two symptoms)	2	1	0
	Asks about associated systemic symptoms such as nausea, fevers, weight loss, pain elsewhere, sweating, vomiting (2=any three symptoms, 1=any two symptoms)	2	1	0
	Asks about risk factors for venous thromboembolic events (VTE): recent surgery, long haul flights, past history of VTE, family history of clotting disorders, history of malignancy (2=any three risk factors, 1=any two risk factors)	2	1	0
	Asks about risk factors for heart disease: diabetes, high cholesterol, high blood pressure, family history of cardiac disease, previous heart disease etc. (2=any three risk factors, 1=any two risk factors)	2	1	0
	Enquires after previous similar episodes (and treatments for this)		1	0
	Explores patient's ideas and concerns regarding the presenting complaint	2	1	0
	Other relevant history:			
	Relevant past medical and surgical history	2	1	0
	Medication history (1) including allergies and the nature of the allergy (1)	2	1	0
	Relevant family history (especially of respiratory/cardiac disease, atopy)		1	0
	Smoking, alcohol and drug use (2=all three, 1=any two factors)	2	1	0
	Relevant social history e.g. recent infective contacts, exercise, lifestyle, diet, housing circumstances, dependents, occupation, pets etc.		1	0
	Appropriate closure (e.g. explains next step, thanks patient and summarises) (2=does well, 1=adequately, 0=poorly or not done)	2	1	0
	Communication Skills			
	Appropriate questioning style (mix of open and closed questions) (2=does well, 1=adequately, 0=poorly or not done)	2	1	0
	Invites questions (1). Listens actively (1).	2	1	0
	Organised approach to history-taking (e.g. systematic, summarises, signposts change in focus of question)	2	1	0
	Simulated patient score (2=very good, 1=satisfactory, 0=poor)	2	1	0
	Examiner to ask: 'What are your differential diagnoses?'			
	Candidate states an appropriate diagnosis (1) and offers a differential (1) (see patient scenarios for possible diagnoses)	2	1	0
	Examiner to ask: 'What investigations/management would you recommend?'			
	Candidate suggests appropriate investigations (1) followed by a sensible line of management (1) (see patient scenarios for possible management options)	2	1	0
	Total Score			

Global Rating	1 Clear Fail	2 Borderline	3 Clear Pass	4 Very Good	5 Outstanding

Candidate Number:	University:
Date:	Year of Study:

STATION 8 – SWOLLEN LEGS

		2	1	0
	Appropriate introduction (1=full name and role), checks relative's name (1)	2	1	0
	Explains purpose of interview and checks consent (2=does well, 1=adequately, 0=poorly or not done)	2	1	0
	Starts with an open question and listens without interrupting (1=both)		1	0
	Presenting Complaint:			
	Establishes the presenting complaint of swollen limbs (1) and classifies the extent of the swelling i.e. one or both legs, whether this extends to the sacrum (1)	2	1	0
	Enquires about factors that make the symptoms better or worse i.e. worse after a long day walking around, better when putting feet up at the end of the day		1	0
	Enquires about how long the symptoms have been developing (1) and their progression (1)	2	1	0
	Establishes that the nature of the swelling is 'pitting oedema'		1	0
	Establishes if patient has suffered previous similar episodes (1) and what treatment they have received before (1)	2	1	0
	Specifically asks about orthopnoea (1) and paroxysmal nocturnal dyspnea (1)	2	1	0
	Asks about associated cardio-respiratory symptoms such as shortness of breath, palpitations, haemoptysis, sputum production (2=any three symptoms, 1=any two symptoms)	2	1	0
	Asks about associated systemic symptoms such as nausea, fevers, weight loss, pain elsewhere, sweating, vomiting (2=any three symptoms, 1=any two symptoms)	2	1	0
	Asks about risk factors for venous thromboembolic events (VTE): recent surgery, long haul flights, past history of VTE, family history of clotting disorders, history of malignancy (2=any three risk factors, 1=any two risk factors)	2	1	0
	Asks about risk factors for heart disease: diabetes, high cholesterol, high blood pressure, family history of cardiac disease, previous heart disease, recent cardiac interventions etc. (2=any three risk factors, 1=any two risk factors)	2	1	0
	Explores patient's ideas and concerns regarding the presenting complaint	2	1	0
	Other relevant history:			
	Relevant past medical and surgical history (especially about cardiac and renal diseases)	2	1	0
	Medication history (1) including allergies and the nature of the allergy (1)	2	1	0
	Relevant family history		1	0
	Smoking, alcohol and drug use (2=all three, 1=any two factors)	2	1	0
	Relevant social history (e.g. carers, exercise, lifestyle, diet, housing circumstances, dependents, occupation, pets etc.)		1	0
	Appropriate closure (e.g. explains next step, thanks patient and summarises) (2=does well, 1=adequately, 0=poorly or not done)	2	1	0
	Communication Skills			
	Appropriate questioning style (mix of open and closed questions) (2=does well, 1=adequately, 0=poorly or not done)	2	1	0
	Invites questions (1). Listens actively (1).	2	1	0
	Organised approach to history-taking (e.g. systematic, summarises, signposts change in focus of question)	2	1	0
	Simulated patient score (2=very good, 1=satisfactory, 0=poor)	2	1	0
	Examiner to ask: 'What are your differential diagnoses?'			
	Candidate states an appropriate diagnosis (1) and offers a differential (1) (see patient scenarios for possible diagnoses)	2	1	0
	Examiner to ask: 'What investigations/management would you recommend?'			
	Candidate suggests appropriate investigations (1) followed by a sensible line of management (1) (see patient scenarios for possible management options)	2	1	0
	Total Score			

Global Rating	**1** Clear Fail	**2** Borderline	**3** Clear Pass	**4** Very Good	**5** Outstanding

Candidate Number:	University:
Date:	Year of Study:

STATIONS 9, 10 & 11 – VOMITING

		2	1	0
	Appropriate introduction (1=full name and role), checks patient's name (1)	2	1	0
	Explains purpose of interview and checks consent (2=does well, 1=adequately, 0=poorly or not done)	2	1	0
	Starts with an open question and listens without interrupting (1=both)		1	0
	Presenting Complaint:			
	Establishes the onset and number of times vomited (1) and the content (1) of the vomitus	2	1	0
	Enquires whether there was any bile (1) or blood (1) in the vomit	2	1	0
	Enquires after the severity of the vomiting (1) and whether the patient has taken any medication already to alleviate the symptoms (1)	2	1	0
	Asks about associated symptoms such as abdominal pain, change in bowel habit, blood passage per rectum, fainting episodes, retching etc. (2=does well, 1=adequately, 0=poorly)	2	1	0
	Candidate explores whether anything caused the vomiting to start (e.g. any food eaten, foreign travel)		1	0
	Enquires after previous similar episodes		1	0
	Explores patient's ideas and concerns regarding the presenting complaint		1	0
	Other relevant history:			
	Systemic features: pregnancy, weight change, appetite, urinary symptoms, fevers, rigors, night sweats etc. (2=all three, 1=two items, 0=one only or none)	2	1	0
	Relevant past medical and surgical history		1	0
	Drug history (1) including allergies (1)	2	1	0
	Relevant family history		1	0
	Smoking (1) and alcohol (1)	2	1	0
	Relevant social history (e.g. housing circumstances, dependents, occupation etc.)		1	0
	Appropriate closure (e.g. explains next step, thanks patient and summarises) (2=does well, 1=adequately, 0=poorly or not done)	2	1	0
	Communication Skills			
	Appropriate questioning style (mix of open and closed questions) (2=does well, 1=adequately, 0=poorly or not done)	2	1	0
	Invites questions (1). Listens actively (1).	2	1	0
	Organised approach to history-taking (e.g. systematic, summarises, signposts change in focus of question)	2	1	0
	Simulated patient score (2=very good, 1=satisfactory, 0=poor)	2	1	0
	Examiner to ask: 'What are your differential diagnoses?'			
	Candidate states an appropriate diagnosis (1) and offers a differential (1) (see patient scenarios for possible diagnoses)	2	1	0
	Examiner to ask: 'What investigations/management would you recommend?'			
	Candidate suggests appropriate investigations (1) followed by a sensible line of management (1) (see patient scenarios for possible management options)	2	1	0
	Total Score			

Global Rating	1 Clear Fail	2 Borderline	3 Clear Pass	4 Very Good	5 Outstanding

Candidate Number:	University:
Date:	Year of Study:

STATION 12 – DIFFICULTY SWALLOWING

		2	1	0
	Appropriate introduction (1=full name and role), checks patient's name (1)	2	1	0
	Explains purpose of interview and checks consent (2=does well, 1=adequately, 0=poorly or not done)	2	1	0
	Starts with an open question and listens without interrupting (1=both)		1	0
	Presenting Complaint:			
	Establishes the onset (1) of the difficulty swallowing (1)	2	1	0
	Enquires whether the difficulty swallowing is related to food or liquids (1) or whether it is progressive to food and then liquids (1)	2	1	0
	Enquires after the severity of the difficulty swallowing/associated aspiration/coughing (1) and establishes the patient's total oral/nutritional intake (1)	2	1	0
	Asks about associated symptoms such as neck swelling when eating, abdominal pain, vomiting, haematemesis, change in bowel habit etc. (2=three items, 1=two items, 0=one or less)	2	1	0
	Enquires after previous similar episodes		1	0
	Explores patient's ideas and concerns regarding the presenting complaint		1	0
	Other relevant history:			
	Systemic features: weight change, appetite, rigors, fevers, night sweats etc. (2=all three, 1=two items, 0=one only or none)	2	1	0
	Relevant past medical and surgical history		1	0
	Medication history (1) including allergies (1)	2	1	0
	Relevant family history		1	0
	Smoking (1) and alcohol (1)	2	1	0
	Relevant social history (e.g. housing circumstances, dependents, occupation etc.)		1	0
	Appropriate closure (e.g. explains next step, thanks patient and summarises) (2=does well, 1=adequately, 0=poorly or not done)	2	1	0
	Communication Skills			
	Appropriate questioning style (mix of open and closed questions) (2=does well, 1=adequately, 0=poorly or not done)	2	1	0
	Invites questions (1). Listens actively (1).	2	1	0
	Organised approach to history-taking (e.g. systematic, summarises, signposts change in focus of question)	2	1	0
	Simulated patient score (2=very good, 1=satisfactory, 0=poor)	2	1	0
	Examiner to ask: 'What are your differential diagnoses?'			
	Candidate states an appropriate diagnosis (1) and offers a differential (1) (see patient scenarios for possible diagnoses)	2	1	0
	Examiner to ask: 'What investigations/management would you recommend?'			
	Candidate suggests appropriate investigations (1) followed by a sensible line of management (1) (see patient scenarios for possible management options)	2	1	0
	Total Score			

Global Rating	1 Clear Fail	2 Borderline	3 Clear Pass	4 Very Good	5 Outstanding

Candidate Number:	University:
Date:	Year of Study:

STATIONS 13 & 14 – RECTAL BLEEDING

	Appropriate introduction (1=full name and role), checks patient's name (1)	2	1	0
	Explains purpose of interview and checks consent (2=does well, 1=adequately, 0=poorly or not done)	2	1	0
	Starts with an open question and listens without interrupting (1=both)		1	0
	Presenting Complaint:			
	Establishes onset (1) and number of episodes of rectal bleeding (1)	2	1	0
	Establishes the nature of the blood i.e. fresh red, dark, clots (1) and if possible volume of blood (1)	2	1	0
	Establishes where the blood is noticed (e.g. on the toilet paper, mixed with the stool, in the toilet pan)		1	0
	Asks about associated symptoms such as change in bowel habit, nausea, vomiting, urinary symptoms etc. (2=three items, 1=two items, 0=one item or less)	2	1	0
	Candidate explores whether the patient is straining at stool (1) and establishes patient's normal bowel habits i.e. type of stool and frequency (1)	2	1	0
	Establishes whether patient has felt any 'lumps' or 'bumps' around the anus		1	0
	Enquires after previous similar episodes		1	0
	Explores patient's ideas and concerns regarding the presenting complaint		1	0
	Other relevant history:			
	Systemic features: weight change, appetite, bone pain, fevers, rigors, night sweats etc. (2=all three, 1=two items, 0=one only or none)	2	1	0
	Relevant past medical and surgical history		1	0
	Medication history (1) including allergies (1)	2	1	0
	Relevant family history (in particular of bowel cancer or inflammatory bowel disease)		1	0
	Smoking (1) and alcohol (1)	2	1	0
	Relevant social history (e.g. housing circumstances, dependents, occupation etc.)		1	0
	Appropriate closure (e.g. explains next step, thanks patient and summarises) (2=does well, 1=adequately, 0=poorly or not done)	2	1	0
	Communication Skills			
	Appropriate questioning style (mix of open and closed questions) (2=does well, 1=adequately, 0=poorly or not done)	2	1	0
	Invites questions (1). Listens actively (1).	2	1	0
	Organised approach to history-taking (e.g. systematic, summarises, signposts change in focus of question)	2	1	0
	Simulated patient score (2=very good, 1=satisfactory, 0=poor)	2	1	0
	Examiner to ask: 'What are your differential diagnoses?'			
	Candidate states an appropriate diagnosis (1) and offers a differential (1) (see patient scenarios for possible diagnoses)	2	1	0
	Examiner to ask: 'What investigations/management would you recommend?'			
	Candidate suggests appropriate investigations (1) followed by a sensible line of management (1) (see patient scenarios for possible management options)	2	1	0
	Total Score			

Global Rating	1 Clear Fail	2 Borderline	3 Clear Pass	4 Very Good	5 Outstanding

Candidate Number:	University:
Date:	Year of Study:

STATIONS 15, 16 & 17 – ABDOMINAL PAIN

	Appropriate introduction (1=full name and role), checks patient's name (1)	**2**	**1**	**0**
	Explains purpose of interview and checks consent (2=does well, 1=adequately, 0=poorly or not done)	**2**	**1**	**0**
	Presenting Complaint:			
	Establishes the character (1) and location of the pain including any radiation (1)	**2**	**1**	**0**
	Enquires after the onset (1) and duration of the pain (1)	**2**	**1**	**0**
	Enquires after the severity of the pain (1) and whether patient has taken any analgesia or medication already to alleviate the symptoms (1)	**2**	**1**	**0**
	Asks about associated symptoms such as nausea, vomiting, urinary symptoms, change in bowel habit etc. (2=does well, 1=adequately, 0=poorly)	**2**	**1**	**0**
	Candidate explores whether anything causes the pain to worsen (1) or improve (1) e.g. straining, coughing, sneezing or analgesia, lying down etc.	**2**	**1**	**0**
	Enquires after previous similar episodes		**1**	**0**
	Explores patient's ideas and concerns regarding the presenting complaint		**1**	**0**
	Other relevant history:			
	Systemic features: weight change, appetite, bone pain, fevers, rigors etc. (2=all three, 1=two items, 0=one only or none)	**2**	**1**	**0**
	Relevant past medical and surgical history		**1**	**0**
	Medication history (1) including allergies (1)	**2**	**1**	**0**
	Relevant family history		**1**	**0**
	Smoking (1) and alcohol (1)	**2**	**1**	**0**
	Relevant social history (e.g. housing circumstances, dependents, occupation etc.)		**1**	**0**
	Appropriate closure (e.g. explains next step, thanks patient and summarises) (2=does well, 1=adequately, 0=poorly or not done)	**2**	**1**	**0**
	Communication Skills			
	Appropriate questioning style (mix of open and closed questions) (2=does well, 1=adequately, 0=poorly or not done)	**2**	**1**	**0**
	Invites questions (1). Listens actively (1).	**2**	**1**	**0**
	Organised approach to history-taking (e.g. systematic, summarises, signposts change in focus of question)	**2**	**1**	**0**
	Simulated patient score (2=very good, 1=satisfactory, 0=poor)	**2**	**1**	**0**
	Examiner to ask: 'What are your differential diagnoses?'			
	Candidate states an appropriate diagnosis (1) and offers a differential (1) (see patient scenarios for possible diagnoses)	**2**	**1**	**0**
	Examiner to ask: 'What investigations/management would you recommend?'			
	Candidate suggests appropriate investigations (1) followed by a sensible line of management (1) (see patient scenarios for possible management options)	**2**	**1**	**0**
	Total Score			

Global Rating	**1** Clear Fail	**2** Borderline	**3** Clear Pass	**4** Very Good	**5** Outstanding

Candidate Number:	University:
Date:	Year of Study:

STATIONS 18 & 19 – DIARRHOEA

	Appropriate introduction (1=full name and role), checks patient's name (1)	2	1	0
	Explains purpose of interview and checks consent (2=does well, 1=adequately, 0=poorly or not done)	2	1	0
	Starts with an open question and listens without interrupting (1=both)		1	0
	Presenting Complaint:			
	Establishes what the patient's normal bowel habits are	2	1	0
	Establishes how many times they are opening their bowels	2	1	0
	Enquires after the consistency (1) and colour (1) of the stool	2	1	0
	Enquires whether there has been any PR blood loss (1) or melaena (1)	2	1	0
	Asks about associated symptoms such as nausea, vomiting, tiredness, dizziness, urinary symptoms etc. (2=does well, 1=adequately, 0=poorly)	2	1	0
	Candidate explores whether the patient has eaten any new foods (1) or had any recent foreign travel (1)	2	1	0
	Enquires after previous similar episodes		1	0
	Explores patient's ideas and concerns regarding the presenting complaint		1	0
	Other relevant history:			
	Systemic features: weight change, appetite, rigors, fevers, abdominal pains and their character/severity, associated bloating or reflux etc. (2=three or more items, 1=two items, 0=one only or none)	2	1	0
	Relevant past medical and surgical history		1	0
	Medication history (1) including allergies (1)	2	1	0
	Relevant family history		1	0
	Smoking (1) and alcohol (1)	2	1	0
	Relevant social history (e.g. housing circumstances, dependents, occupation etc.)		1	0
	Appropriate closure (e.g. explains next step, thanks patient and summarises) (2=does well, 1=adequately, 0=poorly or not done)	2	1	0
	Communication Skills			
	Appropriate questioning style (mix of open and closed questions) (2=does well, 1=adequately, 0=poorly or not done)	2	1	0
	Invites questions (1). Listens actively (1).	2	1	0
	Organised approach to history-taking (e.g. systematic, summarises, signposts change in focus of question)	2	1	0
	Simulated patient score (2=very good, 1=satisfactory, 0=poor)	2	1	0
	Examiner to ask: 'What are your differential diagnoses?'			
	Candidate states an appropriate diagnosis (1) and offers a differential (1) (see patient scenarios for possible diagnoses)	2	1	0
	Examiner to ask: 'What investigations/management would you recommend?'			
	Candidate suggests appropriate investigations (1) followed by a sensible line of management (1) (see patient scenarios for possible management options)	2	1	0
	Total Score			

Global Rating	1 Clear Fail	2 Borderline	3 Clear Pass	4 Very Good	5 Outstanding

Candidate Number:	University:
Date:	Year of Study:

STATIONS 20, 21, 22 & 23 – HEADACHES

		2	1	0
	Appropriate introduction (1=full name and role), checks patient's name (1)	2	1	0
	Explains purpose of interview and checks consent (2=does well, 1=adequately, 0=poorly or not done)	2	1	0
	Starts with an open question and listens without interrupting (1=both)		1	0
	Presenting Complaint:			
	Establishes the character (1) and location of the pain including any radiation (1)	2	1	0
	Enquires after the onset (1) and duration of the pain (1)	2	1	0
	Enquires after the severity of the pain (1) and whether the patient has taken any analgesia or medication already to alleviate the symptoms (1)	2	1	0
	Asks about associated symptoms such as nausea, fevers, rash, stiff neck, vomiting, neurology, aura etc. (2=does well, 1=adequately, 0=poorly)	2	1	0
	Candidate explores whether anything causes the pain to worsen (1) or improve (1) (e.g. straining, coughing, sneezing or analgesia, lying down etc.)	2	1	0
	Enquires after previous similar episodes		1	0
	Explores patient's ideas and concerns regarding the presenting complaint		1	0
	Other relevant history:			
	Systemic features: weight change, appetite, fever (2=all three, 1=two items, 0=one only or none)	2	1	0
	Relevant past medical and surgical history		1	0
	Medication history (1) including allergies (1)	2	1	0
	Relevant family history		1	0
	Smoking (1) and alcohol (1)	2	1	0
	Relevant social history (e.g. housing circumstances, dependents, occupation etc.)		1	0
	Appropriate closure (e.g. explains next step, thanks patient and summarises) (2=does well, 1=adequately, 0=poorly or not done)	2	1	0
	Communication Skills			
	Appropriate questioning style (mix of open and closed questions) (2=does well, 1=adequately, 0=poorly or not done)	2	1	0
	Invites questions (1). Listens actively (1).	2	1	0
	Organised approach to history-taking (e.g. systematic, summarises, signposts change in focus of question)	2	1	0
	Simulated patient score (2=very good, 1=satisfactory, 0=poor)	2	1	0
	Examiner to ask: 'What are your differential diagnoses?'			
	Candidate states an appropriate diagnosis (1) and offers a differential (1) (see patient scenarios for possible diagnoses)	2	1	0
	Examiner to ask: 'What investigations/management would you recommend?'			
	Candidate suggests appropriate investigations (1) followed by a sensible line of management (1) (see patient scenarios for possible management options)	2	1	0
	Total Score			

Global Rating	1 Clear Fail	2 Borderline	3 Clear Pass	4 Very Good	5 Outstanding

Candidate Number:	University:
Date:	Year of Study:

STATIONS 24 & 25 – COLLAPSE

	Appropriate introduction (1=full name and role), checks patient's name (1)	2	1	0
	Explains purpose of interview and checks consent (2=does well, 1=adequately, 0=poorly or not done)	2	1	0
	Starts with an open question and listens without interrupting (1=both)		1	0
	Presenting Complaint:			
	Establishes presenting complaint of collapse (1) and establishes whether it was witnessed or not and if so, by whom (1)	2	1	0
	Enquires what the patient was doing whilst the collapse occurred		1	0
	Enquires whether patient was aware of any symptoms prior to the collapse e.g. aura, palpitations, nausea, chest pain etc.		1	0
	Establishes whether there was any loss of consciousness (1) and duration (1)	2	1	0
	Establishes previous similar episodes		1	0
	Enquires whether patient injured themselves during the collapse		1	0
	Asks whether patient remembers biting their tongue (1) or being incontinent of urine (1)	2	1	0
	Enquires whether patient was confused, orientated or felt any other symptoms when they regained consciousness (1) and if so, how long it took to feel 'normal' again (1)	2	1	0
	Enquires whether patient was told they suffered from any seizures or fits during the collapse (1) and if so whether they can describe exactly what occurred (1)	2	1	0
	Other relevant history:			
	Systemic features: weight change, appetite, fever (2=all three, 1=two items, 0=one only or none)	2	1	0
	Relevant past medical and surgical history	2	1	0
	Medication history (1) including allergies (1)	2	1	0
	Relevant family history		1	0
	Smoking (1) and alcohol (1)	2	1	0
	Relevant social history (e.g. housing circumstances, dependents, occupation etc.)	2	1	0
	Explores patient's ideas, concerns and expectations		1	0
	Appropriate closure (e.g. explains next step, thanks patient and summarises) (2=does well, 1=adequately, 0=poorly or not done)	2	1	0
	Communication Skills			
	Appropriate questioning style (mix of open and closed questions) (2=does well, 1=adequately, 0=poorly or not done)	2	1	0
	Invites questions (1). Listens actively (1).	2	1	0
	Organised approach to history-taking (e.g. systematic, summarises, signposts change in focus of question)	2	1	0
	Simulated patient score (2=very good, 1=satisfactory, 0=poor)	2	1	0
	Examiner to ask: 'What are your differential diagnoses?'			
	Candidate states an appropriate diagnosis (1) and offers a differential (1) (see patient scenarios for possible diagnoses)	2	1	0
	Examiner to ask: 'What investigations/management would you recommend?'			
	Candidate suggests appropriate investigations (1) followed by a sensible line of management (1) (see patient scenarios for possible management options)	2	1	0
	Total Score			

Global Rating	1 Clear Fail	2 Borderline	3 Clear Pass	4 Very Good	5 Outstanding

Candidate Number:	University:
Date:	Year of Study:

STATION 26 – FALLS

	Appropriate introduction (1=full name and role), checks relative's name (1)	**2**	1	**0**
	Explains purpose of interview and checks consent (2=does well, 1=adequately, 0=poorly or not done)	**2**	1	**0**
	Starts with an open question and listens without interrupting (1=both)		1	**0**
	Presenting Complaint:			
	Establishes presenting complaint of collapse (1) and establishes whether it was witnessed or not and if so, by whom (1)	**2**	1	**0**
	Enquires what the patient was doing (1) and where/when they collapsed (1)	**2**	1	**0**
	Enquires whether patient was aware of any symptoms prior to the collapse		1	**0**
	Establishes whether there was any loss of consciousness associated with the collapse (1) and the duration of this (1)	**2**	1	**0**
	Establishes previous similar episodes		1	**0**
	Enquires whether patient suffered from any seizures or fits during the collapse (1) and if so whether they can describe exactly what occurred (1)	**2**	1	**0**
	Asks whether patient bit their tongue (1) or was incontinent of urine (1)	**2**	1	**0**
	Enquires whether patient injured themselves during the collapse (1) especially whether there was any head injury (1)	**2**	1	**0**
	Enquires whether patient was confused, disorientated or felt any other symptoms when they regained consciousness (1) and if so, how long it took to feel 'normal' again (1)	**2**	1	**0**
	Other relevant history:			
	Systemic features: weight change, appetite, fever (2=all three, 1=two items, 0=one only or none)	**2**	1	**0**
	Relevant past medical and surgical history	**2**	1	**0**
	Medication history especially anticoagulants (1) including allergies (1)	**2**	1	**0**
	Relevant family history		1	**0**
	Smoking (1) and alcohol (1)	**2**	1	**0**
	Relevant social history (e.g. housing circumstances, dependents, mobility etc.)	**2**	1	**0**
	Explores patient's ideas, concerns and expectations		1	**0**
	Appropriate closure (e.g. explains next step, thanks patient and summarises) (2=does well, 1=adequately, 0=poorly or not done)	**2**	1	**0**
	Communication Skills			
	Appropriate questioning style (mix of open and closed questions) (2=does well, 1=adequately, 0=poorly or not done)	**2**	1	**0**
	Invites questions (1). Listens actively (1).	**2**	1	**0**
	Organised approach to history-taking (e.g. systematic, summarises, signposts change in focus of question)	**2**	1	**0**
	Simulated patient score (2=very good, 1=satisfactory, 0=poor)	**2**	1	**0**
	Examiner to ask: 'What are your differential diagnoses?'			
	Candidate states an appropriate diagnosis (1) and offers a differential (1) (see patient scenarios for possible diagnoses)	**2**	1	**0**
	Examiner to ask: 'What investigations/management would you recommend?'			
	Candidate suggests appropriate investigations (1) followed by a sensible line of management (1) (see patient scenarios for possible management options)	**2**	1	**0**
	Total Score			

Global Rating	1 Clear Fail	2 Borderline	3 Clear Pass	4 Very Good	5 Outstanding

Candidate Number:	University:
Date:	Year of Study:

STATIONS 27 & 28 – MEMORY LOSS

	Appropriate introduction (1=full name and role), checks patient's name (1)	2	1	0
	Explains purpose of interview and checks consent (2=does well, 1=adequately, 0=poorly or not done)	2	1	0
	Starts with an open question and listens without interrupting (1=both)		1	0
	Presenting Complaint:			
	Establishes presenting complaint of memory loss (1) and establishes whether this is antegrade or retrograde in nature (1)	2	1	0
	Establishes onset (1) and duration (1) of symptoms	2	1	0
	Enquires after any associated neurology such as paraesthesia, weakness, altered speech, visual disturbances, headaches, hearing loss/tinnitus, difficulty recognising familiar faces or places (2=does well, 1=does adequately, 0=poorly)	2	1	0
	Establishes whether there was any preceding head trauma		1	0
	Establishes previous similar episodes		1	0
	Establishes whether the current memory loss has posed any dangers to the patient (1) or to members of the public/others (1) (e.g. forgetting to look before crossing the road or leaving the gas on at home etc.)	2	1	0
	Screens for possible causes/triggers (e.g. stressors, anxiety, life events)		1	0
	Enquires after patient's mental health (1) specifically after symptoms of depression (1)	2	1	0
	Screens for other psychiatric disorders by enquiring after hallucinations, delusions, personality changes, language problems etc.		1	0
	Other relevant history:			
	Systemic features: weight change, appetite, fever, recent infections (2=all three, 1=two items, 0=one only or none)	2	1	0
	Relevant past medical and surgical history (1) especially enquiring after risk factors for vascular disease such as diabetes, heart disease, high cholesterol (1)	2	1	0
	Medication history (1) including allergies (1)	2	1	0
	Relevant family history (1) specifically of dementia (1)	2	1	0
	Smoking (1) and alcohol (1)	2	1	0
	Relevant social history and support (e.g. housing circumstances, dependents, occupation etc.)	2	1	0
	Explores patient's ideas, concerns and expectations	2	1	0
	Appropriate closure (e.g. explains next step, thanks patient and summarises) (2=does well, 1=adequately, 0=poorly or not done)	2	1	0
	Communication Skills			
	Appropriate questioning style (mix of open and closed questions) (2=does well, 1=adequately, 0=poorly or not done)	2	1	0
	Invites questions (1). Listens actively (1).	2	1	0
	Organised approach to history-taking (e.g. systematic, summarises, signposts change in focus of question)	2	1	0
	Simulated patient score (2=very good, 1=satisfactory, 0=poor)	2	1	0
	Examiner to ask: 'What are your differential diagnoses?'			
	Candidate states an appropriate diagnosis (1) and offers a differential (1)	2	1	0
	Total Score			

Global Rating	1 Clear Fail	2 Borderline	3 Clear Pass	4 Very Good	5 Outstanding

Candidate Number:	University:
Date:	Year of Study:

STATIONS 29 & 30 – WEAKNESS

		2	1	0
	Appropriate introduction (1=full name and role), checks patient's name (1)	2	1	0
	Explains purpose of interview and checks consent (2=does well, 1=adequately, 0=poorly or not done)	2	1	0
	Starts with an open question and listens without interrupting (1=both)		1	0
	Presenting Complaint:			
	Establishes presenting complaint of weakness (1) including distribution (1)	2	1	0
	Enquires after any altered sensations such as numbness or paraesthesia in affecting limbs	2	1	0
	Establishes any other neurological symptoms such as altered speech, visual disturbances, headaches, hearing loss/tinnitus	2	1	0
	Establishes onset (1) and duration (1) of symptoms	2	1	0
	Establishes previous similar episodes		1	0
	Establishes risk factors for cardiovascular accident (CVA):			
	Diabetes		1	0
	High blood pressure		1	0
	Raised cholesterol		1	0
	Other relevant history:			
	Systemic features: weight change, appetite, fever (2=all three, 1=two items, 0=one only or none)	2	1	0
	Relevant past medical and surgical history	2	1	0
	Medication history (1) including allergies (1)	2	1	0
	Relevant family history		1	0
	Smoking (1) and alcohol (1)	2	1	0
	Relevant social history (e.g. housing circumstances, dependents, occupation etc.)	2	1	0
	Explores patient's ideas, concerns and expectations	2	1	0
	Appropriate closure (e.g. explains next step, thanks patient and summarises) (2=does well, 1=adequately, 0=poorly or not done)	2	1	0
	Communication Skills			
	Appropriate questioning style (mix of open and closed questions) (2=does well, 1=adequately, 0=poorly or not done)	2	1	0
	Invites questions (1). Listens actively (1).	2	1	0
	Organised approach to history-taking (e.g. systematic, summarises, signposts change in focus of question)	2	1	0
	Simulated patient score (2=very good, 1=satisfactory, 0=poor)	2	1	0
	Examiner to ask: 'What are your differential diagnoses?'			
	Candidate states an appropriate diagnosis (1) and offers a differential (1) (see patient scenarios for possible diagnoses)	2	1	0
	Examiner to ask: 'What investigations/management would you recommend?'			
	Candidate suggests appropriate investigations (1) followed by a sensible line of management (1) (see patient scenarios for possible management options)	2	1	0
	Total Score			

Global Rating	1 Clear Fail	2 Borderline	3 Clear Pass	4 Very Good	5 Outstanding

Candidate Number:	University:
Date:	Year of Study:

STATION 31 – DELIRIUM TREMENS

	Appropriate introduction (1=full name and role), checks patient's name (1)	2	1	0
	Establishes patient's age and occupation		1	0
	Explains purpose of interview and checks consent (2=does well, 1=adequately, 0=poorly or not done)	2	1	0
	Establishes presenting complaint at beginning of consultation: unwell after stopping drinking		1	0
	History of Presenting Complaint			
	Establishes features: tremor (1), fever (1)	2	1	0
	Establishes features: insomnia (1), panic attack (1)	2	1	0
	Establishes features: paranoia (1), formication/hallucination (1)	2	1	0
	Establishes features: nausea (1), low mood (1)	2	1	0
	Establishes lack of: seizures (1), abdominal pain (1)	2	1	0
	Alcohol History			
	Use of scoring system (e.g. CAGE) (2)	2	1	0
	Establishes: nature and amount of alcohol usage (1), previous attempts to stop (1)	2	1	0
	Establishes: duration of drinking (1), being told to stop by others (1)	2	1	0
	Establishes: small repertoire of alcohol choice (1), drinking in the mornings (1)	2	1	0
	Establishes: alcohol tolerance and cravings (1), family history of alcohol use (1)	2	1	0
	Other History Components			
	Past Medical History (1), especially pancreatitis/alcohol-related admissions (1)	2	1	0
	Drug History (1) and allergies (1)	2	1	0
	Social History: alcohol (1), smoking (1)	2	1	0
	Social History: loss of partner (1), loss of job (1)	2	1	0
	Family History		1	0
	General Communication Skills			
	Maintains eye contact with the patient and persists in taking a good history		1	0
	Begins with open questions, and proceeds to more focused questioning		1	0
	Elicits patient's ideas about diagnosis and concerns		1	0
	Closing Remarks			
	Summarises key points		1	0
	Asks if there is anything else that the patient would like to discuss		1	0
	Examiner to Ask:			
	'What is the diagnosis?': Delirium Tremens		1	0
	'What are the complications of this condition?': seizures, confusion, psychiatric disturbance, arrhythmias, reduced level of consciousness, electrolyte disturbances (1 for each, maximum 2)	2	1	0
	'What is the acute treatment of this patient?': IV Pabrinex, benzodiazepine reducing regime (e.g. chlordiazepoxide, diazepam), rehydration, exclusion of complications (e.g. ECG for arrhythmias or amylase for pancreatitis) (1 for each, maximum 2)	2	1	0
	Simulated patient score (2=very good, 1=satisfactory, 0=poor)	2	1	0
	Total Score			

Global Rating	**1** Clear Fail	**2** Borderline	**3** Clear Pass	**4** Very Good	**5** Outstanding

Candidate Number:	University:
Date:	Year of Study:

STATIONS 32, 33, 34, 35 & 36 – PAINFUL JOINTS

	Appropriate introduction (1=full name and role), checks patient's name (1)	**2**	**1**	**0**
	Explains purpose of interview and checks consent (2=does well, 1=adequately, 0=poorly or not done)	**2**	**1**	**0**
	Starts with an open question and listens without interrupting (1=both)		**1**	**0**
	Presenting Complaint:			
	Establishes the onset (1) and duration (1) of the joint pain	**2**	**1**	**0**
	Establishes pattern of joint pain (e.g. symmetrical, small joints, large joints, single joint)		**1**	**0**
	Establishes presence of joint swelling (1) and the distribution of swollen joints (1)	**2**	**1**	**0**
	Enquires whether the patient has any joint stiffness		**1**	**0**
	Enquires whether there is any diurnal variation in the symptoms		**1**	**0**
	Enquires whether activity (1) or heat (1) makes the symptoms better or worse	**2**	**1**	**0**
	Enquires whether the patient has noticed any other lumps or swellings (e.g. rheumatoid nodules, Bouchard's and Heberden's nodes, skin growths like neurofibromas)		**1**	**0**
	Systemic features: rashes, red eyes, dry eyes/mouth, weight loss, diarrhoea, mouth/genital ulcers, bleeding per rectum (2=any three symptoms, 1=any two, 0=one only or none)	**2**	**1**	**0**
	Enquires whether the patient has any neurological symptoms		**1**	**0**
	Enquires after previous similar episodes		**1**	**0**
	Explores patient's ideas and concerns regarding the presenting complaint		**1**	**0**
	Other relevant history:			
	Relevant past medical and surgical history		**1**	**0**
	Medication history (1) including allergies (1)	**2**	**1**	**0**
	Relevant family history		**1**	**0**
	Smoking (1) and alcohol (1)	**2**	**1**	**0**
	Relevant social history (e.g. housing circumstances, dependents, occupation etc.)		**1**	**0**
	Establishes the effect the joint problems are having on the patient's life (e.g. stopping work, unable to do household chores, making patient depressed etc.)		**1**	**0**
	Appropriate closure (e.g. explains next step, thanks patient and summarises) (2=does well, 1=adequately, 0=poorly or not done)	**2**	**1**	**0**
	Communication Skills			
	Appropriate questioning style (mix of open and closed questions) (2=does well, 1=adequately, 0=poorly or not done)	**2**	**1**	**0**
	Invites questions (1). Listens actively (1).	**2**	**1**	**0**
	Organised approach to history-taking (e.g. systematic, summarises, signposts change in focus of question)	**2**	**1**	**0**
	Simulated patient score (2=very good, 1=satisfactory, 0=poor)	**2**	**1**	**0**
	Examiner to ask: 'What are your differential diagnoses?'			
	Candidate states an appropriate diagnosis (1) and offers a differential (1) (see patient scenarios for possible diagnoses)	**2**	**1**	**0**
	Examiner to ask: 'What investigations/management would you recommend?'			
	Candidate suggests appropriate investigations (1) followed by a sensible line of management (1) (see patient scenarios for possible management options)	**2**	**1**	**0**
	Total Score			

Global Rating	**1** Clear Fail	**2** Borderline	**3** Clear Pass	**4** Very Good	**5** Outstanding

Candidate Number:	University:
Date:	Year of Study:

STATIONS 37 & 38 – FATIGUE

	Appropriate introduction (1=full name and role), checks patient's name (1)	2	1	0
	Explains purpose of interview and checks consent (2=does well, 1=adequately, 0=poorly or not done)	2	1	0
	Starts with an open question and listens without interrupting (1=both)	▨	1	0
	Presenting Complaint:			
	Establishes presenting complaint of fatigue (1) and severity of the fatigue such as whether it prevents patient from performing their normal daily tasks (1)	2	1	0
	Establishes duration (1) and onset (1) of symptoms	2	1	0
	Enquires whether the fatigue is constant or during certain tasks or times of the day	▨	1	0
	Establishes whether there was any associated symptoms such as neurology, change in bowel habits, flu-like symptoms, symptoms of pregnancy etc. (2=any three symptoms, 1=any two symptoms, 0=one or none)	2	1	0
	Enquires after any symptoms indicative of underlying malignancy (e.g. weight loss, change in appetite, night sweats or bony pain)	2	1	0
	Enquires about blood loss such as irregular heavy menses, bleeding per rectum, haematuria, haematemesis or haemoptysis	2	1	0
	Screens about symptoms of depression and life events	2	1	0
	Establishes previous similar episodes	▨	1	0
	Other relevant history:			
	Relevant past medical and surgical history	2	1	0
	Medication history (1) including allergies (1)	2	1	0
	Relevant family history	▨	1	0
	Smoking (1) and alcohol (1)	2	1	0
	Relevant social history (e.g. housing circumstances, dependents, occupation etc.)	2	1	0
	Explores patient's ideas, concerns and expectations	2	1	0
	Appropriate closure (e.g. explains next step, thanks patient and summarises) (2=does well, 1=adequately, 0=poorly or not done)	2	1	0
	Communication Skills			
	Appropriate questioning style (mix of open and closed questions) (2=does well, 1=adequately, 0=poorly or not done)	2	1	0
	Invites questions (1). Listens actively (1).	2	1	0
	Organised approach to history-taking (e.g. systematic, summarises, signposts change in focus of question)	2	1	0
	Simulated patient score (2=very good, 1=satisfactory, 0=poor)	2	1	0
	Examiner to ask: 'What are your differential diagnoses?'			
	Candidate states an appropriate diagnosis (1) and offers a differential (1) (see patient scenarios for possible diagnoses)	2	1	0
	Examiner to ask: 'What investigations/management would you recommend?'			
	Candidate suggests appropriate investigations (1) followed by a sensible line of management (1) (see patient scenarios for possible management options)	2	1	0
	Total Score			

Global Rating	1 Clear Fail	2 Borderline	3 Clear Pass	4 Very Good	5 Outstanding

Candidate Number:	University:
Date:	Year of Study:

STATION 39 – HAEMATURIA

	Appropriate introduction (1=full name and role), checks patient's name (1)	2	1	0
	Explains purpose of interview and checks consent (2=does well, 1=adequately, 0=poorly or not done)	2	1	0
	Starts with an open question and listens without interrupting	▓	1	0
	Assesses present history: asks about			
	Number of episodes of haematuria	▓	1	0
	Onset and progression (2=does well, 1=adequately, 0=poorly or not done)	2	1	0
	Extent of blood loss (1) and smell (1)	2	1	0
	Abdominal pain	2	1	0
	General urological questions			
	Frequency, dysuria, urgency, nocturia (2=three or more, 1=two items, 0=one only or none)	2	1	0
	Hesitancy, dribbling, poor stream (2=all three, 1=two items, 0=one or none)	2	1	0
	Back pain	▓	1	0
	Other relevant history: asks about			
	Systemic features: weight change, appetite, fever (2=all three, 1=two items, 0=one only or none)	2	1	0
	Relevant past medical history	▓	1	0
	Relevant family history	▓	1	0
	Medication (2=asks specifically about anticoagulants, 1=any medication history)	2	1	0
	Occupational history (1=any occupational history, 2=asks specifically about aniline dye/chemical exposure)	2	1	0
	Smoking (1) and alcohol (1)	2	1	0
	Communication Skills			
	Appropriate questioning style (mix of open and closed questions) (2=does well, 1=adequately, 0=poorly or not done)	2	1	0
	Listens actively (e.g. picks up cues, responds appropriately, does not repeat questions)	2	1	0
	Organised approach to history-taking (e.g. systematic, summarises, signposts change in focus of question)	2	1	0
	Appropriate closure (e.g. explains next step, thanks patient) (2=does well, 1=adequately, 0=poorly or not done)	2	1	0
	Simulated patient to mark (see simulated patient instructions)	2	1	0
	Examiner to ask: 'What is your differential diagnosis?'			
	Transitional cell carcinoma, renal cell carcinoma, renal stone disease (1=one or two of the above, 2=three or more)	2	1	0
	Total Score			

Global Rating	1 Clear Fail	2 Borderline	3 Clear Pass	4 Very Good	5 Outstanding

Candidate Number:	University:
Date:	Year of Study:

STATION 40 – TESTICULAR LUMP

		2	1	0
	Appropriate introduction (1=full name and role), checks patient's name (1)	2	1	0
	Establishes patient's age and occupation	▨	1	0
	Establishes presenting complaint at beginning of consultation: scrotal lump (1), left side (1)	2	1	0
	History of Presenting Complaint			
	Establishes features: not painful (1), but 'dragging' sensation (1)	2	1	0
	Establishes features: when first noticed (1), current size and not increasing in size (1)	2	1	0
	Establishes features: possible gynaecomastia (1), recent trauma (1)	2	1	0
	Establishes lack of: sexual dysfunction (1), urinary dysfunction (1)	2	1	0
	Establishes lack of: skin changes (e.g. discolouration/eczema) (1), weight loss (1)	2	1	0
	Establishes lack of: fever (1), gastrointestinal symptoms (1)	2	1	0
	Enquires about risk factors: surgery to that testicle in past due to maldescent, family history, infertility (1 mark for each feature, up to a maximum of 2 marks)	2	1	0
	Systemic features: weight change, appetite, fever (2=all three, 1=two items, 0=one only or none)	2	1	0
	Other relevant history:			
	Relevant past medical and surgical history	2	1	0
	Medication history (1) including allergies (1)	2	1	0
	Relevant family history	▨	1	0
	Smoking (1) and alcohol (1)	2	1	0
	Relevant social history (e.g. housing circumstances, dependents, occupation etc.)	2	1	0
	Explores patient's ideas, concerns and expectations	2	1	0
	Appropriate closure (e.g. explains next step, thanks patient and summarises) (2=does well, 1=adequately, 0=poorly or not done)	2	1	0
	Communication Skills			
	Appropriate questioning style (mix of open and closed questions) (2=does well, 1=adequately, 0=poorly or not done)	2	1	0
	Invites questions (1). Listens actively (1).	2	1	0
	Organised approach to history-taking (e.g. systematic, summarises, signposts change in focus of question)	2	1	0
	Simulated patient score (2=very good, 1=satisfactory, 0=poor)	2	1	0
	Examiner to ask: 'What are your differential diagnoses?'			
	Seminoma, teratoma, other tumour (lymphoma, non-germ cell testicular tumours), hydrocele, epididymal cyst, infection (epididymo-orchitis, tuberculosis, syphilis, mumps), torsion (2=any three suggestions, 1=any two suggestions, 0=one or none)	2	1	0
	Examiner to ask: 'What initial investigations would you recommend?'			
	Ultrasound scan, beta-HCG, alphafetoprotein (2=all three, 1=any two, 0=one or none)	2	1	0
	Examiner to Ask: 'How is orchidectomy performed and why?'			
	Via the inguinal approach (1), in order to prevent seeding (1)	2	1	0
	Total Score			

Global Rating	1 Clear Fail	2 Borderline	3 Clear Pass	4 Very Good	5 Outstanding

Candidate Number:	University:
Date:	Year of Study:

STATION 41 – LOWER URINARY TRACT SYMPTOMS (LUTS)

	2	1	0
Appropriate introduction (1=full name and role), checks patient's name (1)	2	1	0
Establishes patient's age and occupation		1	0
Establishes presenting complaint at beginning of consultation: frequent urination with poor stream		1	0
History of Presenting Complaint			
Establishes features: quantifies frequency (1), nocturia (1)	2	1	0
Establishes features: terminal dribbling (1), incomplete voiding (1)	2	1	0
Establishes features: straining (1), hesitancy (1)	2	1	0
Establishes lack of: urgency (1), incontinence (1)	2	1	0
Establishes lack of: haematuria (1), dysuria (1)	2	1	0
Establishes lack of: abdominal/pelvic pain (1), constipation (1)	2	1	0
Establishes lack of: fever (1) back pain (1)	2	1	0
Enquires: about sexual problems (1), previous urinary retention (1)	2	1	0
Systemic features: weight change, appetite, bone pain (2=all three, 1=two items, 0=one only or none)	2	1	0
Rules out previous surgery or interventions		1	0
Other relevant history:			
Relevant past medical and surgical history	2	1	0
Medication history (1) including allergies (1)	2	1	0
Relevant family history		1	0
Smoking (1) and alcohol (1)	2	1	0
Relevant social history (e.g. housing circumstances, dependents, occupation etc.)	2	1	0
Explores patient's ideas, concerns and expectations	2	1	0
Appropriate closure (e.g. explains next step, thanks patient and summarises) (2=does well, 1=adequately, 0=poorly or not done)	2	1	0
Communication Skills			
Appropriate questioning style (mix of open and closed questions) (2=does well, 1=adequately, 0=poorly or not done)	2	1	0
Invites questions (1). Listens actively (1).	2	1	0
Organised approach to history-taking (e.g. systematic, summarises, signposts change in focus of question)	2	1	0
Simulated patient score (2=very good, 1=satisfactory, 0=poor)	2	1	0
Examiner to ask: 'What are your differential diagnoses?'			
Benign prostatic hypertrophy, prostate cancer, bladder/urethral cancer, urinary tract infection, urinary tract stones, detrusor muscle weakness, chronic prostatitis, polyuria (e.g. due to diabetes), neurological (e.g. multiple sclerosis) (2=any three suggestions, 1=any two suggestions, 0=one or none)	2	1	0
Examiner to ask: 'What initial examinations and investigations would you perform?'			
Urine dipstick and cytology, microscopy and sensitivities Blood tests: U&Es, PSA Urinary frequency charting, flow-rate and post-void residual volume measurement Imaging: renal ultrasound scan, KUB, prostatic MRI scan (2=any three suggestions, 1=any two suggestions)	2	1	0
Total Score			

Global Rating	**1** Clear Fail	**2** Borderline	**3** Clear Pass	**4** Very Good	**5** Outstanding

Candidate Number:	University:
Date:	Year of Study:

STATION 42 – BREAST LUMP

		2	1	0
	Appropriate introduction (1=full name and role), checks patient's name (1)	2	1	0
	Establishes patient's age and occupation		1	0
	Establishes presenting complaint at beginning of consultation: breast lump		1	0
	History of Presenting Complaint			
	Establishes features: painlessness (1), current size and whether increasing or changing (1)	2	1	0
	Establishes features: exact site of lump (upper outer quadrant) (1), when first noticed (1)	2	1	0
	Establishes lack of previous breast cancer/breast lumps		1	0
	Establishes lack of: nipple discharge (1), nipple changes (e.g. inversion, discolouration) (1)	2	1	0
	Establishes lack of: skin changes (e.g. discolouration/eczema) (1), axillary lymphadenopathy (1)	2	1	0
	Establishes risk factors: smoking, menstrual history (early menarche and late menopause), family history, childless or late children, not having breast-fed, oestrogens and HRT, radiation to chest (2=any three suggestions, 1=any two suggestions)	2	1	0
	Rules out previous surgery or interventions (e.g. radiation exposure) to the breasts		1	0
	Systemic features: weight change, appetite, fever, bone pain (2=all three, 1=two items, 0=one only or none)	2	1	0
	Other relevant history:			
	Relevant past medical and surgical history	2	1	0
	Medication history (1) including allergies (1)	2	1	0
	Relevant family history		1	0
	Smoking (1) and alcohol (1)	2	1	0
	Relevant social history (e.g. housing circumstances, dependents, occupation etc.)	2	1	0
	Explores patient's ideas, concerns and expectations	2	1	0
	Appropriate closure (e.g. explains next step, thanks patient and summarises) (2=does well, 1=adequately, 0=poorly or not done)	2	1	0
	Communication Skills			
	Appropriate questioning style (mix of open and closed questions) (2=does well, 1=adequately, 0=poorly or not done)	2	1	0
	Invites questions (1). Listens actively (1).	2	1	0
	Organised approach to history-taking (e.g. systematic, summarises, signposts change in focus of question)	2	1	0
	Simulated patient score (2=very good, 1=satisfactory, 0=poor)	2	1	0
	Examiner to ask: 'What are your differential diagnoses?'			
	Candidate states an appropriate diagnosis (1) and offers a differential (1) (see patient scenarios for possible diagnoses)	2	1	0
	Examiner to ask: 'What investigations/management would you recommend?'			
	Candidate suggests appropriate investigations (1) followed by a sensible line of management (1) (see patient scenarios for possible management options)	2	1	0
	Examiner to ask: 'How soon should this patient be seen by a breast specialist?'			
	Candidate states: within 2 weeks		1	0
	Total Score			

Global Rating	1 Clear Fail	2 Borderline	3 Clear Pass	4 Very Good	5 Outstanding

Candidate Number:	University:
Date:	Year of Study:

STATION 43 – NIPPLE DISCHARGE

	Appropriate introduction (1=full name and role), checks patient's name (1)	2	1	0
	Establishes patient's age and occupation		1	0
	Establishes presenting complaint at beginning of consultation: nipple discharge		1	0
	History of Presenting Complaint			
	Establishes features of the discharge: bloody (1), unilateral (1)	2	1	0
	Enquires about quantity of discharge (1) and that patient is not currently breast-feeding (1)	2	1	0
	Establishes lack of pain (1), breast lumps (1)	2	1	0
	Establishes lack of previous breast cancer		1	0
	Establishes lack of nipple changes (e.g. inversion, discolouration)		1	0
	Establishes lack of skin changes (e.g. discolouration/eczema) (1), axillary lymphadenopathy (1)	2	1	0
	Establishes risk factors for cancer: smoking, menstrual history (early menarche and late menopause), family history, childless or late children, oestrogens and HRT, radiation to chest (1 mark for 1, 2 marks for 2)	2	1	0
	Systemic features: weight change, appetite, fever, bone pain (2=all three, 1=two items, 0=one only or none)	2	1	0
	Rules out previous surgery or interventions (e.g. radiation exposure) to the breasts		1	0
	Other relevant history:			
	Relevant past medical and surgical history	2	1	0
	Medication history (1) including allergies (1)	2	1	0
	Relevant family history		1	0
	Smoking (1) and alcohol (1)	2	1	0
	Relevant social history (e.g. housing circumstances, dependents, occupation etc.)	2	1	0
	Explores patient's ideas, concerns and expectations	2	1	0
	Appropriate closure (e.g. explains next step, thanks patient and summarises) (2=does well, 1=adequately, 0=poorly or not done)	2	1	0
	Communication Skills			
	Appropriate questioning style (mix of open and closed questions) (2=does well, 1=adequately, 0=poorly or not done)	2	1	0
	Invites questions (1). Listens actively (1).	2	1	0
	Organised approach to history-taking (e.g. systematic, summarises, signposts change in focus of question)	2	1	0
	Simulated patient score (2=very good, 1=satisfactory, 0=poor)	2	1	0
	Examiner to ask: 'What are your differential diagnoses?'			
	Candidate states: intraductal papilloma, duct ectasia, ductal carcinoma in situ (2=any two suggestions, 1=any suggestion, 0=none)	2	1	0
	Examiner to ask: 'What are your initial investigations?'			
	Candidate states 'triple assessment' with full clinical examination, imaging with mammography or ultrasound, cytology of the nipple discharge or fine needle aspiration/biopsy of any masses found on examination/imaging (2=all three suggestions, 1=any two suggestions, 0=one or none)	2	1	0
	Total Score			

Global Rating	1 Clear Fail	2 Borderline	3 Clear Pass	4 Very Good	5 Outstanding

Candidate Number:	University:
Date:	Year of Study:

STATION 44 – GROIN LUMP

	Appropriate introduction (1=full name and role), checks patient's name (1)	2	1	0
	Establishes patient's age and occupation		1	0
	Establishes presenting complaint at beginning of consultation: groin lump (1)		1	0
	History of Presenting Complaint			
	Establishes features: exact site of lump (1), when first noticed (1)	2	1	0
	Establishes features: associated pain (1), whether it changes/comes and goes (1)	2	1	0
	Establishes features: size (1), unilateral (1)	2	1	0
	Establishes whether it is associated with physical activity		1	0
	Establishes lack of previous breast groin lumps		1	0
	Establishes lack of: irreducibility (1), symptoms of obstruction (pain/vomiting/constipation) (1)	2	1	0
	Establishes risk factors for hernias: coughing, obesity, heavy lifting, constipation (2=any three factors, 1=any two factors, 0=one or none)	2	1	0
	Systemic features: weight change, appetite, fever, bone pain (2=all three, 1=two items, 0=one only or none)	2	1	0
	Rules out previous surgery in this area		1	0
	Other relevant history:			
	Relevant past medical and surgical history	2	1	0
	Medication history (1) including allergies (1)	2	1	0
	Relevant family history		1	0
	Smoking (1) and alcohol (1)	2	1	0
	Relevant social history (e.g. housing circumstances, dependents, occupation etc.)	2	1	0
	Explores patient's ideas, concerns and expectations	2	1	0
	Appropriate closure (e.g. explains next step, thanks patient and summarises) (2=does well, 1=adequately, 0=poorly or not done)	2	1	0
	Communication Skills			
	Appropriate questioning style (mix of open and closed questions) (2=does well, 1=adequately, 0=poorly or not done)	2	1	0
	Invites questions (1). Listens actively (1).	2	1	0
	Organised approach to history-taking (e.g. systematic, summarises, signposts change in focus of question)	2	1	0
	Simulated patient score (2=very good, 1=satisfactory, 0=poor)	2	1	0
	Examiner to ask:			
	'What is your differential diagnosis?': hernia, lymph node, lipoma, abscess, vascular structure (e.g. femoral artery pseudoaneurysm), psoas abscess, disorder of the testicular cord	2	1	0
	'What features of a hernia might make you admit this patient to hospital as an emergency?': tender, irreducible hernia, abdominal pain/vomiting/constipation, changes in skin colour (red/blue/black)	2	1	0
	'What management options are available for hernias?': conservative (e.g. truss) (1), surgical open approach (1), surgical laparoscopic approach (1)	2	1	0
	Simulated patient score (2=very good, 1=satisfactory, 0=poor)	2	1	0
	Total Score			

Global Rating	**1** Clear Fail	**2** Borderline	**3** Clear Pass	**4** Very Good	**5** Outstanding

Candidate Number:	University:
Date:	Year of Study:

STATION 45 – EPISTAXIS

	Appropriate introduction (1=full name and role), checks patient's name (1)	2	1	0
	Establishes patient's age and occupation		1	0
	Establishes presenting complaint at beginning of consultation: frequent epistaxis		1	0
	History of Presenting Complaint			
	Establishes features: frequency (almost daily for 14 days) (1), one or both nostrils (1)	2	1	0
	Establishes features: severity (amount and duration of bleeding) (1), A&E attendances (1)	2	1	0
	Establishes lack of: trauma to nose (including nose-picking/nose-blowing) (1), symptoms of rhinosinusitis (e.g. blocked nose) and of anaemia (e.g. pale, faint, tachycardic, chest pain) (1)	2	1	0
	Establishes risk factors: drugs (aspirin, warfarin, other anticoagulants), bleeding disorders (such as idiopathic thrombocytopenic purpura or hereditary haemorrhagic telangiectasia), nasal sprays (especially steroids) (2=any three aspects, 1=any two, 0=one or none)	2	1	0
	Rules out previous surgery or interventions to the nose		1	0
	Other relevant history:			
	Relevant past medical and surgical history	2	1	0
	Medication history (1) including allergies (1)	2	1	0
	Smoking (1) and alcohol (1)	2	1	0
	Enquires specifically about recreational drugs especially over nasal inhalation of cocaine		1	0
	Relevant family history		1	0
	Relevant social history (e.g. housing circumstances, dependents, occupation etc.)	2	1	0
	Explores patient's ideas, concerns and expectations	2	1	0
	Appropriate closure (e.g. explains next step, thanks patient and summarises) (2=does well, 1=adequately, 0=poorly or not done)	2	1	0
	Communication Skills			
	Appropriate questioning style (mix of open and closed questions) (2=does well, 1=adequately, 0=poorly or not done)	2	1	0
	Invites questions (1). Listens actively (1).	2	1	0
	Organised approach to history-taking (e.g. systematic, summarises, signposts change in focus of question)	2	1	0
	Simulated patient score (2=very good, 1=satisfactory, 0=poor)	2	1	0
	Examiner to ask: 'What are the common causes for epistaxis?'			
	Trauma (nose-picking or facial trauma), mucosal irritation (sprays, hot dry weather, cocaine use), septal abnormalities, rhinosinusitis, tumours, blood disorders (2=any three suggestions, 1=any two suggestions, 0=one or none)	2	1	0
	Examiner to ask: 'What initial investigation would you perform?'			
	Complete head and neck examination, examination of the nose using nasal speculum, rigid or flexible nasendoscopy, blood tests including clotting and haematological screen (2=any three suggestions, 1=any two suggestions)	2	1	0
	Examiner to ask: 'What is the emergency treatment for epistaxis?'			
	Nasal packing, intravenous access with intravenous fluid infusion or blood transfusion if blood loss severe, keep patient nil by mouth in rare cases where surgery may be required (2=any two sensible suggestions, 1=any sensible suggestion)	2	1	0
	Total Score			

Global Rating	1 Clear Fail	2 Borderline	3 Clear Pass	4 Very Good	5 Outstanding

Candidate Number:	University:
Date:	Year of Study:

STATION 46 – HEARING LOSS

		2	1	0
	Appropriate introduction (1=full name and role), checks patient's name (1)	2	1	0
	Establishes patient's age and occupation		1	0
	Establishes presenting complaint at beginning of consultation: hearing loss		1	0
	History of Presenting Complaint			
	Establishes features: progressive gradual loss (1), bilateral (1)	2	1	0
	Establishes how it is affecting patient's life (i.e. needs to turn TV up, family members have noticed and are getting annoyed)		1	0
	Establishes use of cotton buds to 'clean' ears		1	0
	Establishes lack of: tinnitus (1), vertigo/nausea (1)	2	1	0
	Establishes lack of: ear pain (1), discharge or wax (1)	2	1	0
	Establishes lack of: facial weakness (1), headache (1)	2	1	0
	Establishes lack of: recent trauma (e.g. fall, ear syringing) (1), recent upper respiratory tract infection/otitis media (1)	2	1	0
	Establishes risk factors: noise exposure, ototoxic drugs (e.g. aminoglycosides, NSAIDs, furosemide), family history, HTN/cholesterol/diabetes/obesity, smoking (2=any three aspects, 1=any two suggestions, 0=one or none)	2	1	0
	Rules out previous surgery or interventions to the ear		1	0
	Other relevant history:			
	Relevant past medical and surgical history	2	1	0
	Medication history (1) including allergies (1)	2	1	0
	Relevant family history		1	0
	Smoking (1) and alcohol (1)	2	1	0
	Relevant social history (e.g. housing circumstances, dependents, occupation etc.)	2	1	0
	Explores patient's ideas, concerns and expectations	2	1	0
	Appropriate closure (e.g. explains next step, thanks patient and summarises) (2=does well, 1=adequately, 0=poorly or not done)	2	1	0
	Communication Skills			
	Appropriate questioning style (mix of open and closed questions) (2=does well, 1=adequately, 0=poorly or not done)	2	1	0
	Invites questions (1). Listens actively (1).	2	1	0
	Organised approach to history-taking (e.g. systematic, summarises, signposts change in focus of question)	2	1	0
	Simulated patient score (2=very good, 1=satisfactory, 0=poor)	2	1	0
	Examiner to ask: 'What are your differential diagnoses?'			
	Presbyacusis, wax impaction, cerebrovascular disease, otosclerosis, acoustic neuroma, cholesteatoma, chronic inflammation/infection, tympanic membrane perforation, noise-induced hearing loss, autoimmune disorder (2=any three suggestions, 1=any two suggestions, 0=one or none)	2	1	0
	Examiner to ask: 'What are the different types of hearing loss? What clinical test can help you differentiate between the two types?'			
	Hearing loss can be: conductive versus sensorineural (1) Clinical tests may include the: Rinne's and Weber's tests (performed together) (1)	2	1	0
	Examiner to ask: 'What investigations can be performed to investigate this symptom further?'			
	Otoscopy, audiometry, tympanometry (2=all three items, 1=any two items)	2	1	0
	Total Score			

Global Rating	1 Clear Fail	2 Borderline	3 Clear Pass	4 Very Good	5 Outstanding

Candidate Number:		University:
Date:		Year of Study:

STATION 47 – DIZZINESS

Appropriate introduction (1=full name and role), checks patient's name (1)	**2**	**1**	**0**
Establishes patient's age and occupation		**1**	**0**
Establishes and clarifies the presenting complaint at beginning of consultation: i.e. vertigo		**1**	**0**
History of Presenting Complaint			
Establishes features: vertigo with a rotational component (1), sudden onset provoked by certain head movements (1)	**2**	**1**	**0**
Establishes features: episodic (1), severity (1)	**2**	**1**	**0**
Establishes features: duration (less than a minute) (1), slight nausea (1)	**2**	**1**	**0**
Establishes lack of: hearing loss (1), tinnitus (1)	**2**	**1**	**0**
Establishes lack of: severe nausea/vomiting (1) otalgia (1)	**2**	**1**	**0**
Rules out head injury (1) meningism (headache, photophobia, stiff neck) (1)	**2**	**1**	**0**
Other relevant history:			
Relevant past medical and surgical history	**2**	**1**	**0**
Medication history (1) including allergies (1)	**2**	**1**	**0**
Relevant family history		**1**	**0**
Smoking (1) and alcohol (1)	**2**	**1**	**0**
Relevant social history (e.g. housing circumstances, dependents, occupation etc.)	**2**	**1**	**0**
Explores patient's ideas, concerns and expectations	**2**	**1**	**0**
Appropriate closure (e.g. explains next step, thanks patient and summarises) (2=does well, 1=adequately, 0=poorly or not done)	**2**	**1**	**0**
Communication Skills			
Appropriate questioning style (mix of open and closed questions) (2=does well, 1=adequately, 0=poorly or not done)	**2**	**1**	**0**
Invites questions (1). Listens actively (1).	**2**	**1**	**0**
Organised approach to history-taking (e.g. systematic, summarises, signposts change in focus of question)	**2**	**1**	**0**
Simulated patient score (2=very good, 1=satisfactory, 0=poor)	**2**	**1**	**0**
Examiner to ask: 'What are your differential diagnoses?'			
Benign paroxysmal positional vertigo, Ménière's disease, vestibular neuritis, viral labyrinthitis, acoustic neuroma, neurological (cerebrovascular disease, multiple sclerosis, vertebrobasilar insufficiency, brainstem lesions), otosclerosis (2=any three suggestions, 1=any two suggestions, 0=one or none)	**2**	**1**	**0**
Examiner to ask: 'What clinical examinations would you perform?'			
Otoscopy, cranial nerve examinations, Hallpike test	**2**	**1**	**0**
Examiner to ask: 'What is the treatment for benign paroxysmal positional vertigo?'			
Avoid provocation by reducing head movements and moving slowly, Epley manouevres, anti-emetics in the short-term (2=any two suggestions, 1=any one suggestion, 0=none)	**2**	**1**	**0**
Total Score			

Global Rating	**1** Clear Fail	**2** Borderline	**3** Clear Pass	**4** Very Good	**5** Outstanding

Candidate Number:		University:	
Date:		Year of Study:	

STATION 48 – ACROMEGALY

		2	1	0
	Appropriate introduction (1=full name and role), checks patient's name (1)	2	1	0
	Explains purpose of interview and checks consent (2=does well, 1=adequately, 0=poorly or not done)	2	1	0
	Starts with an open question and listens without interrupting (1=both)		1	0
	Presenting Complaint:			
	Establishes presenting complaint of visual disturbance (1) and nature of this disturbance (1)	2	1	0
	Enquires after duration (1) and onset (1) of visual disturbance	2	1	0
	Establishes previous similar episodes		1	0
	Enquires after triggers, trauma or eye drops/change medication for the symptom		1	0
	Enquires after any associated neurology such as limb weakness, speech disturbance, confusion, headaches or hearing loss (2=any three symptoms, 1=any two symptoms, 0=one or none)	2	1	0
	Enquires after symptoms of a pituitary adenoma such as symptoms of hypo/hyperthyroidism, prolactinoma, acromegaly or Cushing's disease (2=any three conditions, 1=any two, 0=one or none)	2	1	0
	Enquires after complications of acromegaly such as median nerve palsy, high blood pressure, myocardial infarcts, sleep apnoea (2=any three complications, 1=any two, 0=one or none)	2	1	0
	Other relevant history:			
	Relevant past medical and surgical history	2	1	0
	Medication history (1) including allergies (1)	2	1	0
	Relevant family history		1	0
	Smoking (1) and alcohol (1)	2	1	0
	Relevant social history (e.g. housing circumstances, dependents, occupation etc.)	2	1	0
	Explores patient's ideas, concerns and expectations	2	1	0
	Appropriate closure (e.g. explains next step, thanks patient and summarises) (2=does well, 1=adequately, 0=poorly or not done)	2	1	0
	Communication Skills			
	Appropriate questioning style (mix of open and closed questions) (2=does well, 1=adequately, 0=poorly or not done)	2	1	0
	Invites questions (1). Listens actively (1).	2	1	0
	Organised approach to history-taking (e.g. systematic, summarises, signposts change in focus of question)	2	1	0
	Simulated patient score (2=very good, 1=satisfactory, 0=poor)	2	1	0
	Examiner to ask: 'What are your differential diagnoses?'			
	Candidate states an appropriate diagnosis (1) and offers a differential (1) (see patient scenarios for possible diagnoses)	2	1	0
	Examiner to ask: 'What investigations/management would you recommend?'			
	Candidate suggests appropriate investigations (1) followed by a sensible line of management (1) (see patient scenarios for possible management options)	2	1	0
	Total Score			

Global Rating	**1** Clear Fail	**2** Borderline	**3** Clear Pass	**4** Very Good	**5** Outstanding

Candidate Number:	University:
Date:	Year of Study:

STATIONS 49, 50 & 51 – RED EYE

	Appropriate introduction (1=full name and role), checks patient's name (1)	2	1	0
	Establishes rapport with the patient (1) and starts with an open question (1)	2	1	0
	History of Presenting Complaint			
	Establishes whether the patient wears glasses or contact lenses		1	0
	Establishes onset, duration and progression of presenting complaint	2	1	0
	Establishes side of the eye affected and whether unilateral or bilateral and if both, whether one side occurred before the other		1	0
	Establishes any triggers or aggravating factors (e.g. weather, time of day)		1	0
	Enquires after any associated visual disturbances and the nature of the disturbance	2	1	0
	Establishes if there is any history of trauma to the eye		1	0
	Enquires after associated symptoms (e.g. redness, grittiness, discharge, reduced tear formation, nasal irritation, sneezing, watery rhinorrhoea)	2	1	0
	Establishes an adequate pain history for any eye pain		1	0
	Enquires after any contacts with similar symptoms		1	0
	Other relevant history:			
	Past medical and surgical history including previous similar episodes of presenting complaint, autoimmune disease, atopy, previous eye operations (cataract, retinal detachment) or any previous eye problems	2	1	0
	Systemic review of associated symptoms below the head and neck: e.g. skin, nail or hair changes, joint pain, dysuria, fevers, nausea, vomiting, mouth or penile ulcers, recent sexually transmitted infections, recent food poisoning	2	1	0
	Family history especially of eye problems such as glaucoma or atopy affecting the eye (allergic rhinitis, eczema) or any autoimmune disease		1	0
	Obtains a drugs history including any allergies (and nature of allergies)		1	0
	Social history especially of occupation (and whether eye protection is worn if working outdoors or with irritants), smoking, alcohol, pets, recent sexual contacts or transmitted infections	2	1	0
	Communication Skills			
	Explores patient's ideas, concerns and expectations		1	0
	Invites questions (1). Candidate was non-patronising (1).	2	1	0
	Avoids medical jargon		1	0
	Summarises the main points from the consultation (1). Use of signposting (1).	2	1	0
	Checks understanding of what has been explained		1	0
	Simulated patient score (2=very good, 1=satisfactory, 0=poor)	2	1	0
	Examiner to ask: 'What are your differential diagnoses?'			
	Candidate states an appropriate diagnosis (1) and offers a differential (1) (see patient scenarios for possible diagnoses)	2	1	0
	Examiner to ask: 'What investigations/management would you recommend?'			
	Candidate suggests appropriate investigations (1) followed by a sensible line of management (1) (see patient scenarios for possible management options)	2	1	0
	Total Score			

Global Rating	**1** Clear Fail	**2** Borderline	**3** Clear Pass	**4** Very Good	**5** Outstanding

Candidate Number:	University:
Date:	Year of Study:

STATION 52 – VISUAL DISTURBANCE

	Appropriate introduction (1=full name and role), checks patient's name (1)	**2**	**1**	**0**
	Establishes rapport with the patient (1) and starts with an open question (1)	**2**	**1**	**0**
	History of Presenting Complaint			
	Establishes whether the patient wears glasses or contact lenses		**1**	**0**
	Establishes onset, duration and progression of presenting complaint	**2**	**1**	**0**
	Establishes side of the eye affected and whether unilateral or bilateral and if both, whether one side occurred before the other		**1**	**0**
	Establishes nature of the visual disturbance (e.g. blurring, tunnel vision, total loss of sight, halos around the eyes etc.)	**2**	**1**	**0**
	Establishes any triggers or aggravating factors including trauma to the eye(s)		**1**	**0**
	Enquires in detail about any pain within one or both eyes	**2**	**1**	**0**
	Enquires after associated symptoms e.g. redness, grittiness, discharge, reduced tear formation, nasal irritation, sneezing, watery rhinorrhoea (2=three symptoms, 1=two symptoms, 0=one or none)	**2**	**1**	**0**
	Establishes if any difficulty adapting to darkness (indicative of open angle glaucoma)		**1**	**0**
	Excludes symptoms of a stroke or TIA: Enquires about headaches, neurology, weakness, dysphasia, altered consciousness		**1**	**0**
	Excludes symptoms of giant cell arteritis: Enquires about muscle pain, scalp tenderness, jaw claudication		**1**	**0**
	Excludes symptoms of a retinal detachment: Enquires about seeing flashes of light, floaters, straight lines appearing curved		**1**	**0**
	Excludes pituitary lesions: Enquires about excessive growth, weight gain/loss, change in menses/fertility, skin changes, palpitations, gynaecomastia		**1**	**0**
	Other relevant history:			
	Past medical and surgical history including previous similar episodes of presenting complaint, endocrine diseases, risk factors for atherosclerosis, diabetes (last time eyes were checked if diabetic) previous eye operations (cataract, retinal detachment) or any previous eye problems	**2**	**1**	**0**
	Family history especially of eye problems such as glaucoma, diabetes, peripheral vascular disease, stroke, heart disease, cataracts, retinal detachment		**1**	**0**
	Obtains a drugs history including eye drops used (1) and any allergies (1)	**2**	**1**	**0**
	Social history, especially of occupation (and whether eye protection is worn if working outdoors or with irritants), smoking, alcohol	**2**	**1**	**0**
	Communication Skills			
	Explores patient's ideas, concerns and expectations		**1**	**0**
	Invites questions (1). Candidate was non-patronising (1).	**2**	**1**	**0**
	Avoids medical jargon		**1**	**0**
	Summarises the main points from the consultation (1). Use of signposting (1).		**1**	**0**
	Checks understanding of what has been explained		**1**	**0**
	Simulated patient score (2=very good, 1=satisfactory, 0=poor)	**2**	**1**	**0**
	Examiner to ask: 'What is your differential diagnosis?'			
	Candidate states myopia	**2**	**1**	**0**
	Examiner to ask: 'What investigations/management would you recommend?'			
	Candidate offers to check patient's vision with Snellen chart, advises patient to attend local ophthalmologist and advises that glasses may help improve her vision	**2**	**1**	**0**
	Total Score			

Global Rating	**1** Clear Fail	**2** Borderline	**3** Clear Pass	**4** Very Good	**5** Outstanding

CHAPTER 2: PSYCHIATRY

Written by Miss A. Verma

THE STATIONS

STATION 1
Time allowed: 10 minutes

You are a junior doctor working in general practice.

Mrs Ellis is a middle-aged lady who complains of having difficulty sleeping and appears rather withdrawn in her affect.

Please take a focussed history from her and formulate a management plan.

The examiner will stop you at 7 minutes to ask you a few questions.

STATION 2
Time allowed: 10 minutes

You are a junior doctor working in general practice.

Mr Smart has come to see you with his mother, who reports that he is having difficulty sleeping.

Please take a focussed history from him and formulate a management plan.

The examiner will stop you at 7 minutes to ask you a few questions.

STATION 3
Time allowed: 10 minutes

You are a junior doctor working in the Accident and Emergency department.

Miss Jamieson has been brought into the department by her work colleague as she has been causing a nuisance at work and is behaving oddly.

Please take a focussed history from her and formulate a management plan.

The examiner will stop you at 7 minutes to ask you a few questions.

STATION 4
Time allowed: 10 minutes

You are a junior doctor in general practice.

Miss Hutton has been brought to see you by her mother who says she has been behaving oddly at home and she is worried her daughter is taking drugs.

Please take a focussed history from her and formulate a management plan.

The examiner will stop you at 7 minutes to ask you a few questions.

STATION 5
Time allowed: 10 minutes

You are a junior doctor in the Accident and Emergency department.

Miss Edwards is a young lady who been brought into the department after calling the ambulance and reporting she is bleeding from her wrists. She has only very superficial cuts to the ventral aspect of both her wrists and is cardiovascular stable. Her wounds have already been cleaned and dressed – they do not require stitches.

Please take a focussed history from her and formulate a management plan.

The examiner will stop you at 7 minutes to ask you a few questions.

SIMULATED PATIENT BRIEFINGS

STATION 1

Name: Mrs Jane Ellis

Age: 52 years old

Job: Retired administrative assistant

PC:

You have come to the GP to request some sleeping tablets as you report you are having problems sleeping and this is making you very tired. You are quite keen to get the tablets and go home as you did not really want to come to the GP regarding this anyway. You have tried quite a few home remedies (such as taking antihistamines before bedtime, drinking warm milk) but none of these have worked. You do not particularly want to talk to the GP and you are somewhat monosyllabic in your answers. You appear subdued and on further questioning you reveal that this has been going on for six months. You report that you initially could not get to sleep at night but now instead you find that you wake up very early without the need for an alarm clock. Although you say you retired about eight months ago, you reveal on further questioning that you were forced into early retirement as the company you worked for was having financial troubles. You report that you used to socialise with people from work but you no longer do so as you do not feel like it, and you also feel very tired and often have headaches so you do not want to go out.

The headaches are like a tight band across the front of your head with no visual disturbance or aura. They resolve by themselves or sometimes you take a couple of paracetamol. You report that you sometimes cry but you are not sure why and that your husband is getting very fed up with your behaviour and keeps asking what is wrong but you cannot think of a particular thing that is the problem. You report that you have not had sex with your husband for four months as you do not feel like it, but you also feel very guilty and you are now worried that he will leave you as you feel you are both drifting apart. You report that you have lost some weight but you have attributed this to your lowered appetite. You say you have not had any thoughts of self harm or suicide. You have never had anything like this before and have never noticed any seasonal association with low mood. You do not have episodes of feeling elated and restless, and have not experienced any auditory hallucinations. There is no history of depression or other mood disorders in your family.

You do not feel suicidal and this is not something you would ever consider. You just want people to leave you alone and let you get on with your own life. You don't particularly like talking about your personal problems.

Past Medical History and Drug History:

None – NKDA.

Social History:

You do not smoke and only occasionally drink alcohol.

You live with your husband and your children live abroad.

Ideas/Concerns/Expectations:

You are worried about not being able to sleep and keep asking for sleeping tablets as you feel they will solve everything.

Diagnosis:

Moderate to severe depression

Differentials:

Bipolar disorder, seasonal affective disorder

Management:

Explain that the patient is suffering from depression and there is treatment available that can help them.

Start patient on an SSRI e.g. citalopram.

Arrange for the patient to have counselling sessions and suggest that the patient can bring her husband to see you also so that you can explain about depression. Explain that the patient and her husband might like to explore couples counselling sessions in due course.

STATION 2

Patient's name: Mr Jay Smart

Mother's name: Mrs Carol Smart

Age: 19 years old

Job: Mechanic

PC:

You are annoyed that your mother has brought you in today. Your mother says that she is very worried about you as you have not been sleeping well and she often finds you awake at 4am working on your bike. She is worried that this lack of sleep is making you irritable and confused as you often argue with the rest of your family including your younger brother. Your appearance is dishevelled and you keep fidgeting – you tell your mother that she is being stupid and there is nothing wrong with waking up early to get work done – you talk very fast and say that she complains if you lie in and she complains if you wake up early so you cannot win. You ask the GP if there is anything wrong with being productive and say it is not your fault your brother is lazy and that you are clever and fast and are the best mechanic in England and that the Queen wanted you to work on her bike and that as you came here today you noticed Mike the receptionist had a new haircut and you really liked it. You mother is teary and tells the GP that you have been acting like this for the past few days and she does not know if it is because you are not sleeping much.

You are adamant that you would never take drugs and that you have not ever taken any drugs and people who need substances are losers. When asked if you ever hear or see things that might not be real you get offended and tell the GP you are not mad! You and your mother both agree that at the age of 16 you had a prolonged period of 'being down' and you lost interest in your friends and activities and quit school – this lasted a month or so and your mother put it down to growing up and you then slowly went back to your usual self and started training as a mechanic. You report that you have never felt better or had more energy and you want to leave so you can get on with your important work. There is no family history of anything like this.

You have not had any periods of low mood or depression. There is nothing in your life which is particularly causing you any anxiety and you have not had any similar previous episodes before. You do not have any suicidal ideation and you do not have any thoughts of causing harm to any of your friends or family.

Past Medical History:

None.

Drug History:

None – NKDA.

Social History:

You live with your parents but plan to move out as soon as possible as they are annoying you.

You smoke 10 cigarettes a day and have never smoked cannabis or done any other drugs.

You occasionally drink alcohol.

There is no one in the family with a psychiatric history.

Ideas/Concerns/Expectations:

You think this visit is stupid and pointless and say you have many more important things to be getting on with.

Diagnosis:

Bipolar disorder – manic episode

Differentials:

Cyclothymic disorder, schizophrenia, drug-induced

Management:

Explain that this young gentleman is suffering from a mood disorder at present.

Refer the patient to an on-call psychiatrist as he will need admission given that he is having an acute mania episode. If the patient cannot or will not comply then admission under the Mental Health Act may be necessary. During his admission he will likely be treated with antipsychotic drugs and may require sedation with short-acting benzodiazepines.

Arrange for the patient to have blood tests and urine tests. Check routine bloods and also check for illicit drugs.

STATION 3

Patient's name: Miss LaToya Jamieson

Work colleague: Miss Sandra Potter

Age: 26 years old

Job: Fast food restaurant worker

PC:

When asked how you are you say that you are fine. You appear slightly restless and keep pushing your hair behind your ear with your right hand. Your speech is jumbled and you occasionally say things which do not make any sense. When asked to explain yourself you just stare into space as if something else has caught your attention or that you are trying to listen to someone or something.

You say that you are keen to go back to work and that your job is very important to you but last week you had an incident and didn't mean to drop a big plate of chips at work. You say the customer frightened you and you got startled which is why you accidently dropped the chips but your work colleague says that you threw the chips at the customer and shouted 'Stop it!' Your colleague also said that the man was not doing anything out of the ordinary and that you then started saying odd things like 'the lalputs are very annoying' and 'my flat is unguarded'. You appeared more and more restless and agitated.

When asked if you hear voices you say you are not hearing anything that is not there and you know where they are. You say you are sick of them and that they continually talk and you get no peace. They speak as if you are in the third person and make derogatory comments like 'She thinks she is too good for us' and they constantly talk about what you are doing saying things like 'She's changing for work' and 'She's closing the windows'. You say you know that these lalputs want to get your flat and so you have had to be very careful about locking up. Your colleague says you have missed quite a lot of work in the past few weeks and have told colleagues at work that people were trying to evict you.

You explain that as you walk to work you have to constantly change direction depending on the signal sent to your transmitter so sometimes you actually never make it to work as by the time you have walked all the way in the streets then it is time to lock up. You start smiling secretively to yourself and then giggle. When asked why you are smiling you tell your colleague that you know what the doctor is writing down and it is quite funny despite the price of that cake you bought yesterday.

Past Medical History and Drug History:

None and no allergies.

Social History:

You just broke up with your boyfriend and you don't care as he was in on it anyway.

You smoke cannabis now and again, smoke about 15 cigarettes a day and drink alcohol occasionally.

You live alone in a council flat and do not have many friends – your family are in Nigeria and you have not seen them since you arrived here at the age of 18 to live with your aunt and to work. You only lived with your aunt for a short time before running away from home and getting your own place.

Family History:

None significant.

Ideas/Concerns/Expectations:

You are sick of the lalputs and want them to stop controlling you.

Diagnosis:

Schizophrenia

Differentials:

Mania, drug-induced

Management:

Explain that this lady is having delusions at present.

Arrange for the patient to have blood and urine tests. Check routine bloods and check for illicit drugs.

Refer the patient to an on-call psychiatrist as she will require treatment either as an inpatient or day patient. She will likely require antipsychotic drug treatment.

The patient, their family and work colleagues will need to be educated about schizophrenia.

Introduction of the Care Programme Approach is required with a care plan and key worker.

STATION 4

Name: Miss Chloe Hutton

Mother's name: Mrs Lilly Hutton

Age: 17 years old

Job: At school

PC:

You think it is ridiculous that your mother brought you to the GP today but you agreed to come as you know that you are not taking drugs and you do not care if she makes you have a test to prove it. Your mother tells the GP you have been behaving strangely at home and wants you tested for drugs. She says that you spend excessive amounts of time in your room and you hardly interact with your family anymore. You used to be very close to your younger siblings and parents but your mum says you are now very irritable and moody at home and spend all your time alone in your room. You refuse to eat meals at the table with your family anymore and instead eat them in your room.

Your mum says you have lost quite a lot of weight and your ribs are now easily visible even when you are wearing clothes! Your mother also says that you seem to have lost your appetite and are always saying you are feeling full. You say that you are training for the end of year athletic competition and that is why you are preoccupied and you are adamant that you are not taking drugs. You say you have been exercising a lot and that is why you go to your room – so you can do sits ups and exercise in peace. You are annoyed with your mother and say that all you are trying to do is get fit and that she instead thinks you are taking drugs! You ask for a test to prove you are not taking drugs. Your mother says that you pretend to go out running but are gone for hours at a time (often three or four hours) so she thinks you are lying about going running and thinks you are going out and taking drugs. You are getting more and more angry and say that you only go running and tell your mother that if she followed you she would realise.

You are otherwise a high achiever in school and get straight A grades. You are the captain of the athletic team and you are also involved with drama and are usually cast as the lead actress in school productions. Your mother says you are usually very sociable and have lots of friends but she says recently you have been asking her to tell friends you are busy when they call to speak to you. If asked, you admit that you have altered you diet and only want to eat healthily and you say that your mother tries to make you eat more than necessary, so you prefer to eat in your room. You also think you are gaining too much weight which is why you are exercising so much as you want to be fit and ready for the athletic competition. You deny ever vomiting up any food or taking laxatives. You are wearing a warm coat with lots of layers even though it is summer. Your mother says you seem to always be cold.

Past Medical History and Drug History:

None and NKDA.

Social History:

You live at home with your parents and two younger siblings.

You do not drink or smoke. You also say you are not taking any drugs.

Ideas/Concerns/Expectations:

You are sick and tired of your mother constantly hassling you about whether you are doing drugs.

Diagnosis:

Anorexia nervosa

Differentials:

Bulimia

Management:

Discuss with patient and mother regarding anorexia nervosa.

Full examination and tests including FBC, iron studies, cortisol, TFTs, FSH/LH and an ECG.

Referral for individual and family psychotherapy.

If patient is significantly depressed antidepressant medications may be indicated. If the patient is very anxious then low dose antipsychotics may be used.

Mood state and suicidality should be regularly monitored.

STATION 5

Name: Miss Jennifer Edwards

Age: 23 years old

Job: Works in a supermarket

PC:

You report that you cut both your wrists. You report that a small amount of blood was visible when you did this and you then panicked and called the ambulance as you had a sudden realisation of what you had done. You have been feeling very down lately and you consumed two bottles of wine this evening before you cut your wrists. You started thinking about slitting your wrists over the last week but decided to go for it this evening when you got home from work. In order to muster up the courage you spent the evening drinking before you finally did it. You have never done anything like this before and your intent at the time was to kill yourself but you immediately changed your mind when you saw the blood. You no longer want to kill yourself but still feel very down and depressed about your life but deny having sought any medical help about this.

You have never been diagnosed as having any psychiatric disorders and live alone. You hardly ever see your family as they live far away – your mother and her partner live in Birmingham and your sister lives in Cornwall.

You had not planned to harm yourself prior to this week and had not written a suicide note. Your mood has been low for about three months since you broke up with your boyfriend who you used to live with. You had found out he had been cheating on you so you threw him out of your flat and now live alone. You say you feel lonely and have not been sleeping well, usually waking up very early in the morning and are unable to get back to bed. You haven't told any of your friends because you think having their sympathy will only make you feel sorrier for yourself and you really want to try to get over this alone.

Past Medical History and Drug History:

None and NKDA.

Social History:

You smoke 10 cigarettes a day and drink a glass or two of wine most evenings. You do not take drugs.

Ideas/Concerns/Expectations:

You are tearful and feel down. You realise that there is a problem and that trying to cut your wrists was a silly idea but don't know how to get over the end of your last relationship and the loneliness you feel. You would be open to the suggestion of counselling or starting antidepressants.

Diagnosis:

Deliberate self harm with low risk of suicide, but with features suggestive of depression.

Management:

Organise a psychological assessment in hospital. If the patient is deemed fit for discharge then psychosocial support and access to community psychiatric services need to be in place.

They will require treatment for depression and this can be managed by the GP given that the suicide risk is low.

PSYCHIATRY

Candidate Number:	University:
Date:	Year of Study:

STATIONS 1 & 2 – DIFFICULTY SLEEPING

		2	1	0
	Appropriate introduction (1=full name and role), checks patient's name (1)	2	1	0
	Explains purpose of interview and checks consent (2=does well, 1=adequately, 0=poorly or not done)	2	1	0
	Starts with an open question and listens without interrupting (1=both)		1	0
	Presenting Complaint:			
	Establishes the onset (1) of the difficulty sleeping and the duration (1)	2	1	0
	Enquires whether there were any precipitating factors which the patient can identify (e.g. loud noises, anxiety, stress at work, caffeine before bedtime etc.)	2	1	0
	Enquires whether the patient has trouble falling asleep and staying asleep (1) or whether they wake up early (1)	2	1	0
	Enquires about their mood and assesses their affect	2	1	0
	Candidate explores whether anything is worrying or upsetting the patient	2	1	0
	Enquires after previous similar episodes		1	0
	Explores patient's ideas and concerns regarding the presenting complaint		1	0
	Other relevant history:			
	Systemic features: anhedonia, weight change, appetite, energy levels, libido (2=all three or more, 1=two items, 0=one only or none)	2	1	0
	Enquires about self harm, suicidal ideation or whether there are thoughts of harming other people	2	1	0
	Relevant past medical and surgical history		1	0
	Medication history (1) including allergies (1)	2	1	0
	Relevant family history		1	0
	Smoking, alcohol and illicit drug abuse (2=all three, 1=any two)	2	1	0
	Relevant social history (e.g. housing circumstances, dependents, occupation etc.)		1	0
	Appropriate closure (e.g. explains next step, thanks patient and summarises) (2=does well, 1=adequately, 0=poorly or not done)	2	1	0
	Communication Skills			
	Appropriate questioning style (mix of open and closed questions) (2=does well, 1=adequately, 0=poorly or not done)	2	1	0
	Organised approach to history-taking (e.g. systematic, summarises, signposts change in focus of question)	2	1	0
	Simulated patient score (2=very good, 1=satisfactory, 0=poor)	2	1	0
	Examiner to ask: 'What are your differential diagnoses?'			
	Candidate states an appropriate diagnosis (1) and offers a differential (1) (see patient scenarios for possible diagnoses)	2	1	0
	Examiner to ask: 'What investigations/management would you recommend?'			
	Candidate suggests appropriate investigations (1) followed by a sensible line of management (1) (see patient scenarios for possible management options)	2	1	0
	Total Score			

Global Rating	1 Clear Fail	2 Borderline	3 Clear Pass	4 Very Good	5 Outstanding

Candidate Number:	University:
Date:	Year of Study:

STATIONS 3 & 4 – BEHAVING ODDLY

	Appropriate introduction (1=full name and role), checks patient's name (1)	**2**	**1**	**0**
	Explains purpose of interview and checks consent (2=does well, 1=adequately, 0=poorly or not done)	**2**	**1**	**0**
	Starts with an open question and listens without interrupting (1=both)		**1**	**0**
	Presenting Complaint:			
	Establishes the onset (1) of the behaviour and the duration (1)	**2**	**1**	**0**
	Enquires whether there were any precipitating factors which the patient can identify	**2**	**1**	**0**
	Enquires whether the patient perceives their behaviour as unusual	**2**	**1**	**0**
	Enquires about their mood and assesses their affect	**2**	**1**	**0**
	Candidate explores whether anything is worrying or upsetting the patient	**2**	**1**	**0**
	Enquires whether the patient is having any auditory or visual hallucinations		**1**	**0**
	Enquires after previous similar episodes		**1**	**0**
	Explores the hallucinations in greater detail (e.g. what they are saying, how many voices are there, whether they are coming from within or outside the head etc.)	**2**	**1**	**0**
	Enquires about thought broadcast, withdrawal or insertion	**2**	**1**	**0**
	Explores patient's ideas and concerns regarding the presenting complaint		**1**	**0**
	Other relevant history:			
	Systemic features: appetite, weight change, anhedonia (2=all three, 1=two items, 0=one only or none)	**2**	**1**	**0**
	Enquires about self harm, suicidal ideation or whether there are thoughts of harming other people	**2**	**1**	**0**
	Relevant past medical and surgical history		**1**	**0**
	Medication history (1) including allergies (1)	**2**	**1**	**0**
	Relevant family history		**1**	**0**
	Smoking, alcohol and drug use (2=all three, 1=any two)	**2**	**1**	**0**
	Relevant social history e.g. housing circumstances, dependents, occupation etc.		**1**	**0**
	Appropriate closure (e.g. explains next step, thanks patient and summarises) (2=does well, 1=adequately, 0=poorly or not done)	**2**	**1**	**0**
	Communication Skills			
	Appropriate questioning style (mix of open and closed questions) (2=does well, 1=adequately, 0=poorly or not done)	**2**	**1**	**0**
	Organised approach to history-taking (e.g. systematic, summarises, signposts change in focus of question)	**2**	**1**	**0**
	Simulated patient score (2=very good, 1=satisfactory, 0=poor)	**2**	**1**	**0**
	Examiner to ask: 'What are your differential diagnoses?'			
	Candidate states an appropriate diagnosis (1) and offers a differential (1) (see patient scenarios for possible diagnoses)	**2**	**1**	**0**
	Examiner to ask: 'What investigations/management would you recommend?'			
	Candidate suggests appropriate investigations (1) followed by a sensible line of management (1) (see patient scenarios for possible management options)	**2**	**1**	**0**
	Total Score			

Global Rating	**1** Clear Fail	**2** Borderline	**3** Clear Pass	**4** Very Good	**5** Outstanding

Candidate Number:	University:
Date:	Year of Study:

STATION 5 – DELIBERATE SELF HARM

	Appropriate introduction (1=full name and role), checks patient's name (1)	2	1	0
	Explains purpose of interview and checks consent (2=does well, 1=adequately, 0=poorly or not done)	2	1	0
	Starts with an open question and listens without interrupting (1=both)		1	0
	Presenting Complaint:			
	Establishes the nature of the deliberate self harm	2	1	0
	Establishes whether the patient intended to kill herself	2	1	0
	Enquires about previous similar episodes	2	1	0
	Enquires whether the patient planned this in advance	2	1	0
	Establishes whether the patient was found by chance or sought help for herself			
	Asks whether the patient still wants to kill herself	2	1	0
	Asks whether the patient left a suicide note (1) or arranged so that they would not be found (1)	2	1	0
	Explores patient's ideas and concerns regarding the presenting complaint		1	0
	Other relevant history:			
	Establishes whether the patient has features suggestive of depression (e.g. anhedonia, weight loss, reduced appetite)		1	0
	Relevant past medical and surgical history		1	0
	Medication history (1) including allergies (1)	2	1	0
	Relevant family history		1	0
	Smoking, alcohol and illicit drug use (2=all three, 1=any two)	2	1	0
	Relevant social history (e.g. housing circumstances, dependents, occupation etc.)		1	0
	Appropriate closure (e.g. explains next step, thanks patient and summarises) (2=does well, 1=adequately, 0=poorly or not done)	2	1	0
	Communication Skills			
	Appropriate questioning style (mix of open and closed questions) (2=does well, 1=adequately, 0=poorly or not done)	2	1	0
	Invites questions (1). Listens actively (1).	2	1	0
	Organised approach to history-taking (e.g. systematic, summarises, signposts change in focus of question)	2	1	0
	Simulated patient score (2=very good, 1=satisfactory, 0=poor)	2	1	0
	Examiner to ask: 'What is your diagnosis?'			
	Candidate states an appropriate diagnosis		1	0
	Examiner to ask: 'What investigations/management would you recommend?'			
	Candidate suggests appropriate investigations (1) followed by a sensible line of management (1) (see patient scenarios for possible management options)	2	1	0
	Examiner to ask: 'How would you rate this patient's suicide risk?'			
	Candidate suggests patient is low risk of re-attempting suicide		1	0
	Total Score			

Global Rating	1 Clear Fail	2 Borderline	3 Clear Pass	4 Very Good	5 Outstanding

CHAPTER 3: PAEDIATRICS

Written by Dr. S. Shelmerdine & Mr. J. Lynch

THE STATIONS

STATION 1
Time allowed: 10 minutes

You are a junior doctor working in general practice.

Mrs Carter has brought her son, Max, who is 1 year old, to see the doctor today because she is worried that he doesn't seem to be putting on as much weight or growing as he should.

Please take a history from the parent and formulate a differential diagnosis.

STATION 2
Time allowed: 10 minutes

You are a junior doctor working in general practice.

Mr Clarke has come to the clinic to see you today because he is concerned that his son, James, aged 2 years old, is rather 'slow' at picking up new skills and wonders whether he may have a developmental problem.

Please take a history from the parent and formulate a differential diagnosis.

STATION 3
Time allowed: 10 minutes

You are a junior doctor working in the Accident and Emergency department.

Mrs Simpson attends your department today with Luka, her 2 year old son, who has been complaining of severe abdominal pains.

Please take a history from the parent and formulate a differential diagnosis.

STATION 4
Time allowed: 10 minutes

You are a junior doctor working in the Accident and Emergency Department.

Mrs Arooba attends your department today and is extremely anxious. She has noticed that her baby is starting to appear to look yellow and is very upset.

Please take a history from the parent and formulate a differential diagnosis.

STATION 5
Time allowed: 10 minutes

You are a junior doctor working in the Accident and Emergency department.

Mr Kooks has brought his 9 month old daughter into your department today after an episode this afternoon where he witnessed her shaking uncontrollably. He is very anxious and wants to speak to a doctor immediately.

Please take a history from the parent and formulate a differential diagnosis.

STATION 6
Time allowed: 10 minutes

You are a junior doctor working in general practice.

Mrs Jackson has come to clinic today to see you regarding a rather nasty rash that her daughter has developed all over her body.

Please take a history from the parent and formulate a differential diagnosis.

STATION 7
Time allowed: 10 minutes

You are a junior doctor working in the Accident and Emergency department.

Mrs Columbo is concerned about her son, Mikey, who appears to have developed a horrible cough in the last three days.

Please take a history from the parent and formulate a differential diagnosis.

SIMULATED PATIENT BRIEFINGS

STATION 1

Parent's name: Mrs Mary Carter

Child's name: Max Carter

Child's age: 1 year old

PC:

Not putting on weight appropriate to age.

Your son is happy and well-behaved, however, you have had concerns for a while that he is not putting on as much weight as he should be. You keep telling the nurses at all the baby checks that his is not following the lines on the charts he should but they don't seem to be listening. Your child seems to be happy enough, and apart from a recent cold he has been in perfect health since he was born. You have been breast feeding up until 6 months ago and he is eating solid foods now. He is eating these without any obvious swallowing problems but then looks full and refuses more food after only having had a small portion. He has not had any change in bowel habits and does not appear to have any developmental delay to your knowledge.

His current weight is 19 pounds, and height is 27 inches.

Early Life and Developmental History:

Your son was born vaginally at term although he was small on arrival (6 pounds), which was similar to your other son. You have been attending the development checks and he has been consistently in the low centiles for height, weight and head circumference. He has reached his normal developmental and social milestones.

Immunisation History:

Up to date apart from the MMR vaccination, which you have omitted due to your concerns of links to autism.

Past Medical/Surgical History:

Never had and medical or surgical history but did have a healthy neonatal period.

Drug History:

On no medications. NKDA.

Family and Social History:

One brother aged 10, fit and well.

His father left the family soon after Max's birth, and you now live with your boyfriend, an actor called Charlie. You are both non-smokers and non-drinkers.

All members of your family have been small, which you will admit if questioned directly.

You are working part-time in a holistic therapy shop.

Ideas/Concerns/Expectations:

You are concerned that Max might be suffering from a disease which prevents him absorbing food correctly.

Diagnosis:

Constitutionally small child

Differentials:

There is a very wide differential for failure to thrive:

Psycho-social/environmental deprivation

Inadequate feeding

Malabsorptive diseases such as coeliac, cystic fibrosis

Protein-losing enteropathy: cow's milk protein intolerance

Chronic unrecognised illness

Management:

Reassurance and regular follow up for this specific patient. Other management would be situation specific and may include general blood tests or cutting out certain foods in the diet and follow-up to check for any improvement in symptoms.

STATION 2

Parent's name: Mr John Clarke

Child's name: James Clarke

Child's age: 1 year old

PC:

Appears to be slow to learn skills.

Your son appears healthy and happy, but you have concerns that he is not behaving in the same way as your other son. This was picked up by the community nurses, who have referred you to the GP. James is now 1 year old but has not even started standing up and balancing his own weight, let alone walking with assistance. He appears to prefer to crawl everywhere. Your other child was always very quick to develop these skills and you cannot fathom what you are doing differently.

His current weight is 22 pounds, and his height is 29 inches.

Early Life and Developmental History:

Although all the antenatal checks were fine, your child was 8 weeks premature when he was born and had to be put on a ventilator for the first week, although you do not know exactly why this was. He has always been small, although is staying within the same centile.

Gross motor – Sits unsupported but is not weight bearing and just crawling.

Fine motor and vision – Can grasp toys but is not transferring objects and has little interest in small objects. Does not follow objects reliably.

Hearing and speech – Uses incoherent words.

Social – Not responding to his own name. Does not play peek-a-boo. Does not clap hands and cannot hold a cup.

Immunisation History:

Full.

Past Medical/Surgical History:

Jaundiced at birth but this resolved in the first week. Weak and pale for first few months. Has frequent colds.

Drug History:

On no medications. NKDA.

Family and Social History:

Lives with two parents. No family history of illnesses. You are obviously a caring family. You are both non-smokers and social drinkers.

One brother aged 5 who is fit and well.

Ideas/Concerns/Expectations:

Concerned that child might have learning difficulties or a syndrome such as Down's.

Diagnosis:

Non-specific developmental delay

Differentials:

Hypertonia: cerebral palsy

Muscular dystrophy

Undiagnosed syndrome

Delayed motor maturation (often familial): diagnosis of exclusion

Management:

This patient requires referral to a paediatrician for evaluation and diagnosis. Depending on diagnosis the child may require the input of a physiotherapist.

STATION 3

Parent's name: Mrs July Simpson

Child's name: Luka Simpson

Child's age: 2 years old

PC:

Severe abdominal pain.

Your child has been happy and playful up until this morning when he suddenly started complaining of abdominal pain, which has worsened such that you have become very worried about him. The pain seems to get better and worse in waves, and he started vomiting a couple of hours after it started. On feeling his tummy you think there is a lump at the lower aspect.

Earlier he was very irritable but now he just appears pale and lethargic. You noticed a small amount of blood mixed in with the stool earlier. There are no apparent aggravating or relieving factors and the child has not eaten all day. You have not been in contact with other children who have infectious bugs recently.

His current weight is 28 pounds, and his height is 31 inches.

Early Life and Developmental History:

Spontaneous vaginal delivery at term weighing 8 pounds. No medical problems as baby. All his developmental milestones have been satisfactory.

Immunisation History:

Up-to-date.

Past Medical/Surgical History:

Had a cold one month previously, which he got over.

Fit and well prior to this.

Drug History:

On no medications. Allergic to penicillin (anaphylaxis).

Family and Social History:

One brother aged 12 who had appendicitis at age 11.

Luka lives at home with his brother and both parents. His father suffers from multiple sclerosis and is a retired banker.

You work as a teacher.

Ideas/Concerns/Expectations:

You are very worried and anxious about your son and want something done immediately.

Diagnosis:

Intussusception

Differentials:

Appendicitis

Gastroenteritis

Strangulated inguinal hernia

Pyloric stenosis

Management:

Admit child and begin immediate resuscitation: IV fluid and NG tube.

Blood tests including FBC (to check for neutrophilia), U&Es (to determine presence of dehydration).

Abdominal imaging: AXR (distended bowel, fluid levels). Ultrasound (doughnut or target sign is seen). Refer to paediatric surgeons for possible radiographic reduction or surgery.

STATION 4

Parent's name: Mrs Joanne Arooba

Child's name: Oliver

Child's age: 2 weeks old

PC:

You are in hospital today because you think your son is going yellow! The yellow skin started to develop when Oliver was 5 days old and was initially very subtle but now you think it is becoming more noticeable and has not subsided. He has not appeared irritated, febrile or unwell to you other than the change in his skin colour. You have not noticed any vomiting, rashes or odd smell to his nappies. He appears to be growing normally and is putting on weight as expected. You have been breast-feeding Oliver since he was born without giving any formula feeds. His appetite is very good and he feeds well requiring nursing approximately every three hours. You generally feed him seven to eight times a day.

You have not noticed any abdominal distension, change in bowel habits or colour of stools/urine. Oliver does not appear to be in any sort of pain or discomfort.

Early Life History:

Oliver was born at term and of normal weight. The delivery was a spontaneous vaginal delivery. No pregnancy-related complications were noted. No neonatal illnesses have been noted so far until now.

Immunisation History:

None so far.

Past Medical/Surgical History:

None so far.

Drug History:

None so far. No allergies that you are aware of.

Social History:

This is your second child. You have another son aged 6 years old called Jamie who is currently being looked after by your parents. He was a healthy baby and you did not experience this problem with him.

You work as a solicitor in the city and your husband is a saxophone player and song writer. He works from home most of the time and looks after your children.

No one in the home smokes.

Family History:

None significant.

Ideas/Concerns/Expectations:

You are very worried that your son will need to be admitted to paediatric ICU. You have heard stories that yellow babies don't do well and can suffer from permanent brain damage. You are very worried that this is what is going to happen to little Oliver.

Diagnosis:

Breast milk jaundice

Differentials:

Hypothyroidism

Septicaemia

Haemolysis (G6PD deficiency, spherocytosis)

Management:

This is the commonest form of prolonged jaundice in term infants. It is a benign process with no real identifiable cause and is relatively common. Up to 10% of breast-fed infants can remain jaundiced up to one month of age. It should be differentiated from 'breast-feeding jaundice' which is secondary to insufficient intake of breast milk or food. Treatment for breast milk jaundice depends on the child's bilirubin level but may include increasing the number of feeds per day, interrupting feeds with formula solution or even phototherapy treatment. Full recovery is expected.

STATION 5

Parent's name: Mr. Ashlee Kooks

Child's name: Greta

Child's age: 9 months old

PC:

You have brought Greta into the A&E department today after having witnessed her suffering from a seizure. You were in the living room watching television about an hour ago with Greta in her crib when suddenly you noticed she was rather quiet. You walked over to the crib and witnessed her body, legs and arms go completely stiff before she threw her head backwards and began rhythmically jerking her arms and legs. The whole episode lasted for two minutes and you noticed her skin turned rather pale in the process. During the episode you were shouting at her but she did not seem to respond. After the episode, Greta went limp and looked very tired before falling asleep. This is the first episode you have ever witnessed like this.

In the past two days you have noticed that Greta has been a little less active than usual and has been sleeping for longer times throughout the day. Although you have not taken her temperature you noticed that when you held her she has felt warmer than usual. You have not noticed any symptoms of coughing, vomiting, change in bowel habits or funny smell to her nappies. No one in your household is currently unwell. You have not been on any foreign travel lately.

Developmental History:

She is able to sit without support, babble, smile and react to loud noises. She cannot stand or walk yet but has started crawling. You do not have any concerns regarding her development.

Early Life History:

Greta was born at term and of normal weight. The delivery was a spontaneous vaginal delivery. No pregnancy-related complications were noted. No neonatal illnesses were identified and Greta has never been admitted to the paediatric ICU department.

Immunisation History:

Up-to-date with all immunisations.

Past Medical/Surgical History:

None significant.

Drug History:

You have tried to feed her some soluble paracetamol yesterday when you noticed she felt rather warm but she is not on anything regular. To your knowledge Greta does not have any drug allergies.

Social History:

Greta is your first and only child. You live with Greta and your wife in a small cottage in the suburbs of London with one pet cat. You normally work as a travel agent and your wife does not work. Neither of you smoke.

Family History:

You were told by your wife that she suffered from seizures whenever she was ill as a child although she is currently not epileptic.

Ideas/Concerns/Expectations:

You worry that this episode is due to epilepsy and are really worried that Greta will suffer with this condition for the rest of her life. Your wife is currently at home and has suffered from postnatal depression since the birth and you know that if Greta was to become seriously ill your wife might not be able to take the news very well.

Diagnosis:

Febrile convulsions

Differential:

Childhood epilepsy (difficult to differentiate from just one episode)

Management:

Febrile convulsions famously occur in some children between the ages of 6 months to 6 years although the majority occur between 1 and 4 years of age. Fifty percent of children who suffer with their first febrile convulsion will have another seizure the next time they suffer with a fever but the chances do lessen with age. During an episode parents should be advised to not restrain their child, to support their child's head and turn it to one side to both prevent injury and choking. After the convulsion, parents should place their child in the recovery position. It may be advisable to give the child paracetamol or ibuprofen to lower their temperature if they are found to be suffering from a fever and occasionally GPs may offer parents Diazepam to shorten the episodes if they are found to be repetitive. It is thought that there is a genetic predisposition to febrile convulsions but only 1% of children with febrile convulsions do develop epilepsy.

STATION 6

Parent's name: Mrs. Alice Jackson

Child's name: Katrina Jackson

Child's age: 5 years old

PC:

Over the last day or so you have noticed that your daughter Katrina has been suffering with a widespread rash all over her body which looks like lots of tiny little reddish brown raised spots that are irregular in size and shape. They are itchy and predominantly over her face and trunk, but also a few are on her arms and legs. Prior to this rash (for the last two days), Katrina did suffer from a cough and flu-like symptoms and complained that her eyes felt itchy and red.

At present she is feeling rather run down and tired all the time. Her temperature has been very high last night and today (40°C) which prompted you to seek medical advice. She is not hungry and is off her food but she has not lost any significant amount of weight. She has not had any change in bowel habits or seizures. She has missed the last three days of school and you haven't taken her to see any doctors yet thinking that this was just a cold that she would get over it herself. You have given her paracetamol and ibuprofen yesterday and today to try to lower her temperature but it is still quite high.

You have not had any recent travel abroad or alteration in the food you feed Katrina. No one in the household is ill but you are uncertain whether there is something 'going round' at her school.

Developmental History:

Katrina is usually a lively little girl who is very active and playful. She is popular at school and has many friends. She enjoys painting and drawing. She has a good vocabulary, can dance, sing and loves talking and interacting with others. Her teachers do not have concerns regarding her development.

Early Life History:

Katrina was one week post dates but normal weight at delivery. The delivery was by caesarean section because she was lying in a breech orientation. No pregnancy-related complications were noted. No neonatal illnesses were identified. Katrina was taken home after one night in the hospital after the delivery.

Immunisation History:

All immunisations apart from the MMR vaccine as you were not convinced that this vaccination was safe to give to your child (although your older son was vaccinated with the MMR jab before there were concerns regarding its safety).

Past Medical/Surgical History:

None of note.

Drug History:

None regular and no drug allergies that you are aware of.

Social History:

Katrina is your second child. You have one older son, Miles, aged 8 years old. Katrina and Miles get on well together and attend the same primary school.

You are no longer married to their father and divorced two years ago. The children are coping well with the change.

You all live with your mother in the family home by the seaside.

You have two dogs at home and one pet hamster.

No one in the home smokes.

Family History:

None significant.

Ideas/Concerns/Expectations:

You are very worried that Katrina has contracted measles from school. You feel extremely guilty about missing out the MMR vaccine because you didn't want Katrina to develop autism, but feel that you may have been misguided by what you read in the newspapers about the vaccine. If the doctor tells you that measles is a possibility then you start crying and blaming yourself for your daughter's illness.

Diagnosis:

Measles

Differentials:

Chicken pox, rubella, scarlet fever

Management:

There is no treatment for measles and management is largely supportive. Paracetamol or ibuprofen is advised to reduce fevers and for pain relief. Parents should be advised to bring their child to see their GP if they do not appear to be recovering well. Complications from measles may include bronchitis, pneumonia and in severe cases panencephalitis with a mortality rate of up to 15% if this develops.

STATION 7

Parent's name: Mrs. Pauline Columbo

Child's name: Mikey Columbo

Child's age: 4 years old

PC:

You are worried about your youngest son, Mikey, who has been suffering from a bad cough and wheezing over the last 2–3 days. He seems to have contracted a cold from one of his friends at school about four days ago but is now suffering from a dry cough (no sputum) and a wheeze whenever he exerts himself. Last night, for example, he was wheezing all evening after having a 'pillow fight' with his sister and appeared very breathless. When you spoke to him he was also complaining of some chest tightness. This subsequently disappeared when he caught his breath again. He denied any chest pain. He has not taken any days off school for this problem.

He has had a few similar episodes in the past which always seem to occur in conjunction with colds/flu and normally in the winter months. In between episodes he appears well in himself and does not have any significant wheezing or cough.

Developmental History:

He is currently at nursery. The teachers at his school do not have any concerns regarding his progress in class and say he is interacting well with all the other students.

Early Life History:

Mikey was born at term and of normal weight. The delivery was a spontaneous vaginal delivery. No pregnancy-related complications were noted. No neonatal illnesses were identified.

Immunisation History:

All up-to-date.

Past Medical/Surgical History:

Mikey occasionally suffers from dry patches of skin over his elbows and on the backs of his knees. They are usually itchy but do not get inflamed or infected. You believe that these are bouts of eczema and your two other children have the same condition.

Drug History:

No known allergies.

You use an emollient called 'Diprobase' whenever Mikey or his siblings have dry skin and it seems to relieve their eczema.

Social History:

You and your husband have three children, Laura (8 years old), Kris (6 years old) and Mikey (who is the youngest). The children all get on well and play together. Laura and Kris also suffer from eczema but do not have any respiratory symptoms.

No one in the family is currently ill or coughing.

Mikey enjoys school and is a very active and lively boy.

No one in the family smokes.

You all live in a large five bedroom house with a large garden.

Both your husband and yourself run a small internet business from home selling computers and can supervise the children easily.

There are no pets in the house.

Family History:

Your husband suffers from very mild asthma and hay fever during the summer months.

All your three children suffer with eczema.

Ideas/Concerns/Expectations:

You worry that Mikey is having a bad chest infection and that he may pass this on to his siblings. You don't want to have all three of your children ill with the flu at home!

Diagnosis:

Asthma (episodic viral associated)

Differentials:

Lower respiratory tract infection, viral illness, allergic rhinitis

Management:

Childhood asthma is a very common condition and it is worth reading up on this topic in detail. There are many variations to the presentation, however, in general children present with wheeziness, cough, chest tightness and breathlessness. Many children have a family history of atopy and in some cases a trigger may be found. Treatment of childhood asthma should follow the stepwise approach as stated in the BTS (British Thoracic Society) guidelines. In general the principles of asthma treatment are to control the symptoms, prevent exacerbations and maintain the best achievable pulmonary function whilst minimising the side effects of any medication.

PAEDIATRICS

Candidate Number:		University:	
Date:		Year of Study:	

STATION 1 – FAILURE TO THRIVE

		2	1	0
	Appropriate introduction (1=full name and role), checks patient's name (1)	2	1	0
	Establishes rapport with the parent (1) and starts with an open question (1)	2	1	0
	Presenting Complaint			
	Establishes onset, duration and progression of the presenting complaint: small for age (2=detailed history of presenting complaint, 1=adequate history)	2	1	0
	Associated symptoms asks about: vomiting, irritability, poor feeding, frequency of dirty nappies, nature of stool (2=three symptoms, 1=two symptoms, 0=one or none)	2	1	0
	Diet and appetite		1	0
	Risk factors during pregnancy: smoking, alcohol consumption, illness, use of medications (1 mark=2 aspects, 0=one or no aspects asked)		1	0
	Past medical (1) or surgical history or any previous hospitalizations (1)	2	1	0
	Medication history (1) including allergies and nature of allergies (1)	2	1	0
	Family history		1	0
	Social history – siblings, parents' jobs, special dietary requirements, living accommodation, second-hand smoke exposure (2=does well, 1=adequately, 0=poorly)	2	1	0
	Early Life and Developmental History			
	Pregnancy – preterm, spontaneous vaginal delivery, any illnesses during pregnancy (2=any two options, 1=one option)	2	1	0
	Birth – weight at birth, condition at birth, any delivery related complications (2=all three aspects or other equivalent sensible questions relating to birth, 1=any two aspects)	2	1	0
	Illnesses during the neonatal period		1	0
	Current height and weight (and checks whether this is normal for their age)		1	0
	Gross motor function		1	0
	Fine motor function		1	0
	Social function		1	0
	Vision and hearing		1	0
	Immunisation schedule		1	0
	Systems Enquiry			
	Cardiovascular – sweating, cyanosis, pallor, SOB **Respiratory –** cough, wheeze, snoring **Gastrointestinal –** appetite, diet, vomiting, pain, abdominal distention **Neurology –** headaches, fits, weakness **Musculoskeletal –** limp, limb pain, joint swelling, pain (2=explores thoroughly all systems, 1=explores adequately at least 2 systems, 0=poorly or not done)	2	1	0
	Explores parent's ideas, concerns and expectations (2=does well, 1=adequately, 0=not done)	2	1	0
	Invites questions (1). Candidate was non-patronising (1).	2	1	0
	Avoids medical jargon		1	0
	Summarises the main points from the consultation (1). Signposting (1).	2	1	0
	Checks understanding of what has been explained		1	0
	Simulated patient score (2=very good, 1=satisfactory, 0=poor)	2	1	0
	Examiner to ask: 'What is your differential diagnosis?'			
	Candidate suggests a sensible diagnosis (1) and differential (1)	2	1	0
	Total Score			

Global Rating	**1** Clear Fail	**2** Borderline	**3** Clear Pass	**4** Very Good	**5** Outstanding

Candidate Number:	University:
Date:	Year of Study:

STATION 2 – DEVELOPMENTAL DELAY

		2	1	0
	Appropriate introduction (1=full name and role), checks patient's name (1)	2	1	0
	Establishes rapport with the parent (1) and starts with an open question (1)	2	1	0
	Presenting Complaint			
	Establishes the nature of the presenting complaint: slow to pick up skills (1) especially gross motor (1)	2	1	0
	Otherwise fit and well		1	0
	Associated symptoms e.g. irritability, fever, poor feeding, poor sleeping, change in bowel habits, rash (2=three symptoms, 1=two symptoms, 0=one or none)	2	1	0
	Risk factors during pregnancy: smoking, alcohol consumption, illness, use of medications (1 mark=2 aspects, 0=one or no aspects asked)		1	0
	Past medical (1) or surgical history or any previous hospitalizations (1)	2	1	0
	Medication history (1) including allergies and nature of allergies (1)	2	1	0
	Family history		1	0
	Social history – siblings, parents' jobs, special dietary requirements, personality, living accommodation, second-hand smoke exposure (2=does well, 1=adequately, 0=poorly)	2	1	0
	Early Life and Developmental History			
	Pregnancy – preterm, spontaneous vaginal delivery, any illnesses during pregnancy (2=any two options, 1=one option)	2	1	0
	Birth – weight at birth, condition at birth, any delivery-related complications (2=all three aspects or other equivalent sensible questions relating to birth, 1=any two aspects)	2	1	0
	Illnesses during the neonatal period		1	0
	Current height and weight (and checks whether this is normal for their age)		1	0
	Gross motor function		1	0
	Fine motor function		1	0
	Social function		1	0
	Vision and hearing		1	0
	Immunisation schedule		1	0
	Systems Enquiry			
	Cardiovascular – sweating, cyanosis, pallor, SOB **Respiratory –** cough, wheeze, snoring **Gastrointestinal –** appetite, diet, vomiting, pain, abdominal distention **Neurology –** headaches, fits, weakness **Musculoskeletal –** limp, limb pain, joint swelling, pain (2=explores thoroughly all systems, 1=explores adequately at least 2 systems, 0=poorly or not done)	2	1	0
	Explores parent's ideas, concerns and expectations (2= does well, 1=adequately, 0=not done)	2	1	0
	Invites questions (1). Candidate was non-patronising (1).	2	1	0
	Avoids medical jargon (1)		1	0
	Summarises the main points from the consultation (1). Signposting (1).	2	1	0
	Checks understanding of what has been explained		1	0
	Simulated patient score (2=very good, 1=satisfactory, 0=poor)	2	1	0
	Examiner to ask: 'What is your differential diagnosis?'			
	Candidate suggests a sensible diagnosis (1) and differential (1)	2	1	0
	Total Score			

Global Rating	**1** Clear Fail	**2** Borderline	**3** Clear Pass	**4** Very Good	**5** Outstanding

Candidate Number:	University:
Date:	Year of Study:

STATION 3 – ABDOMINAL PAIN

		2	1	0
	Appropriate introduction (1=full name and role), checks patient's name (1)	2	1	0
	Establishes rapport with the parent (1) and starts with an open question (1)	2	1	0
	Presenting Complaint			
	Establishes onset (1), duration and progression (1) of abdominal pain	2	1	0
	Establishes character (1) and severity (1) of abdominal pain	2	1	0
	Associated symptoms: vomiting, irritability, fever, PR bleeding, change in bowel habits, anorexia (2=three symptoms, 1=two symptoms, 0=one or none)	2	1	0
	Aggravating or relieving factors (1)		1	0
	Infectious contacts (1)		1	0
	Past medical (1) or surgical history or any previous hospitalizations (1)	2	1	0
	Medication history (1) including allergies and nature of allergies (1)		1	0
	Family history (1)		1	0
	Social history – siblings, parents' jobs, special dietary requirements, schooling, friends, hobbies, personality, pets, living accommodation, second-hand smoke exposure (2=does well, 1=adequately, 0=poorly)	2	1	0
	Early Life and Developmental History			
	Pregnancy – preterm, spontaneous vaginal delivery, any illnesses during pregnancy	2	1	0
	Birth – weight at birth, condition at birth, any delivery related complications	2	1	0
	Illnesses during the neonatal period		1	0
	Current height and weight (and checks whether this is normal for their age)		1	0
	Gross motor function		1	0
	Fine motor function		1	0
	Social function		1	0
	Vision and hearing		1	0
	Immunisation schedule		1	0
	Systems Enquiry			
	Cardiovascular – sweating, cyanosis, pallor, SOB **Respiratory** – cough, wheeze, snoring **Gastrointestinal** – appetite, diet, vomiting, pain, abdominal distention **Neurology** – headaches, fits, weakness **Urinary system** – **urinary** colour, frequency, smell **Musculoskeletal** – limp, limb pain, joint swelling, pain (2=explores thoroughly, 1=explores adequately, 0=poorly or not done)	2	1	0
	Explores parent's ideas, concerns and expectations (1)		1	0
	Invites questions (1). Candidate was non-patronising (1).	2	1	0
	Avoids medical jargon		1	0
	Summarises the main points from the consultation (1). Signposting (1).	2	1	0
	Checks understanding of what has been explained		1	0
	Simulated patient score (2=very good, 1=satisfactory, 0=poor)	2	1	0
	Examiner to ask: 'What is your differential diagnosis?'			
	Candidate suggests a sensible diagnosis (1) and differential (1)	2	1	0
	Total Score			

Global Rating	1 Clear Fail	2 Borderline	3 Clear Pass	4 Very Good	5 Outstanding

Candidate Number:	University:
Date:	Year of Study:

STATION 4 – JAUNDICE

		2	1	0
	Appropriate introduction (1=full name and role), checks patient's name (1)	2	1	0
	Establishes rapport with the parent (1) and starts with an open question (1)	2	1	0
	Presenting Complaint			
	Establishes onset, duration and progression of the presenting complaint (2=detailed history of presenting complaint, 1=adequate or only vague history obtained)	2	1	0
	Enquires if the child has been complaining of any abdominal pain (1) or distension (1)	2	1	0
	Enquires after any change in bowel habit, dark urine or pale stools		1	0
	Associated symptoms e.g. vomiting, crying, irritability, fever, poor feeding, poor sleeping, change in bowel habits, rash (2=three symptoms, 1=two symptoms, 0=one or none)	2	1	0
	Enquires about any medication that has been given/tried		1	0
	Infectious contacts		1	0
	Past medical (1) or surgical history or any previous hospitalizations (1)	2	1	0
	Medication history (1) including allergies and nature of allergies (1)	2	1	0
	Family history		1	0
	Social history – siblings, parents' jobs, special dietary requirements, schooling, friends, hobbies, personality, pets, living accommodation, second-hand smoke exposure (2=does well, 1=adequately, 0=poorly)	2	1	0
	Early Life History			
	Pregnancy – preterm, spontaneous vaginal delivery, any illnesses during pregnancy (2=any two options, 1=one option)	2	1	0
	Birth – weight at birth, condition at birth, any delivery-related complications (2=all three aspects or other equivalent sensible questions relating to birth, 1=any two aspects)	2	1	0
	Illnesses during the neonatal period		1	0
	Developmental History			
	Establishes that child is currently of normal height and weight and parents are not worried about general development		1	0
	Gross, fine motor function		1	0
	Social, vision and hearing function		1	0
	Immunisation schedule		1	0
	Systems Enquiry			
	Cardiovascular – sweating, cyanosis, pallor, SOB **Respiratory** – cough, wheeze, snoring **Gastrointestinal** – appetite, diet, vomiting, pain, abdominal distention **Neurology** – headaches, fits, weakness **Musculoskeletal** – limp, limb pain, joint swelling, pain (2=explores thoroughly all systems, 1=explores adequately at least 2 systems, 0=poorly or not done)	2	1	0
	Explores parent's ideas, concerns and expectations (2=does well, 1=adequately, 0=not done)	2	1	0
	Invites questions (1). Candidate was non-patronising (1).	2	1	0
	Avoids medical jargon		1	0
	Summarises the main points from the consultation (1). Signposting (1).	2	1	0
	Simulated patient score (2=very good, 1=satisfactory, 0=poor)	2	1	0
	Examiner to ask: 'What is your differential diagnosis?'			
	Candidate suggests a sensible diagnosis (1) and differential (1)	2	1	0
	Total Score			

Global Rating	**1** Clear Fail	**2** Borderline	**3** Clear Pass	**4** Very Good	**5** Outstanding

Candidate Number:	University:
Date:	Year of Study:

STATION 5 – SEIZURES

		2	1	0
	Appropriate introduction (1=full name and role), checks patient's name (1)	2	1	0
	Establishes rapport with the parent (1) and starts with an open question (1)	2	1	0
	Presenting Complaint			
	Establishes onset and duration of the presenting complaint	2	1	0
	Establishes exactly what happened during the seizure (e.g. jerking all four limbs, loss of consciousness, drowsiness after the event etc.) (2=in detail, 1=only a vague impression obtained, 0=not enquired about)	2	1	0
	Enquires about any medication that has been given/tried		1	0
	Associated symptoms (e.g. vomiting, crying, irritability, fever, poor feeding, poor sleeping, change in bowel habits, rash) (2=three symptoms, 1=two symptoms, 0=one or none)	2	1	0
	Enquires whether parent is aware of any particular triggers for the seizure		1	0
	Enquires whether there have been any previous similar episodes		1	0
	Infectious contacts		1	0
	Past medical (1) or surgical history or any previous hospitalizations (1)	2	1	0
	Medication history (1) including allergies and nature of allergies (1)	2	1	0
	Family history (especially of seizures and epilepsy)		1	0
	Social history – siblings, parents' jobs, pets, living accommodation, second-hand smoke exposure (2=does well, 1=adequately, 0=poorly)	2	1	0
	Early Life History			
	Pregnancy – preterm, spontaneous vaginal delivery, any illnesses during pregnancy (2=any two options, 1=one option)	2	1	0
	Birth – weight at birth, condition at birth, any delivery-related complications (2=all three aspects or other equivalent sensible questions relating to birth, 1=any two aspects)	2	1	0
	Illnesses during the neonatal period		1	0
	Developmental History			
	Establishes that child is currently of normal height and weight and parents are not worried about their general development		1	0
	Gross, fine motor function		1	0
	Social, vision and hearing function		1	0
	Immunisation schedule		1	0
	Systems Enquiry			
	Cardiovascular – sweating, cyanosis, pallor, SOB **Respiratory** – cough, wheeze, snoring **Gastrointestinal** – appetite, diet, vomiting, pain, abdominal distention **Neurology** – headaches, fits, weakness **Musculoskeletal** – limp, limb pain, joint swelling, pain (2=explores thoroughly all systems, 1=explores adequately at least 2 systems, 0=poorly or not done)	2	1	0
	Explores parent's ideas, concerns and expectations (2=does well, 1=adequately, 0=not done)	2	1	0
	Invites questions (1). Candidate was non-patronising (1).	2	1	0
	Avoids medical jargon		1	0
	Summarises the main points from the consultation (1). Signposting (1).	2	1	0
	Simulated patient score (2=very good, 1=satisfactory, 0=poor)	2	1	0
	Examiner to ask: 'What is your differential diagnosis?'			
	Candidate suggests a sensible diagnosis (1) and differential (1)	2	1	0
	Total Score			

Global Rating	1 Clear Fail	2 Borderline	3 Clear Pass	4 Very Good	5 Outstanding

Candidate Number:	University:
Date:	Year of Study:

STATION 6 – RASH

	Appropriate introduction (1=full name and role), checks patient's name (1)	**2**	**1**	**0**
	Establishes rapport with the parent (1) and starts with an open question (1)	**2**	**1**	**0**
	Presenting Complaint			
	Establishes onset and progression of the presenting complaint	**2**	**1**	**0**
	Establishes the exact nature of the rash e.g. distribution, description, whether it is itchy, red, blotchy, discharging or if there is any bleeding (2=detailed history, 1=adequate or vague history)	**2**	**1**	**0**
	Enquires about any medication that has been given/tried		**1**	**0**
	Associated symptoms (e.g. vomiting, crying, irritability, fever, poor feeding, poor sleeping, change in bowel habits, rash) (2=three symptoms, 1=two symptoms, 0=one or none)	**2**	**1**	**0**
	Asks whether any evidence of infectious contacts either at school or at home		**1**	**0**
	Past medical (1) or surgical history or any previous hospitalizations (1)	**2**	**1**	**0**
	Medication history (1) including allergies and nature of allergies (1)	**2**	**1**	**0**
	Family history		**1**	**0**
	Social history – siblings, parents' jobs, special dietary requirements, schooling, friends, hobbies, personality, pets, living accommodation, second-hand smoke exposure (2=does well, 1=adequately, 0=poorly)	**2**	**1**	**0**
	Early Life History			
	Pregnancy – preterm, spontaneous vaginal delivery, any illnesses during pregnancy(2=any two options, 1=one option)	**2**	**1**	**0**
	Birth – weight at birth, condition at birth, any delivery-related complications (2=all three aspects or other equivalent sensible questions relating to birth, 1=any two aspects)	**2**	**1**	**0**
	Illnesses during the neonatal period		**1**	**0**
	Developmental History			
	Establishes that child is currently of normal height and weight and parents are not worried about general development		**1**	**0**
	Gross, fine motor function		**1**	**0**
	Social, vision and hearing function		**1**	**0**
	Immunisation schedule (in particular whether the MMR vaccine was given)		**1**	**0**
	Systems Enquiry			
	Cardiovascular – sweating, cyanosis, pallor, SOB **Respiratory** – cough, wheeze, snoring **Gastrointestinal** – appetite, diet, vomiting, pain, abdominal distention **Neurology** – headaches, fits, weakness **Musculoskeletal** – limp, limb pain, joint swelling, pain (2=explores thoroughly all systems, 1=explores adequately at least 2 systems, 0=poorly or not done)	**2**	**1**	**0**
	Explores parent's ideas, concerns and expectations	**2**	**1**	**0**
	Invites questions (1). Candidate was non-patronising (1).	**2**	**1**	**0**
	Avoids medical jargon		**1**	**0**
	Summarises the main points from the consultation (1). Signposting (1).	**2**	**1**	**0**
	Simulated patient score (2=very good, 1=satisfactory, 0=poor)	**2**	**1**	**0**
	Examiner to ask: 'What is your differential diagnosis?'			
	Candidate suggests a sensible diagnosis (1) and differential (1)	**2**	**1**	**0**
	Total Score			

Global Rating	**1** Clear Fail	**2** Borderline	**3** Clear Pass	**4** Very Good	**5** Outstanding

Candidate Number:	University:
Date:	Year of Study:

STATION 7 – COUGH

		2	1	0
	Appropriate introduction (1=full name and role), checks patient's name (1)	2	1	0
	Establishes rapport with the parent (1) and starts with an open question (1)	2	1	0
	Presenting Complaint			
	Establishes onset, duration and progression of the presenting complaint (2=detailed questioning regarding timing and severity of complaint, 1=vague or only adequate history)	2	1	0
	Establishes the character of the cough, triggers and whether any sputum produced (2=detailed history of the cough, 1=vague history of the cough, 0=not done)	2	1	0
	Frequency of cough		1	0
	Enquires about any medication that has been given/tried		1	0
	Associated symptoms e.g. vomiting, crying, irritability, fever, poor feeding, shortness of breath, chest pain/tightness, wheezing (2=three symptoms, 1=two symptoms, 0=one or none)	2	1	0
	Establishes whether there have been any previous similar episodes (1) and how often (1)	2	1	0
	Establishes that child is healthy and asymptomatic in between episodes		1	0
	Asks whether there is any evidence of infectious contacts either at school or at home		1	0
	Past medical or surgical history or any previous hospitalizations	2	1	0
	Medication history (1) including allergies and nature of allergies (1)	2	1	0
	Family history		1	0
	Social history – siblings, parents' jobs, special dietary requirements, schooling, friends, hobbies, personality, pets, living accommodation, second-hand smoke exposure (2=does well, 1=adequately, 0=poorly)	2	1	0
	Early Life History			
	Pregnancy – preterm, spontaneous vaginal delivery, any illnesses during pregnancy (2=any two options, 1=one option)	2	1	0
	Birth – weight at birth, condition at birth, any delivery-related complications (2=all three aspects or other equivalent sensible questions relating to birth, 1=any two aspects)	2	1	0
	Illnesses during the neonatal period		1	0
	Developmental History			
	Establishes that child is currently of normal height and weight and parents are not worried about general development		1	0
	Gross, fine motor function		1	0
	Social, vision and hearing function		1	0
	Immunisation schedule		1	0
	Systems Enquiry			
	Cardiovascular – sweating, cyanosis, pallor, SOB **Respiratory** – cough, wheeze, snoring **Gastrointestinal** – appetite, diet, vomiting, pain, abdominal distention **Neurology** – headaches, fits, weakness **Musculoskeletal** – limp, limb pain, joint swelling, pain (2=explores thoroughly all systems, 1=explores adequately at least 2 systems, 0=poorly or not done)	2	1	0
	Explores parent's ideas, concerns and expectations (2=does well, 1=adequately, 0=not done)	2	1	0
	Invites questions (1). Candidate was non-patronising (1).	2	1	0
	Avoids medical jargon		1	0
	Summarises the main points from the consultation (1). Signposting (1).	2	1	0
	Simulated patient score (2=very good, 1=satisfactory, 0=poor)	2	1	0
	Examiner to ask: 'What is your differential diagnosis?'			
	Candidate suggests a sensible diagnosis (1) and differential (1)	2	1	0
	Total Score			

Global Rating	1 Clear Fail	2 Borderline	3 Clear Pass	4 Very Good	5 Outstanding

CHAPTER 4: GYNAECOLOGY

Written by Dr. T. North

- Menstrual Problems
- Post Menopausal Bleeding
- Pelvic Pain
- Abnormal Vaginal Bleeding
- Abnormal Vaginal Discharge
- Incontinence and Prolapse
- Subfertility

THE STATIONS

STATION 1
Time allowed: 10 minutes

You are a junior doctor working in general practice.

Mrs Olivia Mallet is attending the practice with a history of heavy periods.

Please take a focussed history from her and formulate a management plan.

The examiner will stop you at 7 minutes to ask you for your differential diagnoses.

STATION 2
Time allowed: 10 minutes

You are a junior doctor working in Obstetrics and Gynaecology.

Mrs Janet Simpson is attending the gynaecology clinic because of episodes of post menopausal bleeding.

Please take a focussed history from her and formulate a management plan.

STATION 3
Time allowed: 7 minutes

You are a junior doctor working in Obstetrics and Gynaecology.

Miss Ellie Bull is attending the gynaecology clinic because of ongoing pelvic pain.

Please take a focussed history from her stating your differential diagnoses for her pain after the consultation.

STATION 4
Time allowed: 7 minutes

You are a junior doctor working in Obstetrics and Gynaecology.

Miss Ashley Hanson is attending the gynaecology clinic because of abnormal vaginal bleeding.

Please take a focussed history from her.

STATION 5
Time allowed: 10 minutes

You are a junior doctor working in Accident and Emergency.

Mrs Melody Rose is attending the department because she has been feeling very unwell for the past two days. She is shivery and complaining of 'abnormal' discharge.

Please take a focussed history from her.

The examiner will stop you at 7 minutes to ask you a few questions.

STATION 6
Time allowed: 10 minutes

You are a junior doctor working in Obstetrics and Gynaecology.

Mrs Alison Sampson is attending the gynaecology clinic today complaining of a dragging sensation down below.

Please take a focussed history from her and formulate a management plan discussing the necessary investigations, surgical and non-surgical options for managing her problem.

STATION 7
Time allowed: 10 minutes

You are a junior doctor working in Obstetrics and Gynaecology.

Mrs Lily Whitcroft is attending the gynaecology clinic because despite trying to conceive she has not fallen pregnant. Recently her GP organised a transvaginal ultrasound scan for her which showed that both ovaries were bulky with multiple small follicles on the surface of them.

A friend of Mrs Whitcroft has told her that polycystic ovarian syndrome can make you infertile. She is incredibly anxious and upset.

Take a focused history from Mrs Whitcroft explaining to her what polycystic ovary syndrome is including any lifestyle advice. Please also answer any questions she may have.

SIMULATED PATIENT BRIEFINGS

STATION 1

Name: Mrs Olivia Mallet

Age: 46 years old

Job: Air hostess on private jets

PC:

For the past six months your periods have become heavier and more protracted. They used to only last 2–3 days but recently they are lasting up to one week. You are flooding through pads at night to the point you have to wear a super-size tampon and two pads to bed. Your periods are not particularly painful, nor do you suffer with cyclical pelvic pain. Your periods are still regular, every 28–30 days and your last period ended 10 days ago. You have no bleeding between periods or after intercourse. You are sexually active and use condoms as your main form of contraception. You have had no abnormal discharge and your bowels are opening normally. You have noticed in the last two months you have been suffering with urinary urgency and frequency. You have no dysuria, and your GP has checked your urine twice for an infection and both times it has been negative.

Obstetric and Gynaecological History:

In your obstetric history you have been pregnant three times. You had a termination at the age of 21 and you have two sons who are both grown up now. Both of these deliveries were vaginal. You are up-to-date with your smears. You had an abnormal smear when you were in your twenties but did not undergo any treatment because of it. You have had no further problems since.

Past Medical History:

Hypothyroidsim

Drug History:

You are allergic to plasters as they give you a rash.

Thyroxine – dose uncertain but it is 2 pills a day.

Social History:

You are an ex-smoker who gave up about 10 years ago (in the past you smoked 5 cigarettes a day for 20 years) and you drink socially.

Ideas/Concerns/Expectations:

You work as an air hostess on a private jet and the symptoms are really beginning to affect your quality of life and job. You are desperate to know what is wrong with you and if this can be cured.

At the end of the consultation ask the candidate what they think is going on and what sort of tests you will need to have in order for a definite diagnosis.

STATION 2

Name: Mrs Janet Simpson

Age: 63 years old

Job: Retired nurse

PC:

Your periods ended when you were 52 years old and went through the menopause. You have had three episodes of vaginal bleeding over the past month which really surprised you. The first one was very light. However, the last two have been heavier to the point that you had to wear a pad for the whole day. When you went to change the pads you found that they were completely soaked each time. Your GP has been very efficient and referred you under the two week rule.

You have had no abdominal pain or weight loss. You are sexually active but the bleeding has not occurred after intercourse. Sometimes you can feel quite dry down below but you often use lubricants that you buy off the internet. You have no pain on intercourse. You have no bowel or urinary problems.

Obstetric and Gynaecological History:

You previously had an endometrial polyp which gave you very heavy periods when you were younger, which was removed in your thirties. Otherwise you have had no gynaecological problems. You had abnormal smears in your twenties but never had any treatment for them and they resolved on their own. You did take HRT for a short while at the time of your menopause (perhaps about two years). It was given as a patch but you can't remember what it was called or what the active ingredient in it was.

You had a termination when you were 23 years old but do not have any children and did not have any miscarriages.

Past Medical History:

Hypercholesterolaemia

Left total hip replacement last year for osteoarthritis

Drug History:

You have an allergy to latex which makes your skin itchy and sore.

Simvastatin 20mg po on

Social History:

You do not drink or smoke. Your mother died of endometrial cancer at 73 years old and your sister was diagnosed with breast cancer at 35 years old but the cancer was removed and treated successfully. She is still alive now.

Ideas/Concerns/Expectations:

You are incredibly anxious as having been a nurse you know what post menopausal bleeding means until proven otherwise.

At the end of the consultation ask the candidate:
1)   What do they think the diagnosis is?
2)   What tests do they need to run?

STATION 3

Name: Miss Ellie Bull

Age: 19 years old

Job: Student

PC:

You have always had problems with your periods since you started them at age 13. They have always been particularly painful and you used to have time off school because of it. However, recently it is beginning to affect your life to the point you are behind on deadlines at college.

The pain tends to start a week before your period is due. It is generally low down in your pelvis, not particularly more on one side than the other. The pain persists and gets progressively worse until your period ends. It is cramp-like in nature and can range from being on a pain scale of 6 to 10 out of 10. The problem is that your periods have recently got longer, now lasting up to 10 days, so you are beginning to feel like you spend more of the month in pain than not. You take regular paracetamol and ibuprofen for the pain, but if you forget to take it you find yourself doubled over in pain. The pain can be so severe that you have to sit over the toilet because you think you are going to vomit, however, you have not been sick.

Your last period was 11 days ago and it is only just finishing. You do pass large blood clots and sometimes they can be very heavy, but you do not flood your pads on a regular basis. You do not get bleeding in between your cycles or after intercourse and you have not had any abnormal discharge.

Obstetric and Gynaecological History:

You are sexually active and have been taking the pill (Microgynon) since the age of 16. Sometimes you suffer with deep pain on intercourse but not on a regular basis and not severe enough to stop you from having intercourse. You do not think that the pill has helped the pain and you mainly take it as a form of contraception although you are not good at remembering to take it and frequently miss a pill.

You are sexually active and have multiple partners. You do not tend to use barrier methods of contraception and were treated for chlamydia when you were 17 years old. You have never had a cervical smear as you are only 19 years old.

You have had two terminations in the past, one at the age of 16 and one six months ago. Both were surgical terminations and there were no related procedural complications.

Past Medical History:

Nil of note.

Drug History:

No allergies

Microgynon contraceptive pill

Social History:

You are currently at college doing an art foundation course. You smoke about 20 cigarettes a day and on average drink at least a couple of pints of beer a day.

Ideas/Concerns/Expectations:

You are worried that you may have contracted another sexually transmitted infection but you are not sure. At the end of the consultation you ask the doctor what they think the diagnosis is.

STATION 4

Name: Miss Ashley Hanson

Age: 28 years old

Job: Film producer

PC:

You started a new relationship a few months ago and on three occasions after having intercourse you have had some spotting of fresh red blood. The bleeds were heavy enough for you to need to wear a panty liner for the next 12 hours or so. At the moment you do not experience any abnormal vaginal discharge, nor do you have any pain on intercourse.

Obstetric and Gynaecological History:

You had your first cervical smear at the age of 25 and it was normal. You have been previously tested for sexually transmitted infections, the last time was two years ago and the results were negative.

You have had no bleeding between your periods and your periods are regular, every 28 days. You used to have very heavy periods when you were a teenager, but after a termination at the age of 22 your periods have become not too heavy and are only three days long. Every now and again you suffer with painful periods, but not on a regular basis and it doesn't really affect your life.

At present you are not using any method of contraceptive, but were thinking about going back on the pill. Apart from your termination at age 23 (which was medically terminated) you had a normal vaginal delivery of a baby girl when you were 17 years old. She was given up for adoption and you do not have any contact with her.

Past Medical History:

Removal of right lower wisdom teeth six months ago.

Recurrent urinary tract infections as a child but they have not been a problem in adulthood.

You are currently suffering with a chest infection and are on antibiotics.

Drug History:

You are not allergic to any medication as far you know.

You are currently taking a course of antibiotics for a chest infection but cannot remember what they are called. You think it might be Augmentin.

Family History:

You grandmother died of ovarian cancer at age 80 and your older sister had previous treatment to her cervix for abnormal cells.

Social History:

You are a very busy film producer who travels all over the world. You have quite a stressful life but really enjoy your job. You smoke 20–30 cigarettes a day and drink a couple of glasses of wine a night during the week, more at the weekends. You find it hard to quantify exactly how much this is though.

Ideas/Concerns/Expectations:

You are very anxious to know what could be causing this bleeding, especially because you have a family history of cancer. At the end of the consultation ask the candidate what sort of things might be responsible for the bleeding.

STATION 5

Name: Mrs Melody Rose

Age: 47 years old

Job: Supermarket cashier

PC:

Two weeks ago you had quite a raunchy weekend away with a new partner who you just met. A week or so later you started feeling unwell. First you noticed some yellow vaginal discharge, which is now green. At certain times you thought the discharge looked like chunks of gristle. It was also quite foul-smelling and you noticed moderate amounts of the discharge so that you have to wear a panty liner to stop this from soiling your underwear. You felt quite shivery and shaky the other day and when you took your temperature last night you noticed that this was high at about 39°C.

You have also been vomiting and had a few episodes of diarrhoea in the last week. You do not have any severe pelvic pains but do have mild generalised abdominal pains – nothing severe enough to need painkillers for though. They do not radiate and you would rate them about 4 out of 10 in pain severity. In addition to this, over the last 24 hours you have noticed you are becoming more yellow. You deny any increased frequency of your urine or any dysuria. You do not have flank pain.

You have never had bleeding after intercourse. However, you have noticed some superficial pain on intercourse after that weekend. You have been wondering if there is a cut down below because that is what the pain feels like.

Obstetric and Gynaecological History:

You have four children, all normal vaginal deliveries. You have never had sexually transmitted infections before and have a Mirena coil in situ which was only inserted six weeks ago. You are very keen to keep this in if the candidate suggests removing it. Prior to the Mirena coil you were on the progesterone-only pill, for this reason you are not too sure when your last true period was.

You were told many years ago that your doctor thought you have fibroids but you have never had an ultrasound scan or seen a gynaecologist about it.

Past Medical History:

You suffer with Gilbert's syndrome, which has not previously caused you any problems.

Drug History:

You are not taking any regular medications but are allergic to Septrin, it makes you vomit. It is a rather old antibiotic which you don't think is prescribed now but the allergy occurred when you were a child and had the flu.

Social History:

You got divorced a year and a half ago after 20 years of marriage. You smoke about 20 a day and have been drinking in excess ever since your divorce. You are not dependent on alcohol but think you definitely binge drink where you could take in excess of three bottles of red wine in one Saturday night on your own. You did use illicit drugs as a teenager and have recently started using cocaine again, but not on a regular basis, and only as a bit of fun.

At the end of the consultation the examiner is to ask the candidate the following questions:

1)   Give a differential diagnosis for the cause of the patient's sepsis.

2)   Give a differential diagnosis for the cause of the patient's jaundice.

STATION 6

Name: Mrs Alison Sampson

Age: 58 years old

Job: Charity worker

PC:

You have come to the gynaecology clinic today because your GP has referred you after you complained to him with a lump you had noticed 'down below' just at the region of where your vagina is. It is difficult to describe as it doesn't look like a spot or a growth but as if something inside you is 'popping out'. You have noticed it there for the last six months but think it has got bigger and more uncomfortable in the last six months. It seems to get bigger at the end of the day when you have been particularly active and also when you strain, like when you cough or laugh out loud.

You have had no problems opening your bowels but in the last three months have suffered a little with the leakage of urine. Although the nature of your work means you live in Africa for most of the time, whenever you visit the UK you are a keen golfer and find that when you go to swing at the golf ball you also leak a little bit of urine. This also occurs mostly when you strain. You rarely get symptoms of leakage without straining and you never get any warning that it will happen. You do not suffer from any urgency and can hold onto your urine until you find a toilet if you are desperate (i.e. you rarely get 'caught out').

You don't suffer with any urgency, dysuria, frequency, nocturia or problems when opening your bowels.

Obstetric and Gynaecological History:

You went through the menopause about six years ago and can't remember when your last period was. You have never taken any hormone replacement therapy. You are not sexually active and haven't been since you were widowed seven years ago. You cannot remember when your last smear was but have never had an abnormal one.

You have three children. The first two were delivered by normal vaginal delivery and you had an emergency hysterectomy with the delivery of your third child. Your memory of this is vague but you think it was because the placenta was embedded very deep and they could not stop you bleeding. They did not remove your ovaries.

Past Medical History:

Hysterectomy (aged 37)

Cholecystectomy (aged 42)

Hypertension

Hypercholesterolaemia

Drug History:

No allergies to medication but true anaphylactic reaction to bee stings.

Frusemide 10mg po od

Simvastatin 20mg po on

Social History:

You volunteer for a charity abroad and spend almost half the year in Africa. You only returned to the UK about a month ago. You do not smoke but like to have a small shot of brandy before going to bed because it helps you sleep better.

Ideas/ Concerns/ Expectations:

You are keen to know what options are available to you and where you go from here as you feel this is beginning to affect your life so much you cannot cope with it for much longer.

STATION 7

Name: Mrs Lily Whitcroft

Age: 31 years old

Job: Banker

PC:

About seven months ago you and your husband decided you wanted to have children so you had your Mirena coil removed. You have not managed to conceive despite trying with your partner at least three times a week for the last six months.

You recently visited your GP because you had been having some non-specific pelvic pain. A transvaginal ultrasound scan was performed which revealed that you had polycystic ovaries. The GP did not discuss this in great deal with you and did not know at the time you were trying to conceive. All he said to you was that it wasn't dangerous and there was no need to have anything done about it. He mentioned it was quite 'common'. No blood tests were performed. When you later spoke to a close friend about the results, she told you that this could be a cause for your infertility and that there was no cure for it. She scared you when she said that it would be likely you would never conceive!

You have read a little about polycystic ovaries on the internet but do not feel you have any of the common symptoms with it, for example you do not suffer with hirsutism or acne. You had spots as a teenager but never took any medication for it. However, you do sometimes struggle with your weight and because of your busy job you do not get as much time to go to the gym as you would like. Your diet is not healthy, and you snack on junk food when hungry.

Obstetric and Gynaecological History:

Your periods were regular, every 28–30 days, although in the last three years you think they are becoming lighter and less regular occurring about every 34–38 days. You bleed for about four days each cycle. The periods are not painful. You started your periods at the age of 14.

You had a termination at the age of 22 because you were still training in your job and your ex-boyfriend had left to work abroad. You have never had any miscarriages and your husband does not have any children from a previous relationship. Your last cervical smear test was normal and was three years ago.

For contraception you used to have a Mirena coil in situ until seven months ago. You are currently not on any contraception.

Past Medical History:

Hyperthyroidism

Torn Achilles tendon at age of 24 – repaired surgically

Drug History:

Allergy to cyclizine which makes you feel light-headed and funny.

Carbimazole 15mg po od

Social History:

You are a career woman who recently got married.

You used to smoke socially but stopped this when you were trying to conceive seven months ago. Your partner does not smoke and is the same age as yourself. Both of you drink socially but rarely get drunk.

Ideas/Concerns/ Expectations:

You have an immense amount of guilt surrounding your termination. You remember at the time wondering whether this was your one chance to have a child. You blame yourself and although at the time you didn't want the child and you are petrified that you blew your only chance.

You have been doing some reading on the internet and you have heard that there are some medications that you could take, but are really struggling to understand what this 'illness' is. You were hoping to get a clear explanation and answers today!

The questions you would most like answered today include:
1)   What is polycystic ovarian syndrome?
2)   Does having polycystic ovaries on an ultrasound scan mean that you are infertile?
3)   Is there any medication or treatment for this 'illness'?

GYNAECOLOGY

Candidate Number:	University:
Date:	Year of Study:

STATION 1 – MENSTRUAL PROBLEMS

Appropriate introduction (1=full name and role), checks patient's name (1)	2	1	0
Explains purpose of interview and checks consent (2=does well, 1=adequately, 0=poorly or not done)	2	1	0
Presenting Complaint:			
Establishes onset, duration (1) and nature of presenting complaint (1)	2	1	0
Enquires after frequency (1) and volume (1) of bleeding (i.e. constant, number of pads, passage of clots etc.)	2	1	0
Enquires after dysmenorrhea (1) and presence of pelvic pain (1)	2	1	0
Establishes date of last menstrual period (1) and length of cycles (1)	2	1	0
Establishes if there is any other presence of abnormal bleeding i.e. post coital bleeding (1) or inter-menstrual bleeding (1)	2	1	0
Asks after presence of vaginal discharge		1	0
Enquires after presence of bowel (1) or urinary (1) symptoms	2	1	0
Asks about associated symptoms such as pallor, flushing, fainting episodes, bleeding elsewhere such as haemoptysis/per rectum/haematuria, weight loss etc. (2=offers 3 symptoms, 1=offers 2 symptoms, 0=less than 2 other symptoms)	2	1	0
Enquires after previous similar episodes and/or treatments		1	0
Explores patient's ideas and concerns regarding the presenting complaint		1	0
Previous obstetric and gynaecology history:			
Enquires after sexual history/activity (1) and previous sexually acquired infections (1)	2	1	0
Contraceptive usage (1) and type of contraception used (1)	2	1	0
Last cervical smear test date (1) and result of the smear test (1)	2	1	0
Previous pregnancies and method of delivery, including related complications		1	0
Previous terminations (1) and miscarriages (1)	2	1	0
Other relevant history:			
Relevant past medical and surgical history (1) especially of bleeding disorders (1)	2	1	0
Medication history (1) including allergies (1)	2	1	0
Relevant family history (especially of bleeding disorders)		1	0
Smoking (1) and alcohol (1)	2	1	0
Appropriate closure (e.g. explains next step, thanks patient and summarises) (2=does well, 1=adequately, 0=poorly or not done)	2	1	0
Communication Skills			
Appropriate questioning style (mix of open and closed questions) (2=does well, 1=adequately, 0=poorly or not done)	2	1	0
Invites questions (1). Listens actively (1).	2	1	0
Organised approach to history-taking (e.g. systematic, summarises, signposts change in focus of question)	2	1	0
Simulated patient score (2=very good, 1=satisfactory, 0=poor)	2	1	0
Examiner to ask: 'What are your differential diagnoses?'			
Candidate states an appropriate diagnosis (1) (fibroids or endometrial/cervical polyp) and offers a differential (1) (endometriosis or exclusion of malignancy – cervical/endometrial/ovarian)	2	1	0
Examiner to ask: 'What investigations would you recommend?'			
Candidate suggests transvaginal ultrasound scan (1) and hysteroscopy and biopsy (1)	2	1	0
Total Score			

Global Rating	1 Clear Fail	2 Borderline	3 Clear Pass	4 Very Good	5 Outstanding

Candidate Number:	University:
Date:	Year of Study:

STATION 2 – POST MENOPAUSAL BLEEDING

	Appropriate introduction (1=full name and role), checks patient's name (1)	2	1	0
	Explains purpose of interview and checks consent (2=does well, 1=adequately, 0=poorly or not done)	2	1	0
	Presenting Complaint:			
	Establishes age of patient (1) and what age patient went through the menopause/date of last menstrual period (1)	2	1	0
	Establishes how many episodes of bleeding patient has had (1) and volume/heaviness (1)	2	1	0
	Enquires after the presence of abdominal/pelvic pain (1) or bowel/urinary symptoms (1)	2	1	0
	Enquires after presence of dyspareunia (1) or post coital bleeding (1)	2	1	0
	Enquires after vaginal dryness during intercourse		1	0
	Asks about associated symptoms such as pallor, unexplained fatigue, bone pain, weight loss, other sites of abnormal bleeding such as haemoptysis/per rectal bleeding, haematuria (2=offers 3 symptoms, 1=offers 2 symptoms, 0=less than 2 other symptoms)	2	1	0
	Previous obstetric and gynaecology history:			
	Enquires after sexual history/activity (1) and previous sexually acquired infections (1)	2	1	0
	Last cervical smear test date (1) and result of the smear test (1)	2	1	0
	Establishes history of gynaecological problems – fibroids/polyps/prolapse		1	0
	Previous pregnancies and method of delivery including related complications		1	0
	Previous terminations (1) and miscarriages (1)	2	1	0
	Other relevant history:			
	Relevant past medical and surgical history		1	0
	Medication history (1) including allergies (1)	2	1	0
	Establishes history of HRT use – What type (i.e. combined tablet) (1) and for how many years has it been taken? (1)	2	1	0
	Establishes family history of ovarian/breast cancer (1) and type of relative (i.e. 1st/2nd degree on mother's side) (1)	2	1	0
	Smoking (1) and alcohol (1)	2	1	0
	Appropriate closure (e.g. explains next step, thanks patient and summarises) (2=does well, 1=adequately, 0=poorly or not done)	2	1	0
	Communication Skills			
	Appropriate questioning style (mix of open and closed questions) (2=does well, 1=adequately, 0=poorly or not done)	2	1	0
	Invites questions (1). Listens actively (1).	2	1	0
	Explores patient's ideas, concerns and expectations (2=does well, 1=adequately, 0=not done)	2	1	0
	Organised approach to history-taking (e.g. systematic, summarises, signposts change in focus of question)		1	0
	Simulated patient score (2=very good, 1=satisfactory, 0=poor)	2	1	0
	Examiner to ask: 'What are your differential diagnoses?'			
	Candidate states an appropriate diagnosis (1) (endometrial cancer/endometrial polyp) and offers a differential (1) (cervical cancer/atrophic vaginitis)	2	1	0
	Examiner to ask: 'What investigations would you recommend?'			
	Candidate suggests transvaginal/pelvic ultrasound scan to determine endometrial thickness (if <5mm then biopsy not required)		1	0
	Endometrial biopsy – pipelle (1) (if endometrial thickness between 5mm and 9mm) and hysteroscopy and dilation and curettage (1) (if endometrial thickness >10mm, because possibility of endometrial polyp)	2	1	0
	Total Score			

Global Rating	1 Clear Fail	2 Borderline	3 Clear Pass	4 Very Good	5 Outstanding

Candidate Number:	University:
Date:	Year of Study:

STATION 3 – PELVIC PAIN

		2	1	0
	Appropriate introduction (1=full name and role), checks patient's name (1)	2	1	0
	Explains purpose of interview and checks consent (2=does well, 1=adequately, 0=poorly or not done)	2	1	0
	Presenting Complaint:			
	Establishes onset, duration (1) and cyclical nature of presenting complaint (1)	2	1	0
	Obtains a full pain history of the pelvic pain (i.e. site, character, radiation, pain scale)	2	1	0
	Enquires after the progression of the pain (worsening/improving) (1) and types of medication or therapy already attempted (1)	2	1	0
	Establishes date of last menstrual period (1) and length of cycles (1)	2	1	0
	Establishes history of dysmenorrhea (1) and menorrhagia (1)	2	1	0
	Establishes length of periods (1) and nature of associated bleeding (1) (i.e. volume/passage of clots and whether there is any relationship to pain severity)	2	1	0
	Establishes if there is any other presence of abnormal bleeding (i.e. post coital bleeding (1) or inter-menstrual bleeding (1))	2	1	0
	Establishes history of dyspareunia (1) and if superficial or deep (1)	2	1	0
	Enquires after presence of bowel (1) or urinary (1) symptoms	2	1	0
	Asks about associated symptoms such as pallor, flushing, fainting episodes, bleeding elsewhere such as haemoptysis/per rectum/haematuria, weight loss etc. (2=offers 3 symptoms, 1=offers 2 symptoms, 0=less than 2 other symptoms)	2	1	0
	Explores patient's ideas and concerns regarding the presenting complaint including affect on life	2	1	0
	Previous obstetric and gynaecology history:			
	Enquires after sexual history/activity (1) and previous sexually acquired infections (1)	2	1	0
	Contraceptive usage (1) and type of contraception used including patient compliance (1)	2	1	0
	Last cervical smear test date (1) and result of the smear test (1)	2	1	0
	Previous pregnancies and method of delivery, including related complications		1	0
	Previous terminations (1) and miscarriages (1)	2	1	0
	Establishes history of other gynaecological problems, in particular – ovarian cysts	2	1	0
	Other relevant history:			
	Relevant past medical and surgical history		1	0
	Medication history (1) including allergies (1)	2	1	0
	Relevant family history		1	0
	Smoking (1) and alcohol (1)	2	1	0
	Appropriate closure (e.g. explains next step, thanks patient and summarises) (2=does well, 1=adequately, 0=poorly or not done)	2	1	0
	Communication Skills			
	Appropriate questioning style (mix of open and closed questions) (2=does well, 1=adequately, 0=poorly or not done)	2	1	0
	Invites questions (1). Listens actively (1).	2	1	0
	Organised approach to history-taking (e.g. systematic, summarises, signposts change in focus of question)		1	0
	Simulated patient score (2=very good, 1=satisfactory, 0=poor)	2	1	0
	Examiner to ask: 'What are your differential diagnoses?'			
	Candidate states an appropriate diagnosis (1) (endometriosis) and offers a differential (1) (chronic pelvic inflammatory disease)	2	1	0
	Total Score			

Global Rating	1 Clear Fail	2 Borderline	3 Clear Pass	4 Very Good	5 Outstanding

Candidate Number:		University:
Date:		Year of Study:

STATION 4 – ABNORMAL VAGINAL BLEEDING

	Appropriate introduction (1=full name and role), checks patient's name (1)	2	1	0
	Explains purpose of interview and checks consent (2=does well, 1=adequately, 0=poorly or not done)	2	1	0
	Presenting Complaint:			
	Establishes onset (1) and nature of presenting complaint (post coital bleeding) (1)	2	1	0
	Enquires after volume (1) and number of episodes of bleeding (1) (i.e. number of pads, passage of clots etc.)	2	1	0
	Establishes date of last menstrual period (1) and length of cycles (1)	2	1	0
	Establishes if there is any other presence of abnormal vaginal bleeding (i.e. inter-menstrual)		1	0
	Enquires after presence of bowel (1) or urinary (1) symptoms	2	1	0
	Asks after presence of vaginal discharge (1) or dyspareunia (1)	2	1	0
	Enquires after dysmenorrhea (1) and menorrhagia (1)	2	1	0
	Enquires after previous similar episodes and/or treatments		1	0
	Explores patient's ideas and concerns regarding the presenting complaint	2	1	0
	Previous obstetric and gynaecology history:			
	Enquires after sexual history/activity (1) and previous sexually acquired infections (1)	2	1	0
	Contraceptive usage (1) and type of contraception used including patient compliance (1)	2	1	0
	Last cervical smear test date (1) and result of the smear test (1)	2	1	0
	Previous pregnancies and method of delivery, including related complications		1	0
	Previous terminations (1) and miscarriages (1)	2	1	0
	Other relevant history:			
	Relevant past medical and surgical history		1	0
	Medication history (1) including allergies (1)	2	1	0
	Relevant family history (especially of gynaecological cancers)		1	0
	Smoking (1) and alcohol (1)	2	1	0
	Appropriate closure (e.g. explains next step, thanks patient and summarises) (2=does well, 1=adequately, 0=poorly or not done)	2	1	0
	Communication Skills			
	Appropriate questioning style (mix of open and closed questions) (2=does well, 1=adequately, 0=poorly or not done)	2	1	0
	Invites questions (1). Listens actively (1).	2	1	0
	Organised approach to history-taking (e.g. systematic, summarises, signposts change in focus of question)		1	0
	Simulated patient score (2=very good, 1=satisfactory, 0=poor)	2	1	0
	Examiner to ask: 'What are your differential diagnoses?'			
	Candidate states an appropriate diagnosis (1) (cervical ectropion/cervical polyp) and offers a differential (1) (cervical carcinoma/vaginitis/cervicitis)	2	1	0
	Total Score			

Global Rating	1 Clear Fail	2 Borderline	3 Clear Pass	4 Very Good	5 Outstanding

Candidate Number:	University:
Date:	Year of Study:

STATION 5 – ABNORMAL VAGINAL DISCHARGE

	Appropriate introduction (1=full name and role), checks patient's name (1)	2	1	0
	Explains purpose of interview and checks consent (2=does well, 1=adequately, 0=poorly or not done)	2	1	0
	Presenting Complaint:			
	Establishes onset, duration (1) and nature of presenting complaint (1)	2	1	0
	Enquires after amount (1) and colour/smell/consistency of discharge (1)	2	1	0
	Asks about and takes a thorough history of any associated pelvic pain (i.e. site, radiation, triggering factors, character of pain and pain scale) (2=done well, 1=adequately)	2	1	0
	Enquires after dysmenorrhea (1) and menorrhagia (1)	2	1	0
	Establishes date of last menstrual period (1) and length of cycles (1)	2	1	0
	Establishes if there is any other presence of abnormal bleeding (i.e. post coital bleeding) (1) or inter-menstrual bleeding (1)	2	1	0
	Enquires after presence of bowel (1) or urinary (1) symptoms	2	1	0
	Asks about associated symptoms such as fevers, rigors, weight loss, loss of appetite, vomiting, night sweats, jaundice, collapse (2=offers 3 symptoms, 1=offers 2 symptoms)	2	1	0
	Enquires after previous similar episodes and/or treatments		1	0
	Explores patient's ideas and concerns regarding the presenting complaint	2	1	0
	Previous obstetric and gynaecology history:			
	Enquires after sexual history/activity (1) and previous sexually acquired infections (1)	2	1	0
	Contraceptive usage (1) and type of contraception used including compliance (1)	2	1	0
	Last cervical smear test date (1) and result of the smear test (1)	2	1	0
	Previous pregnancies and method of delivery, including related complications		1	0
	Previous terminations (1) and miscarriages (1)	2	1	0
	Previous significant gynaecological disorders or history of gynaecological surgery		1	0
	Other relevant history:			
	Relevant past medical and surgical history		1	0
	Medication history (1) including allergies (1)	2	1	0
	Relevant family history (especially of bleeding disorders)		1	0
	Smoking (1) and alcohol (1)	2	1	0
	Appropriate closure (e.g. explains next step, thanks patient and summarises) (2=does well, 1=adequately, 0=poorly or not done)	2	1	0
	Communication Skills			
	Appropriate questioning style (mix of open and closed questions) (2=does well, 1=adequately, 0=poorly or not done)	2	1	0
	Invites questions (1). Listens actively (1).	2	1	0
	Explores patient's ideas, concerns and expectations (2=does well, 1=adequately, 0=not done)	2	1	0
	Organised approach to history-taking (e.g. systematic, summarises, signposts change in focus of question)		1	0
	Simulated patient score (2=very good, 1=satisfactory, 0=poor)	2	1	0
	Examiner to ask: 'What are your differential diagnoses?'			
	Candidate states an appropriate diagnosis relating to gynaecological problems – sepsis – endometritis secondary to pelvic inflammatory disease (1) or fibroid degeneration (1)	2	1	0
	Candidate suggests reason for the jaundice – perihepatitis, viral hepatitis (1) or due to underlying Gilbert's syndrome (1)	2	1	0
	Total Score			

Global Rating	1 Clear Fail	2 Borderline	3 Clear Pass	4 Very Good	5 Outstanding

Candidate Number:	University:
Date:	Year of Study:

STATION 6 – INCONTINENCE AND PROLAPSE

	Appropriate introduction (1=full name and role), checks patient's name (1)	2	1	0
	Explains purpose of interview and checks consent (2=does well, 1=adequately, 0=poorly or not done)	2	1	0
	Presenting Complaint:			
	Establishes onset, duration (1) and nature of presenting complaint (dragging sensation) (1)	2	1	0
	Establishes presence and description of a lump (1) and its location (1)	2	1	0
	Enquires after factors which worsen the symptoms (i.e. end of day) (1) and whether lump interferes with sexual intercourse (1)	2	1	0
	Establishes history of associated urinary symptoms i.e. urge incontinence/stress incontinence/dysuria/haematuria/increased frequency (2=asks 3 symptoms or more, 1=asks only 2 symptoms)	2	1	0
	Establishes history of nocturia (1) and disruption to patient's sleep (1)	2	1	0
	Enquires whether urinary symptoms have ever resulted in patient being 'caught out' (1) and enquires after triggers affecting her urinary symptoms (1)	2	1	0
	Establishes history of other bowel/urinary symptoms – constipation/diarrhoea/faecal incontinence (1) and if has to digitalise the vagina to open bowels or pass urine (1)	2	1	0
	Enquires after previous similar episodes and/or treatments		1	0
	Establishes history of daily fluid intake: type of fluid intake (i.e. large amount of caffeine-based drinks such as tea/coffee/coke) (1) and volume and timing of fluid intake (i.e. how much and when during the day) (1)	2	1	0
	Explores patient's ideas and concerns regarding the presenting complaint including how this affects her life	2	1	0
	Previous obstetric and gynaecology history:			
	Enquires after age of menopause (1) and date of last menstrual period (1)	2	1	0
	Last cervical smear test date (1) and result of the smear test (1)	2	1	0
	Previous pregnancies and method of delivery, including related complications	2	1	0
	Previous terminations (1) and miscarriages (1)	2	1	0
	Establishes history of previous gynaecology problems		1	0
	Other relevant history:			
	Relevant past medical and surgical history (1)	2	1	0
	Medication history (1) including allergies (1)	2	1	0
	Smoking (1) and alcohol (1)	2	1	0
	Appropriate closure (e.g. explains next step, thanks patient and summarises) (2=does well, 1=adequately, 0=poorly or not done)	2	1	0
	Communication Skills			
	Appropriate questioning style (mix of open and closed questions) (2=does well, 1=adequately, 0=poorly or not done)	2	1	0
	Invites questions (1). Listens actively (1).	2	1	0
	Organised approach to history-taking (e.g. systematic, summarises, signposts change in focus of question)		1	0
	Simulated patient score (2=very good, 1=satisfactory, 0=poor)	2	1	0
	Examiner to ask: 'What are your differential diagnoses?'			
	Candidate states an appropriate diagnosis (prolapse) (1) and differential diagnosis (stress incontinence) (1)	2	1	0
	Examiner to ask: 'What investigations could be carried out?'			
	Urodynamic studies for stress incontinence (1) and urinalysis/random blood glucose to exclude diabetes and urinary tract infections (1)	2	1	0
	Examiner to ask: 'What non-surgical interventions could be considered?'			
	Prolapse – physiotherapy and weight reduction and pessary (1) Stress incontinence – treat underlying infection/diabetes and pelvic floor exercise and physiotherapy (1)	2	1	0
	Examiner to ask: 'What surgical interventions could be considered?'			
	Prolapse – anterior/posterior wall repairs and hysterectomy (1) Stress incontinence – Burch colposuspension and tension-free vaginal tape (1)	2	1	0
	Total Score			

Global Rating	**1** Clear Fail	**2** Borderline	**3** Clear Pass	**4** Very Good	**5** Outstanding

Candidate Number:	University:
Date:	Year of Study:

STATION 7 – FERTILITY ISSUES

		2	1	0
	Appropriate introduction (1=full name and role), checks patient's name (1)	2	1	0
	Explains purpose of interview and checks consent (2=does well, 1=adequately, 0=poorly or not done)	2	1	0
	Presenting Complaint:			
	Establishes presenting complaint (subfertility) (1) and recent ultrasound result of polycystic ovaries (1)	2	1	0
	Enquires after frequency of intercourse (1) and length of time patient and partner have been attempting to conceive (1)	2	1	0
	Enquires after method of contraceptive used prior to attempting to conceive		1	0
	Establishes and confirms patient is not on any contraception at the moment		1	0
	Establishes age of menarche (1) and history of oligomenorrhea/amenorrhea (1)	2	1	0
	Establishes history of hirsutism (1) and diabetes (1)	2	1	0
	Establishes history of weight problems (1) and acne (1)	2	1	0
	Enquires after previous treatments/ investigations for subfertility undertaken by patient		1	0
	Enquires after previous treatments/ investigations for subfertility undertaken by partner		1	0
	Asks whether partner has fathered any children previously from another relationship		1	0
	Explores patient's ideas and concerns regarding the presenting complaint	2	1	0
	Previous obstetric and gynaecology history:			
	Enquires after previous sexually acquired infections		1	0
	Last cervical smear test date (1) and result of the smear test (1)	2	1	0
	Previous pregnancies and method of delivery, including related complications		1	0
	Previous terminations (1) and miscarriages (1)	2	1	0
	Other relevant history:			
	Relevant past medical and surgical history		1	0
	Medication history (1) including allergies (1)	2	1	0
	Smoking and alcohol history for patient (1) and partner (1)	2	1	0
	Appropriate closure (e.g. explains next step, thanks patient and summarises) (2=does well, 1=adequately, 0=poorly or not done)	2	1	0
	Explanation of Polycystic Ovarian Syndrome			
	Explains that polycystic ovary syndrome exists as a spectrum (1) and just because she has these appearances on her ultrasound scan does not mean she has the 'syndrome' unless biochemical tests are done and she has clinical symptoms (1)	2	1	0
	Explains that patients with PCOS can vary in both their clinical symptoms (1) and their biochemical abnormalities (1)	2	1	0
	Explains that because of hormonal changes – (hypersecretion of luteinising hormone and androgens) some patients do not ovulate (1) and this can lead to difficulty conceiving although not always (1)	2	1	0
	Advises patient on lifestyle changes such as a healthy diet (1) and weight loss (1)	2	1	0
	Medications which are started for PCOS sufferers can include starting Metformin (1) and Clomiphene (1) to help conceive	2	1	0
	Reassures patient that she is not 'infertile' (1) and there is no need at present to start medication but that further tests may be performed to rule out PCOS (1)	2	1	0
	Communication Skills			
	Appropriate questioning style (mix of open and closed questions) (2=does well, 1=adequately, 0=poorly or not done)	2	1	0
	Invites questions (1). Listens actively (1).	2	1	0
	Organised approach to history-taking (e.g. systematic, summarises, signposts change in focus of question)		1	0
	Simulated patient score (2=very good, 1=satisfactory, 0=poor)	2	1	0
	Total Score			

Global Rating	1 Clear Fail	2 Borderline	3 Clear Pass	4 Very Good	5 Outstanding

CHAPTER 5: OBSTETRICS

Written by Dr. T. North

- Antepartum Haemorrhage
- Pre-eclampsia
- Hyperemesis Gravidarum
- Gestational Diabetes
- Booking Visit
- Puerperal Pyrexia
- Twin Pregnancy
- Breech Pregnancy
- Early Pregnancy Complications
- Post-Dates Pregnancy
- Intra-uterine Growth Retardation
- Abdominal Pain in Pregnancy

THE STATIONS

STATION 1
Time allowed: 7 minutes

You are a junior doctor working in obstetrics and gynaecology.

You are asked to see Mrs Morton on the antenatal ward. When passing urine a few hours ago she noticed some blood in the toilet bowl. She is incredibly anxious as she has not felt the baby move for the last hour or so.

Please take a focussed history from her and formulate a management plan.

STATION 2
Time allowed: 7 minutes

You are a junior doctor working in general practice.

Your next patient is a Mrs Altweg. She is a 31 year old lady who is 37 weeks pregnant. She has been feeling generally unwell for the past few days but also has a severe headache today. She has come today to find out if she is allowed to take any painkillers for her headache as she is scared of harming the baby.

Please take a focussed history from her and formulate a management plan.

The examiner will stop you at 5 minutes to ask you a few questions.

STATION 3
Time allowed: 7 minutes

You are a junior doctor working in the Accident and Emergency department.

Sally Gibbs is 10 weeks pregnant. She is attending the department because she has been suffering with intractable vomiting. She is at her wits' end and is desperate for something to make her feel better.

Please take a focussed history from her and formulate a management plan.

The examiner will stop you at 5 minutes to ask you a few questions.

STATION 4
Time allowed: 10 minutes

You are a junior doctor working in obstetrics and gynaecology.

Today you are working in the antenatal clinic. Josephine Lovelock is a woman who has been sent to the clinic by the community midwife because she has had a glucose tolerance test result of 10. She has a body mass index of 41. She is feeling well in herself and does not understand what all the fuss is about.

Take a history from Josephine and explain what the test results mean for both herself and her baby.

STATION 5
Time allowed: 7 minutes

You are a junior doctor working in general practice.

The community midwife has had to go home sick and you have been asked to take over her clinic for the morning. Mrs Janet Wiley is attending for her booking visit.

Please take a full history from her. The examiner will stop you at 5 minutes to ask you if you think this patient is high or low risk and what her appropriate management should be.

STATION 6
Time allowed: 7 minutes

You are a junior doctor working in the Accident and Emergency department.

Mrs Estelle Ford is attending with a high fever and abdominal pain. It has been seven days since she gave birth to her baby girl.

Take a history from Estelle and at the end of the consultation suggest a differential diagnosis.

STATION 7
Time allowed: 7 minutes

You are a junior doctor working in obstetrics and gynaecology.

Mrs Imogen Ward is 14 weeks pregnant with dichorionic, dizygotic twins. She has come to the antenatal clinic because she has lots of questions regarding her twin pregnancy.

Please explain to Mrs Ward the risks and complications associated with twin pregnancies and answer any questions she may have.

STATION 8
Time allowed: 7 minutes

You are a junior doctor working in obstetrics and gynaecology.

Miss Louise Paul is 36 weeks pregnant. She has had an ultrasound scan today which has confirmed that baby is extended breech.

Please take a full antenatal history from Miss Paul and explain her options for management and delivery.

STATION 9
Time allowed: 7 minutes

You are a junior doctor working in the Accident and Emergency department.

Miss Sally Graham is 26 years old and is attending the department today with symptoms of abdominal pain and PV spotting. She had a positive pregnancy test two days ago.

Take a history from Sally and at the end of the consultation offer a differential diagnosis.

STATION 10
Time allowed: 7 minutes

You are a junior doctor working in obstetrics and gynaecology.

Today Mrs Sumita Patel has come to the antenatal clinic because she is one week overdue.

Please take a history from Sumita and discuss the plans for her further management, which will now include a cervical sweep and booking for induction of labour.

STATION 11
Time allowed: 7 minutes

You are a junior doctor working in obstetrics and gynaecology.

Mrs Katherine Warner has been sent to the antenatal clinic because her baby has been measuring 'small for dates'. An ultrasound scan today confirms that the estimated foetal weight is below the 10th centile. She has also been told her baby has reduced growth velocity.

Please take a focussed history from her and formulate a management plan.

STATION 12
Time allowed: 7 minutes

You are a junior doctor working in general practice.

Mrs Jessica Woodstock is 34 weeks into her pregnancy. She has developed abdominal pain this morning and is incredibly anxious something has happened to her baby.

Please take a focussed history from her and state your differential diagnoses.

SIMULATED PATIENT BRIEFINGS

STATION 1

Name: Mrs Morton

Age: 34 years old

Job: Personal assistant

You are 35 weeks into your first pregnancy. You have had two previous miscarriages over the past five years. Work has been particularly stressful today and you have been looking forward to going on maternity leave next week. When going to the toilet this afternoon you noticed about a cup full of fresh red blood in the toilet bowl (only give amount and colour if asked specifically). You are still bleeding now and have soaked through two further pads.

You had a little bit of spotting at 10 weeks but have had no further problems with bleeding this pregnancy. At your anomaly scan you were noted to have a low-lying placenta and are due for a repeat scan next week to see if it has moved 'upwards'. You are rhesus negative. On the way to the hospital you have had some mild cramping, 'like period pain' but nothing severe.

Your last smear was about two years ago and you have never had any abnormal smears in the past. There is no past medical or family history of bleeding disorders. You have been taking iron tablets for the past few weeks which your community midwife gave you. You do not drink, smoke or take recreational drugs.

You are incredibly scared and anxious. You have not felt the baby move for the past few hours!

STATION 2

Name: Mrs Altweg

Age: 31 years old

Job: Betting shop attendant

You are a 31 year old lady who is 37 weeks into her first pregnancy. Apart from suffering with some lower back pain, for which you are seeing the physiotherapist, this pregnancy had been uneventful. A few days ago you started feeling tired and sick. Today you have a severe frontal headache which has made you vomit twice already this morning. Just after you had vomited you became very light-headed and had to sit down. It was then that you noticed flashing lights in your vision. You think this lasted on and off for a good hour.

Your partner also commented this morning that you face was looking a lot more swollen. You think your mother had something called 'pre-eclampsia' when she had you. You remember her telling you about her having to have an emergency caesarean section because she had very high blood pressure. You are incredibly anxious about this as you have been told pre-eclampsia can run in families. You really do not want to have a caesarean section and in your birth plan you wanted to use the birthing pool. You are worried that now you are feeling unwell you will no longer be able to do this.

You are not currently taking any medications and are not allergic to anything. You smoke about two cigarettes a day, but do not drink or take any drugs. As far as you know you have had no problems with your blood pressure prior to pregnancy. Your dad has diabetes but you have been tested this pregnancy and the results were all normal.

You feel fairly confident that if you could get rid of the headache you would feel a lot better. You are keen to know what you could take. Normally for headaches you take ibuprofen and this makes you feel a lot better, but you are very concerned about it affecting the baby. (Ask the candidate what you could take for your headache.)

At the end of the scenario ask the candidate for their diagnosis.

STATION 3

Name: Mrs Sally Gibbs

Age: 25 years old

Job: House wife

You are 10 weeks into your third pregnancy. For the past nine days you have been vomiting uncontrollably. You have no abdominal pain or headache but feel very dehydrated and are worried as you are barely passing any urine and what there has been was very concentrated and smelly. Otherwise you have not had any urinary symptoms and no pain passing urine. You are not able to tolerate any liquids and are now feeling incredibly weak. You don't feel strong enough to look after your 18 month old daughter.

You have had no bleeding or admissions to hospital so far this pregnancy. You had a similar problem with your first pregnancy but it was never this bad. Your mum is one of a twin, you have not had an ultrasound scan so far this pregnancy, but have a date for your 12 week scan in a fortnight.

This is your third pregnancy, all were by natural conception. You had a termination when you were 19 and also have your daughter, Poppy, who is 18 months old. Your husband is in the army and is currently abroad. You do not have any other family support which is why it has taken you so long to seek help. There is nobody to look after your daughter – this makes you very worried. If the candidate offers reasonable suggestions for help then you should appear more at ease. If they are unable to reassure you that it will be okay, you become more and more concerned and refuse to have any investigations.

At the end of the scenario you should ask the candidate if they wish to do any investigations on you and if so which ones.

STATION 4

Name: Miss Josephine Lovelock

Age: 21 years old

Job: Unemployed

You have been sent into the consultant clinic by your community midwife because your glucose tolerance test result is high. You feel well in yourself and have had no symptoms of diabetes. You have already been told that you have something called 'impaired glucose tolerance' but know very little about what this means or involves. All you were told was that the results weren't the same as diabetes because it wasn't high enough but you may develop diabetes later. If the candidate tells you the test result shows you have diabetes then tell them that the community midwife said you did not have diabetes – use the term 'impaired glucose tolerance'.

This is your first pregnancy and you are now 25 weeks pregnant. Up until now you have had no problems. You have no social support and live in a council flat. You are not sure who the father of your child is. You enjoy comfort eating and get very upset if you are told you need to cut out sugar from your diet. If the candidate mentions diet control and weight gain in a gentle and softly approached manner then you respond well to the idea of losing weight – engage with them about ways this could be done. If the candidate is not sensitive with regards to your weight and not empathic you become very defensive.

You grandfather is diabetic, but up until now you have had no medical problems. You smoke 20 cigarettes a day and have no intentions of giving up smoking. You drink alcohol socially (about 6 small glasses of wine or cocktails per week) and have not stopped this in the pregnancy as you feel it is 'within the limits'. You do not take any recreational drugs.

Notes:

In impaired glucose tolerance, patients are asked to keep a diary of their blood sugar readings and show these at all antenatal visits. The readings should be taken three times daily, before and after meals. Only if blood sugars are not well controlled then either oral hypoglycaemics or insulin injections may be started. Patients are required to have more frequent appointments with their midwife, obstetrician and diabetic specialist nurse. They also have a greater risk of developing diabetes in the future and will need to have a further glucose tolerance test after delivery.

Most diabetic patients are induced early at 38–39 weeks because there is a risk the baby could suffer from 'macrosomia'. When the baby is first born it is necessary to also monitor their blood sugars. Other complications relating to the child include a slightly higher risk of breathing problems and jaundice.

Overall gestational diabetes has a lot of implications for both mum and baby and it is very important that candidates understand this.

STATION 5

Name: Mrs Janet Wiley

Age: 43 years old

Job: Lawyer

You are a high flying lawyer who has a very poor obstetric history. By your dates you are 11 weeks and 2 days and your last menstrual period was the 3rd August. You are not very sure of your dates as you often have quite short cycles lasting about 20 to 22 days.

This is your third pregnancy. You had a termination aged 22. You tried to get pregnant for many years with no success and two years ago conceived with the help of IVF. Sadly you had premature labour at 24 weeks. Your little girl Katie was delivered vaginally but died at just one day old. This pregnancy has been conceived naturally – you think it is a miracle baby and you see it as your last chance. Last time the consultant mentioned possibly putting a stitch into the cervix to help prevent the premature labour, but since then you have moved house and are longer in the same area.

In 1995 you had a LLETZ for CIN 2 and it is thought your premature labour could have been as a result of this treatment. You also had a myomectomy in 2001 because it was thought your subfertility might be because of your fibroids.

You do not suffer with diabetes, autoimmune disease or thromboembolic diseases. As a child you suffered with acute renal failure which was secondary to dehydration when you had a burst appendix, but no history of cardiac disease. However, you have always been told your blood pressure is 'borderline high' but have never been treated for it.

You are currently taking folic acid and are not allergic to any medications. Your mother suffered with pre-eclampsia with you and because of this had to have an emergency caesarean section. Apart from this you have no other relevant family history.

You are an ex-smoker who gave up about 15 years ago. You have the occasional drink and have not taken any recreational drugs since you left university over 20 years ago.

Overall you know that this pregnancy is high risk, appear relieved when the candidate suggests they refer you to the hospital to see the consultant as soon as possible. If the candidate does not suggest this and feels you can be managed in the community you become anxious and upset.

STATION 6

Name: Mrs Estelle Ford

Age: 31 years old

Job: Playwright

It is seven days ago since you gave birth to your daughter, Poppy. It was your first ever pregnancy and was uncomplicated antenatally. You had a vaginal delivery with what you were told was a second degree tear and an episiotomy. Unfortunately after having a lovely natural birth you had to go to theatre for a manual removal of placenta. You were given some antibiotics afterwards which are now finished. You cannot remember the name of them but you think they started with an 'A'.

You have been feeling unwell for the last 24 hours. Last night you noticed you were incredibly shaky and couldn't stop sweating. You feel really unwell and have had a recorded temperature at home of 38.7°C after some paracetamol. You have some pain in your lower abdomen, which has only really developed over the last few hours and you also feel a little sore in your left flank. Your lochia has increased in the last 12 hours and you have been soaking pads every 5 hours or so. You also passed some large 50p size clots when you last went to the toilet. You don't think you have any urinary symptoms but everything down there is very sore anyway and you have prevented yourself going to the toilet as often as a result. You have had no smelly vaginal discharge. Your last cervical smear test was two years ago and was normal.

You are normally very fit and do not drink or smoke; there is no family history to note. Apart from the antibiotics you were given when you left hospital you are taking your iron tablets. You are allergic to strawberries and shellfish, but no medications that you know of. When you eat these foods you come up in a rash but you have never had any hospital admission and do not carry an EpiPen.

At the end of the scenario you should ask the candidate what they think the diagnosis is.

STATION 7

Name: Mrs Imogen Ward

Age: 32 years old

Job: Actress

You are 15 weeks into your first pregnancy and have been referred into the consultant in the antenatal clinic because you are pregnant with twins. On the 12 week scan they told you the twins were dichorionic and dizygotic.

You are incredibly anxious about the pregnancy because you have been told by so many people that having twins is a lot more complicated than singleton pregnancies. You are hoping to find out today what all these increased risks are. All you know is that there is an increased risk that both of them might not make it and that there is a risk that both may also die. This obviously frightens you a lot.

You have always dreamed of having a home water birth and want to know if this is still going to be possible. If the candidate is empathetic towards your desire then respond to them well explaining that if it is safer for the babies to be delivered in hospital then it is probably the better idea. If the candidate fails to show an understanding then you demand to speak to the consultant.

If a home birth is not an option then you would really like to at least have a normal delivery. You would like to know if this is possible and what the prerequisites are for having a vaginal delivery with twins. You would also like to know what 'dizygotic' and 'dichorionic' means. You have tried to look it up on the internet but could not really understand it.

You are fit and well and do not take any regular medications. You have no drug allergies and do not smoke or drink. You have never been pregnant before and have never had any miscarriages or terminations. The pregnancy was planned and you have a good relationship with your partner, who is very supportive. You do not have a family history of twin pregnancies.

STATION 8

Name: Miss Louise Paul

Age: 18 years old

Job: Unemployed

You are 36 weeks into your second pregnancy. You have had no previous miscarriages or terminations. You have been attending the antenatal clinic on a regular basis because you are a type 1 diabetic. Your control has not been ideal and the diabetic team has agreed to increase your insulin. You also had a fulminant eclamptic episode with your first baby. This manifested itself after a spontaneous vaginal delivery at 37 weeks where you had a seizure and were admitted to intensive care. So far in this pregnancy your blood pressure and urinalysis have been normal. The consultant has instructed you from 36 weeks to have twice weekly blood pressure checks and daily testing of your urine.

Within your current pregnancy you have been told that the baby is 'head up' since 32 weeks, and an ultrasound scan today has confirmed it is still breech. Your first pregnancy was cephalic. You are keen to have a normal vaginal delivery. Your placenta is high and posterior and you have never been told you have fibroids. Apart from the diabetes, this pregnancy has been uncomplicated so far with no antepartum haemorrhage or premature rupture of membranes. Apart from your insulin you are not taking any medications and are not allergic to anything. There is no family history to note.

You do not smoke or drink any alcohol. You live at home with your partner who is a builder and your first child who is now 2 years old. You do not work full-time but do the odd shift in the pub down the road for some spending money on child nappies/food/clothes.

If the candidate does not instigate the discussion about external cephalic version, ECV, then ask what is going to happen to you when you deliver and whether vaginal delivery is still a safe option despite the 'head up'. You have heard of ECV and are keen to give it a go. You would like to know what percentage of ECVs are successful and what will happen if it fails. You would also like to know what will happen between now and the ECV booking if you suddenly go into labour and your waters break.

STATION 9

Name: Miss Sally Graham

Age: 26 years old

Job: Policewoman

Today you have attended A&E because you have developed a colicky type of pain in your lower abdomen on the left-hand side. You are very anxious as you and your partner have been trying for a baby for the last 6 months and 2 days ago you had a positive pregnancy test and don't want anything to happen to the baby. Your last menstrual period was 8 weeks ago and you normally have 28 day cycles.

The pain woke you last night and has been very severe ever since. You have tried taking some paracetamol, but this did not really help. It is worse when you move, cough and laugh and better when you lie still. In the last hour you have developed pain at the bottom of your shoulder on the left-hand side. You have not felt sick with the pain and your bowels are opening normally. You have no urinary symptoms. In the last few hours you have noticed a few spots of dark blood on your knickers but no clots or soft tissue residues.

You had a surgical termination when you were 22 years old and have never had any miscarriages. Your last cervical smear was one year ago and normal. You were diagnosed with Chlamydia when you were 19 years old and treated with antibiotics but never had any complications from this that you know of. You have never had any 'pelvic' surgery as such, but had a perforated appendix when you were 12 years old, which was removed and you have always been worried this might affect your fertility.

At present you are taking folic acid because you have been told this helps the baby stay strong and healthy. You are allergic to penicillin, from which you develop an itchy rash. You used to smoke 20 a day but gave up when you met your partner three years ago. You haven't drunk since you found out you were pregnant but otherwise normally drink a glass of wine in an evening.

At the end of consultation ask the candidate what they think the diagnosis is.

STATION 10

Name: Mrs Sumita Patel

Age: 32 years old

Job: Social worker

You are a 32 year old who is 41 weeks into your second pregnancy. You had an early first trimester miscarriage one year ago for which a cause was not found. In this pregnancy you are beginning to become very uncomfortable as you have been suffering with symphysis pubis dysfunction (SPD) for the past two months. The pregnancy has been reasonably uncomplicated although you did have a couple of episodes of bleeding in the first trimester which were quite anxiety-provoking because of your previous miscarriage.

You are normally fit and well. Your only surgical history is a cholecystectomy performed with 'keyhole surgery' about 6 years ago for gallstones. You do not drink or smoke. You have been taking Co-codamol regularly because of the pain in your pelvis. However, you are not allergic to any medications. Your last cervical smear test was three years ago and normal.

If the candidate raises the possibility of induction you are very keen to go ahead with this as your SPD is causing you so much pain. You are happy to have a cervical sweep but would like to know what this entails and if there are any risks to the baby. Specifically ask the candidate if there are any risks of infection to the baby. You would also like to know what the induction of labour involves.

STATION 11

Name: Mrs Katherine Warner

Age: 38 years old

Job: Geologist

You have been sent in to the antenatal clinic today because your community midwife measured you at 31 cm when you are actually 35 weeks and 4 days pregnant. This is your fourth pregnancy in total. You had a medical termination when you were 19 years old and a first trimester miscarriage at 31 years of age. You also have a son called Joseph who is now four and a half. You measured small for dates with him and were induced at 36 weeks because his growth had drastically dropped off the charts and the doctors were worried about the blood supply to him not being adequate. Although you were induced you ended up having an emergency caesarean section because of foetal distress, which was also very distressing for you! Joseph weighed 4.2 lbs at birth and was monitored on the paediatric intensive care unit for a week before you were able to take him home. He was very tiny and fragile but is now fit and healthy and did not suffer from any neonatal illnesses.

You have had no real problems with this pregnancy so far. Your anomaly scans so far have been normal as far as you understand. The last one was performed at 20 weeks and you have not had another one since then. Your baby has had measurements which are on the 25th centile and you were told they were slightly small but not to worry and that no congenital abnormalities were seen. You have slightly raised blood pressure for which you take methyldopa 250mg four times a day. Essential hypertension was diagnosed in your first pregnancy and you have been taking the methyldopa ever since. You measure your blood pressure at home and it has been well controlled so far, measuring on average 130/85.

You do not drink, smoke or take any kind of recreational drugs. In your first pregnancy you remember being told you had quite low platelets, but apart from that you have no kidney problems or clotting disorders that you know of. You have never been told you suffered with pre-eclampsia and you think you have a very good diet including fresh fruit and vegetables.

You had your tonsils out when you were 10 years old and apart from the caesarean section you have never had any other operations. You had a kidney infection at the age of 21 for which you were admitted to hospital for intravenous antibiotics but this cleared up and has caused you no problems. You are not allergic to any medications.

STATION 12

Name: Mrs Jessica Woodstock

Age: 35 years old

Job: Recruitment consultant

You are 34 weeks into your first pregnancy. You have had no previous terminations or miscarriages. In the middle of the night you were woken by severe abdominal pain. It is constant with frequent episodes of severe exacerbations. Initially it was over the whole of the lower abdomen, but it has also spread round to the lower back now. You got up to go to the toilet and noticed a few spots of dark brown blood on your pyjama bottoms, but have not had any PV bleeding until this point or since. You were unable to get back to sleep because the pain was so severe.

Since the pain started you have only felt a few foetal movements which concerns you as your baby is normally very active first thing in the morning. Besides this you have not noticed any gushes of fluid or had your waters break. You have not been vomiting, nauseated or had any fevers or shivers. You last opened your bowels yesterday and it was normal. You have only passed a small amount of urine this morning and it was not painful.

You have smoked about 20 cigarettes a day since you were 17 years old. You have been drinking the odd glass of wine in the evening during the pregnancy but do not take any recreational drugs. Your community midwife has been keeping a close eye on you because you have had the odd high blood pressure reading and a little bit of protein in the urine. You haven't been diagnosed as having pre-eclampsia. As far as you know the baby is growing fine but your last scan was at 20 weeks and you haven't had any other scans since this time. The sonographer during the scan did mention something about a low placenta but told you not to worry because she said the placenta could still 'move' before delivery and it wasn't something you should be concerned over. Apart from the abdominal pain last night your pregnancy has been uneventful.

You had recurrent urinary tract infections as a teenager. At the age of 11 you had an operation on your right wrist which was fixed with pins. You are not taking any medications nor are you allergic to anything.

At the end of the consultation ask the candidate what they think is going on. Your last cervical smear test was last year and it was normal.

OBSTETRICS

Candidate Number:	University:
Date:	Year of Study:

STATION 1 – ANTEPARTUM HAEMORRHAGE

	Appropriate introduction (1=full name and role), checks patient's name, age and number of weeks pregnant (1)	2	1	0
	Explains purpose of interview and checks consent (2=does well, 1=adequately, 0=poorly or not done)	2	1	0
	Establishes Presenting Complaint:			
	Establishes volume (1) and colour (1) (dark brown/fresh red) of blood loss	2	1	0
	Takes a detailed history of associated abdominal pain (2=does well, 1=adequate)	2	1	0
	Previous bleeding in this pregnancy – number of weeks (1) and outcome (1)	2	1	0
	Asks after precipitating factors to the bleeding (e.g. intercourse, recent surgery)		1	0
	Asks whether patient is aware of the position of their placenta from previous scans		1	0
	Asks whether patient is aware of their blood group and rhesus status		1	0
	Establishes history of pregnancy to date (any current pregnancy-related problems such as pre-eclampsia, gestational diabetes, pregnancy-related hypertension etc.)	2	1	0
	Previous obstetric and gynaecology history:			
	Establishes history of previous pregnancies: • number of weeks when delivered (1) • method of delivery (1)	2	1	0
	Establishes history of previous pregnancies: • bleeding (APH/PPH) (1) • problems during pregnancy (i.e. pre-eclampsia, GDM) (1)	2	1	0
	Establishes history of previous miscarriages (1) and/or terminations (1)	2	1	0
	Establishes history of cervical smears: previous abnormal smears (1) and when last smear was taken (1)	2	1	0
	Previous general medical history:			
	Establishes personal (1) or family history (1) of bleeding disorder	2	1	0
	Relevant past medical (1) and surgical (1) history	2	1	0
	Establishes medications taken during (1) and prior to pregnancy (1)	2	1	0
	Establishes history of known drug allergies (1) and how they manifest (1)	2	1	0
	Smoking, alcohol and history of substance abuse (2=done well, 1=adequate)	2	1	0
	Relevant social history (e.g. housing circumstances, dependents, occupation etc.)		1	0
	Appropriate closure (e.g. explains next step, thanks patient and summarises) (2=does well, 1=adequately, 0=poorly or not done)	2	1	0
	Communication Skills			
	Appropriate questioning style (mix of open and closed questions) (2=does well, 1=adequately, 0=poorly or not done)	2	1	0
	Invites questions (1). Listens actively (1).	2	1	0
	Organised approach to history-taking (e.g. systematic, summarises, signposts change in focus of question)	2	1	0
	Simulated patient score (2=very good, 1=satisfactory, 0=poor)	2	1	0
	Total Score			

Global Rating	**1** Clear Fail	**2** Borderline	**3** Clear Pass	**4** Very Good	**5** Outstanding

Candidate Number:	University:
Date:	Year of Study:

STATION 2 – PRE-ECLAMPSIA

		2	1	0
	Appropriate introduction (1=full name and role), checks patient's name, age and number of weeks pregnant (1)	2	1	0
	Explains purpose of interview and checks consent (2=does well, 1=adequately, 0=poorly or not done)	2	1	0
	Presenting Complaint:			
	Enquires about nature of the headache (1) elicits complete history of nature of headache (1)	2	1	0
	Establishes presence of visual disturbances/flashing lights		1	0
	Elicits that patient has epigastric pain (1) and asks specifically about vomiting (1)	2	1	0
	Establishes history of swelling (1) specifically about face and hands (1)	2	1	0
	Asks after other systemic features: weight change, appetite, fever, rigors, seizures (2=three items; 1=two items; 0=one only or none)	2	1	0
	Previous obstetric and gynaecology history:			
	Asks about previous pregnancies and deliveries		1	0
	Establishes history of previous miscarriages (1) or terminations (1)	2	1	0
	Establishes history of cervical smears		1	0
	Other relevant history:			
	Relevant past medical history in particular regarding hypertension and diabetes	2	1	0
	Relevant family history of pre-eclampsia		1	0
	Establishes medications taken during (1) and prior to pregnancy (1)	2	1	0
	Establishes history of known drug allergies (1) and how they manifest (1)	2	1	0
	Relevant social history (e.g. housing circumstances, dependents, occupation etc.)		1	0
	Explores patient's ideas, concerns and expectations	2	1	0
	Candidate to explain to patient that NSAIDs are not appropriate to use in pregnancy (1) however, paracetamol is considered safe for use (1)	2	1	0
	Appropriate closure (e.g. explains next step, thanks patient and summarises) (2=does well, 1=adequately, 0=poorly or not done)	2	1	0
	Communication Skills			
	Appropriate questioning style (mix of open and closed questions) (2=does well, 1=adequately, 0=poorly or not done)	2	1	0
	Invites questions (1). Listens actively (1).	2	1	0
	Organised approach to history-taking (e.g. systematic, summarises, signposts change in focus of question)	2	1	0
	Simulated patient score (2=very good, 1=satisfactory, 0=poor)	2	1	0
	Examiner to ask: 'What are your differential diagnoses?'			
	Candidate states an appropriate diagnosis of pre-eclampsia (1) and offers an appropriate differential diagnosis (e.g. migraine, tension headache, gastritis) (1)	2	1	0
	Examiner to ask: 'What investigations/management would you recommend?'			
	Candidate suggests referral to hospital under obstetric care for close monitoring, administration of antihypertensives, CTG to assess the foetus and consideration of anticonvulsants (magnesium sulphate) and early delivery with possible induction of labour or caesarean section if thought appropriate by specialist (2=any three suggestions, 1=any two suggestions)	2	1	0
	Investigations to include: regular blood pressure monitoring, blood tests including liver function, platelets, clotting, renal function and urate. Urine protein levels may also be requested (urinalysis and protein creatine ratio, with possible 24 hour urine collection being required) (2=any three suggestions, 1=any two suggestions)	2	1	0
	Total Score			

Global Rating	1 Clear Fail	2 Borderline	3 Clear Pass	4 Very Good	5 Outstanding

Candidate Number:		University:		
Date:		Year of Study:		

STATION 3 – HYPEREMESIS GRAVIDARUM

	Appropriate introduction (1=full name and role), checks patient's name, age and number of weeks pregnant (1)	**2**	**1**	**0**
	Explains purpose of interview and checks consent (2=does well, 1=adequately, 0=poorly or not done)	**2**	**1**	**0**
	Presenting Complaint:			
	Establishes history of vomiting: how long the patient has been vomiting for (1) and whether the patient is tolerating any food or water (1)	**2**	**1**	**0**
	Establishes history of abdominal pain (1) or headache (1)	**2**	**1**	**0**
	Establishes history of urinary symptoms (1) and volume and colour of urine (1)	**2**	**1**	**0**
	Enquires as to whether patient has had an ultrasound scan so far this pregnancy (important to exclude molar pregnancy and twins)		**1**	**0**
	Establishes history of any bleeding in early pregnancy		**1**	**0**
	Asks for history of foreign travel, food poisoning, infective contacts		**1**	**0**
	Asks after other systemic features: weight change, appetite, fever, rigors, seizures (2=three items; 1=two items; 0=one only or none)	**2**	**1**	**0**
	Previous obstetric and gynaecology history:			
	Establishes history of similar symptoms in previous pregnancy: • antenatal history, asks specifically about hyperemesis (1) • problems with delivery and postpartum (1)	**2**	**1**	**0**
	Establishes history of previous miscarriages (1) or terminations (1)	**2**	**1**	**0**
	Establishes history of cervical smears		**1**	**0**
	Other relevant history:			
	Relevant past medical history	**2**	**1**	**0**
	Relevant family history of twins (1) or hyperemesis (1)	**2**	**1**	**0**
	Establishes medications taken during (1) and prior to pregnancy (1)	**2**	**1**	**0**
	Establishes history of known drug allergies		**1**	**0**
	Relevant social history (e.g. housing circumstances, dependents, occupation etc.)		**1**	**0**
	Explores patient's ideas, concerns and expectations and reassures appropriately	**2**	**1**	**0**
	Appropriate closure (e.g. explains next step, thanks patient and summarises) (2=does well, 1=adequately, 0=poorly or not done)	**2**	**1**	**0**
	Communication Skills			
	Appropriate questioning style (mix of open and closed questions) (2=does well, 1=adequately, 0=poorly or not done)	**2**	**1**	**0**
	Invites questions (1). Listens actively (1).	**2**	**1**	**0**
	Organised approach to history-taking (e.g. systematic, summarises, signposts change in focus of question)	**2**	**1**	**0**
	Simulated patient score (2=very good, 1=satisfactory, 0=poor)	**2**	**1**	**0**
	Examiner to ask: 'What are your differential diagnoses?'			
	Candidate states an appropriate diagnosis of hyperemesis gravidarum (1) and offers an appropriate differential diagnosis (e.g. twin pregnancy, food poisoning, dehydration) (1)	**2**	**1**	**0**
	Examiner to ask: 'What investigations/management would you recommend?'			
	Candidate suggests admission to hospital for blood tests checking FBC, U&Es, LFTs, glucose, CRP; urine dipstick for ketones and infection and an ultrasound scan to exclude twin or molar pregnancy (2=any three suggestions, 1=any two suggestions)	**2**	**1**	**0**
	Management would include close observation of blood pressure, pulse, renal function, administration of anti-emetic medication and resuscitation with intravenous fluids (2=any three suggestions, 1=any two suggestions)	**2**	**1**	**0**
	Total Score			

Global Rating	**1** Clear Fail	**2** Borderline	**3** Clear Pass	**4** Very Good	**5** Outstanding

Candidate Number:	University:
Date:	Year of Study:

STATION 4 – GESTATIONAL DIABETES

Appropriate introduction (1=full name and role), checks patient's name, age and number of weeks pregnant (1)	2	1	0
Explains purpose of interview and checks consent (2=does well, 1=adequately, 0=poorly or not done)	2	1	0
Explanation of test results:			
Establishes what patient understands about the recent investigation performed (1) and if she is aware of the results (1)	2	1	0
Explanation of diagnosis of 'impaired glucose tolerance' (1) because GTT result <11.1 but >7.9 (1)	2	1	0
Explains that the diagnosis stems from a lack of resistance of the body to insulin (1) causing blood sugar levels to rise (1)	2	1	0
Reassures patient that although the results are not normal, there are ways of managing the condition		1	0
Advises patient on diet control (1) in particular to cut down on sugar intake (1)	2	1	0
Explains that if blood sugars are poorly controlled with diet she may require tablets (1) or insulin injections (1)	2	1	0
Explains to patient that she will need to check her blood sugar levels at home regularly to monitor her progress (1), three times a day before and after meals (1)	2	1	0
Advises patient of increased frequency of antenatal visits (1) and also to see diabetic specialist teams (physicians and nurses) (1)	2	1	0
Implications for the baby:			
Explains that most patients with blood sugar problems have an induction of labour (1) at 38–39 week' gestation (1)	2	1	0
Explains that if sugar levels are poorly controlled then the baby is at risk of developing macrosomia (1) and risk of shoulder dystocia at birth (1)	2	1	0
Tells patient that the baby may also have problems with their blood sugar levels too at first (1) but reassures that the paediatric doctors will check this regularly (1)	2	1	0
Candidate mentions that the baby may also suffer from jaundice or with breathing problems (1) and the paediatric doctors will be present when it is born (1)	2	1	0
Obstetric history:			
Asks how the patient is progressing with current pregnancy and any problems encountered so far specifically symptoms of polyuria (1) and polydypsia (1)	2	1	0
Enquires after previous miscarriages (1) or terminations (2)	2	1	0
Other relevant history:			
Relevant past medical history	2	1	0
Relevant family history, in particular of diabetes or gestational diabetes		1	0
Establishes medications taken during (1) and prior to pregnancy (1)	2	1	0
Establishes history of known drug allergies (1)		1	0
Establishes smoking, alcohol and recreational drug history	2	1	0
Relevant social history (e.g. housing circumstances, dependents, occupation etc.)		1	0
Explores patient's ideas, concerns and expectations and reassures appropriately	2	1	0
Appropriate closure (e.g. explains next step, thanks patient and summarises) (2=does well, 1=adequately, 0=poorly or not done)	2	1	0
Communication Skills			
Appropriate questioning style (mix of open and closed questions) (2=does well, 1=adequately, 0=poorly or not done)	2	1	0
Invites questions (1). Listens actively (1).	2	1	0
Organised approach to history-taking (e.g. systematic, summarises, signposts change in focus of question)	2	1	0
Simulated patient score (2=very good, 1=satisfactory, 0=poor)	2	1	0
Total Score			

Global Rating	1 Clear Fail	2 Borderline	3 Clear Pass	4 Very Good	5 Outstanding

Candidate Number:	University:
Date:	Year of Study:

STATION 5 – BOOKING VISIT

		2	1	0
	Appropriate introduction (1=full name and role), checks patient's name, age and number of weeks pregnant (1)	2	1	0
	Explains purpose of interview and checks consent (2=does well, 1=adequately, 0=poorly or not done)	2	1	0
	Obstetric History:			
	Establishes last menstrual period (1) and accuracy of dates (1)	2	1	0
	Establishes number of previous pregnancies (1) and pregnancy-related complications (1) e.g. premature labour or foetal loss	2	1	0
	Enquires after previous miscarriages (1) or terminations (2)	2	1	0
	Establishes mode of delivery with previous pregnancies		1	0
	Establishes history of cervical smears – date of last smear (1) and history of abnormal smears and previous treatment (1)	2	1	0
	Establishes history of previous uterine surgery (1) or other surgery (1)	2	1	0
	Past medically relevant history:			
	Establishes history of hypertension (1) and diabetes (1)	2	1	0
	Establishes history of autoimmune disease (1) and thromboembolic disease (1)	2	1	0
	Establishes history of cardiac (1) and renal disease (1)	2	1	0
	Establishes family history of chromosomal abnormalities/birth defects		1	0
	Establishes history of gestational diabetes (1) and pre-ecplampsia (1)	2	1	0
	Establishes history of hypertension		1	0
	Establishes relevant any other past medical history		1	0
	Establishes medications taken during (1) and prior to pregnancy (1)	2	1	0
	Establishes history of known drug allergies		1	0
	Establishes smoking, alcohol and recreational drug history	2	1	0
	Relevant social history (e.g. housing circumstances, dependents, occupation etc.)		1	0
	Explores patient's ideas, concerns and expectations and reassures appropriately	2	1	0
	Appropriate closure (e.g. explains next step, thanks patient and summarises) (2=does well, 1=adequately, 0=poorly or not done)	2	1	0
	Communication Skills			
	Appropriate questioning style (mix of open and closed questions) (2=does well, 1=adequately, 0=poorly or not done)	2	1	0
	Invites questions (1). Listens actively (1).	2	1	0
	Organised approach to history-taking (e.g. systematic, summarises, signposts change in focus of question)	2	1	0
	Simulated patient score (2=very good, 1=satisfactory, 0=poor)	2	1	0
	Examiner to ask: 'How would you stratisfy the risk of this pregnancy?'			
	Candidate establishes that pregnancy is high (1) and the patient should be referred for specialist lead services during the course of the pregnancy in hospital (1)	2	1	0
	Total Score			

Global Rating	1 Clear Fail	2 Borderline	3 Clear Pass	4 Very Good	5 Outstanding

Candidate Number:		University:	
Date:		Year of Study:	

STATION 6 – PUERPERAL PYREXIA

	Appropriate introduction (1=full name and role), checks patient's name, age and time since delivery (1)	2	1	0
	Explains purpose of interview and checks consent (2=does well, 1=adequately, 0=poorly or not done)	2	1	0
	Establishes Presenting Complaint:			
	Establishes length of time of presenting complaint	▓	1	0
	Establishes mode of delivery (1) and complications at delivery – retained placenta/prolonged rupture of membranes/pyrexia in labour (1)	2	1	0
	Takes a detailed history of any associated pain (2=does well, 1=adequate)	2	1	0
	Establishes history of lochia: number of pads being soaked over what time (1) and passage of clots (1)	2	1	0
	Establishes history of urinary symptoms: dysuria (1) and urinary frequency (1)	2	1	0
	Establishes history of perineal wound (1) and offensive vaginal discharge (1)	2	1	0
	Asks after other systemic features: weight change, appetite, fever, rigors, seizures (2=three items; 1=two items; 0=one only or none)	2	1	0
	Enquires after other features of infection such as cough, sputum production, change in bowel habits, diarrhoea, other skin wounds such as recent cannula sites (2=any three, 1=any two)	2	1	0
	Previous obstetric and gynaecology history:			
	Establishes history of previous pregnancies and pregnancy-related complications	▓	1	0
	Establishes history of previous miscarriages (1) or terminations (1)	2	1	0
	Establishes history of cervical smears: previous abnormal smears and when last smear was taken	2	1	0
	Previous general medical history:			
	Relevant past medical (1) and surgical (1) history	2	1	0
	Establishes medications taken during (1) and prior to pregnancy (1)	2	1	0
	Establishes history of known drug allergies (1) and how they manifest (1)	2	1	0
	Smoking, alcohol and history of substance abuse (2=done well, 1=adequate)	2	1	0
	Appropriate closure (e.g. explains next step, thanks patient and summarises) (2=does well, 1=adequately, 0=poorly or not done)	2	1	0
	Communication Skills			
	Appropriate questioning style (mix of open and closed questions) (2=does well, 1=adequately, 0=poorly or not done)	2	1	0
	Invites questions (1). Listens actively (1).	2	1	0
	Organised approach to history-taking (e.g. systematic, summarises, signposts change in focus of question)	2	1	0
	Simulated patient score (2=very good, 1=satisfactory, 0=poor)	2	1	0
	Examiner to ask: 'What do you think the diagnosis is?'			
	Candidate suggests the diagnosis of endometritis (1) and a differential diagnosis of pyelonephritis (1)	2	1	0
	Total Score			

Global Rating	1 Clear Fail	2 Borderline	3 Clear Pass	4 Very Good	5 Outstanding

Candidate Number:	University:
Date:	Year of Study:

STATION 7 – TWIN PREGNANCY

Appropriate introduction (1=full name and role), checks patient's name, age and number of weeks pregnant (1)	**2**	**1**	**0**
Explains purpose of interview and checks consent (2=does well, 1=adequately, 0=poorly or not done)	**2**	**1**	**0**
Establishes Antepartum Complications of Twin Pregnancy:			
Starts by asking patient what they hope to gain from the interview and their specific concerns		**1**	**0**
Explains that pregnancy care will be consultant-led in cases of twin pregnancies		**1**	**0**
Explains increased risk of preterm labour (1) and miscarriage (1)	**2**	**1**	**0**
Explains increased risk of congenital abnormalities (1) and intra-uterine growth restriction (1)	**2**	**1**	**0**
Explains increased risk of medical complications for mum: gestational diabetes, hyperemesis (1), pre-eclampsia (1) and anaemia (1) (maximum any 2 marks)	**2**	**1**	**0**
Establishes Intrapartum Complications of Twin Pregnancy:			
Explains caesarean section is more likely (1) because of malpresentation of second twin (1)	**2**	**1**	**0**
Explains that with vaginal delivery there is more risk to the second twin (1) – cord prolapse/breech presentation (1)	**2**	**1**	**0**
Explains increased risk of postpartum haemorrhage (1) reassures patient that hormone drip will be started straight after delivery to help reduce risk (1)	**2**	**1**	**0**
Explanation of dichorionic dizygotic twin pregnancy:			
Explains term 'dizygotic' – meaning different oocytes (1) are fertilised by different sperm (1)	**2**	**1**	**0**
Explains term 'dichorionic' – meaning each foetus has its own placenta (1) and twins will not be identical (1)	**2**	**1**	**0**
Mode of twin delivery:			
Explains to patient that home birth is not appropriate in a twin pregnancy		**1**	**0**
If a vaginal delivery is an option, twins are normally induced at 38–39 weeks		**1**	**0**
When the twin which is presenting to the cervix first is cephalic in presentation, then (as long as there are no other complications), vaginal delivery is an option	**2**	**1**	**0**
When the twin who is presenting to the cervix first is lying in a 'breech' or 'transverse' position (1) then caesarean section is the best choice of delivery (1)	**2**	**1**	**0**
The presentation and lie of the foetuses are likely to change during the course of the pregnancy as they grow (1) so it's too early to determine the mode of delivery (1)	**2**	**1**	**0**
Previous obstetric history:			
Establishes history of previous pregnancies, in particular twin pregnancies		**1**	**0**
Establishes history of previous miscarriages (1) or terminations (1)	**2**	**1**	**0**
Establishes history of cervical smears: previous abnormal smears and when last smear was taken	**2**	**1**	**0**
Previous general medical history:			
Relevant past (1) medical and surgical (1) history	**2**	**1**	**0**
Establishes medications taken during (1) and prior to pregnancy (1)	**2**	**1**	**0**
Establishes history of known drug allergies		**1**	**0**
Smoking, alcohol and history of substance abuse (2=done well, 1=adequate)	**2**	**1**	**0**
Relevant social history (e.g. housing circumstances, dependents, occupation etc.)		**1**	**0**
Appropriate closure (e.g. explains next step, thanks patient and summarises) (2=does well, 1=adequately, 0=poorly or not done)	**2**	**1**	**0**
Communication Skills			
Appropriate questioning style (mix of open and closed questions) (2=does well, 1=adequately, 0=poorly or not done)	**2**	**1**	**0**
Invites questions (1). Listens actively (1).	**2**	**1**	**0**
Organised approach to history-taking (e.g. systematic, summarises, signposts change in focus of question)	**2**	**1**	**0**
Simulated patient score (2=very good, 1=satisfactory, 0=poor)	**2**	**1**	**0**
Total Score			

Global Rating	**1** Clear Fail	**2** Borderline	**3** Clear Pass	**4** Very Good	**5** Outstanding

Candidate Number:	University:
Date:	Year of Study:

STATION 8 – BREECH PREGNANCY

	Appropriate introduction (1=full name and role), checks patient's name, age and number of weeks pregnant (1)	2	1	0
	Explains purpose of interview and checks consent (2=does well, 1=adequately, 0=poorly or not done)	2	1	0
	Establishes Presenting Complaint:			
	Asks patient how their current pregnancy is progressing so far		1	0
	Discusses recent ultrasound scan results (1) and asks patient what they understand about the findings (e.g. breech lie) (1)	2	1	0
	Establishes what patient understands regarding breech deliveries		1	0
	Establishes aetiology for breech and contraindications to ECV:			
	Asks about history of uterine fibroids		1	0
	Asks about the position of the placenta		1	0
	Establishes history of antepartum haemorrhage (1) or premature rupture of membranes (1)	2	1	0
	Previous history of breech delivery		1	0
	Previous obstetric and gynaecology history:			
	Establishes history of complications in previous pregnancies (e.g. fulminant pre-eclampsia) (1) and enquires as to management of this pregnancy – patient is to dipstick her urine daily and have twice weekly blood pressures taken from 36 weeks (1)	2	1	0
	Establishes mode of delivery of previous pregnancies		1	0
	Establishes history of previous miscarriages (1) or terminations (1)	2	1	0
	Explanation of management and delivery:			
	Confirms patient has no absolute contraindications to an external cephalic version (1) despite having a high risk pregnancy i.e. breech (1)	2	1	0
	Candidate explains not all ECV is successful (1), there is a 50% chance of failure or baby turning back to original position (1)	2	1	0
	Explains if ECV fails or patient chooses not to have ECV we would recommend an elective caesarean section (1) at 38 weeks (1)	2	1	0
	Candidate explains to patient that if she goes into labour she needs to attend the hospital as a matter of urgency (1) as there is an increased risk of cord prolapse (1)	2	1	0
	Previous general medical history:			
	Relevant past medical (1) and surgical (1) history	2	1	0
	Establishes medications taken during (1) and prior to pregnancy (1)	2	1	0
	Establishes history of known drug allergies		1	0
	Smoking, alcohol and history of substance abuse (2=done well, 1=adequate)	2	1	0
	Relevant social history (e.g. housing circumstances, dependents, occupation etc.)		1	0
	Appropriate closure (e.g. explains next step, thanks patient and summarises) (2=does well, 1=adequately, 0=poorly or not done)	2	1	0
	Communication Skills			
	Appropriate questioning style (mix of open and closed questions) (2=does well, 1=adequately, 0=poorly or not done)	2	1	0
	Invites questions (1). Listens actively (1).	2	1	0
	Organised approach to history-taking (e.g. systematic, summarises, signposts change in focus of question)	2	1	0
	Simulated patient score (2=very good, 1=satisfactory, 0=poor)	2	1	0
	Total Score			

Global Rating	1 Clear Fail	2 Borderline	3 Clear Pass	4 Very Good	5 Outstanding

Candidate Number:		University:	
Date:		Year of Study:	

STATION 9 – EARLY PREGNANCY COMPLICATIONS

	Appropriate introduction (1=full name and role), checks patient's name, age and number of weeks pregnant (1)	**2**	**1**	**0**
	Explains purpose of interview and checks consent (2=does well, 1=adequately, 0=poorly or not done)	**2**	**1**	**0**
	Establishes Presenting Complaint:			
	Establishes length of time of presenting complaint		**1**	**0**
	Takes a detailed history of any associated pain (2=does well, 1=adequate)	**2**	**1**	**0**
	Establishes history of PV bleeding: volume, colour (1) and if passing large clots (1)	**2**	**1**	**0**
	Establishes history of nausea/vomiting (1) and bowel symptoms (1)	**2**	**1**	**0**
	Establishes history of urinary symptoms: frequency (1) and dysuria (1)	**2**	**1**	**0**
	Asks after other systemic features: weight change, appetite, fever, rigors, seizures (2=three items; 1=two items; 0=one only or none)	**2**	**1**	**0**
	Previous obstetric and gynaecology history:			
	Establishes last menstrual period (1) and usual length of cycles (1)	**2**	**1**	**0**
	Establishes history of previous pregnancies		**1**	**0**
	Establishes history of previous miscarriages (1) or terminations (1)	**2**	**1**	**0**
	Establishes history of cervical smears: previous abnormal smears (1) and when last smear was taken (1)	**2**	**1**	**0**
	Risk factors for ectopic pregnancy:			
	Establishes history of previous ectopic pregnancy (1) and if so, management (1)	**2**	**1**	**0**
	Establishes history of pelvic inflammatory disease		**1**	**0**
	Establishes history of assisted conception		**1**	**0**
	Establishes history of previous pelvic surgery		**1**	**0**
	Previous general medical history:			
	Relevant past medical (1) and surgical (1) history	**2**	**1**	**0**
	Establishes medications taken during (1) and prior to pregnancy (1)	**2**	**1**	**0**
	Establishes history of known drug allergies (1) and nature of allergy (1)	**2**	**1**	**0**
	Smoking, alcohol and history of substance abuse (2=done well, 1=adequate)	**2**	**1**	**0**
	Appropriate closure (e.g. explains next step, thanks patient and summarises) (2=does well, 1=adequately, 0=poorly or not done)	**2**	**1**	**0**
	Communication Skills			
	Appropriate questioning style (mix of open and closed questions) (2=does well, 1=adequately, 0=poorly or not done)	**2**	**1**	**0**
	Invites questions (1). Listens actively (1).	**2**	**1**	**0**
	Organised approach to history-taking (e.g. systematic, summarises, signposts change in focus of question)	**2**	**1**	**0**
	Simulated patient score (2=very good, 1=satisfactory, 0=poor)	**2**	**1**	**0**
	Examiner to ask: 'What do you think the diagnosis is?'			
	Candidate suggests the diagnosis of ectopic pregnancy (1) or threatened miscarriage (1)	**2**	**1**	**0**
	Examiner to ask: 'Name one blood test and imaging investigation you would request.'			
	Candidate suggests beta-HCG blood levels (1) and transvaginal ultrasound scan (1)	**2**	**1**	**0**
	Total Score			

Global Rating	**1** Clear Fail	**2** Borderline	**3** Clear Pass	**4** Very Good	**5** Outstanding

Candidate Number:		University:		
Date:		Year of Study:		

STATION 10 – POST-DATES PREGNANCY

Appropriate introduction (1=full name and role), checks patient's name, age and number of weeks pregnant (1)	2	1	0
Explains purpose of interview and checks consent (2=does well, 1=adequately, 0=poorly or not done)	2	1	0
Enquires after Current Pregnancy-Related Issues:			
Enquires about any complications in current pregnancy		1	0
Establishes that patient will be post-dates if pregnancy is prolonged after 42 weeks (1) and that this may hold risks to the baby (1)	2	1	0
Explains that risks to baby in post-dates pregnancy include malnutrition or chest-related complications (2=explains well and in sensitive manner, 1=adequate)	2	1	0
Cause for post-dates delivery is not always clearly established		1	0
Previous obstetric and gynaecology history:			
Establishes history of previous pregnancies and related complications	2	1	0
Establishes history of previous miscarriages (1) or terminations (1)	2	1	0
Establishes history of cervical smears: previous abnormal smears and when last smear was taken	2	1	0
Explanation of cervical sweep:			
Establishes that to advance the delivery a cervical sweep or induction is performed (1) and pregnancy will not be allowed to go over 42 weeks (1)	2	1	0
Candidate explains to patient that a cervical sweep should be performed (1) and this increases the chances of labour happening in the next 48 hours (1)	2	1	0
Candidate explains that a cervical sweep entails a vaginal examination and assessment of favourability (1) after which two fingers are used to sweep between membranes and cervix (1)	2	1	0
Explains risks of cervical sweep: small amount of bleeding after (1) and risk of rupture of membranes (1)	2	1	0
Candidate warns patient it could painful		1	0
Candidate explains there are no risks of infection to the baby		1	0
Explanation of induction of labour:			
Candidate explains to patient that an internal examination is performed to assess favourability of cervix		1	0
If the cervix is favourable then the membranes will be ruptured (1) and hormone drip started to induce contractions (1)	2	1	0
If the cervix is unfavourable then patient will be given a vaginal tablet called Prostin to ripen the cervix (1) and this may have to be repeated (1)	2	1	0
Candidate explains that Prostin can cause the uterus to stimulate too much (1) if this happens they will be given another medicine to help it relax (1)	2	1	0
Candidate explains if a hormone drip is used then baby will have to be monitored (1) continuously (1) with a CTG	2	1	0
Previous general medical history:			
Relevant past medical (1) and surgical (1) history	2	1	0
Establishes medications taken during (1) and prior to pregnancy (1)	2	1	0
Establishes history of known drug allergies (1) and nature of allergy (1)	2	1	0
Smoking, alcohol and history of substance abuse (2=done well, 1=adequate)	2	1	0
Enquires after patient's ideas/concerns and expectations of procedure		1	0
Appropriate closure (e.g. explains next step, thanks patient and summarises) (2=does well, 1=adequately, 0=poorly or not done)	2	1	0
Communication Skills			
Appropriate questioning style (mix of open and closed questions) (2=does well, 1=adequately, 0=poorly or not done)	2	1	0
Invites questions (1). Listens actively (1).	2	1	0
Organised approach to history-taking (e.g. systematic, summarises, signposts change in focus of question)		1	0
Simulated patient score (2=very good, 1=satisfactory, 0=poor)	2	1	0
Total Score			

Global Rating	1 Clear Fail	2 Borderline	3 Clear Pass	4 Very Good	5 Outstanding

Candidate Number:	University:
Date:	Year of Study:

STATION 11 – INTRA-UTERINE GROWTH RETARDATION

	Appropriate introduction (1=full name and role), checks patient's name, age and time since delivery (1)	**2**	**1**	**0**
	Explains purpose of interview and checks consent (2=does well, 1=adequately, 0=poorly or not done)	**2**	**1**	**0**
	Establishes Presenting Complaint:			
	Enquires about progress and any complications relating to current pregnancy		**1**	**0**
	Establishes whether any abnormal results on anomaly scans to date		**1**	**0**
	Enquires specifically about growth of current baby on charts in the anomaly scans		**1**	**0**
	Previous obstetric and gynaecology history:			
	Establishes history of previous pregnancies and establishes patient's history of essential hypertension (1) and pre-eclampsia (1) in last pregnancy	**2**	**1**	**0**
	Establishes IUGR in first pregnancy (1) and enquires regarding outcomes (1)	**2**	**1**	**0**
	Establishes history of previous mode of delivery – emergency caesarean section (1) and reason for it (1)	**2**	**1**	**0**
	Establishes weight at delivery of first child		**1**	**0**
	Establishes history of previous miscarriages (1) or terminations (1)	**2**	**1**	**0**
	Establishes history of cervical smears: previous abnormal smears and when last smear was taken	**2**	**1**	**0**
	Previous general medical history:			
	Relevant past medical of kidney disease (1) and clotting disorders (1)	**2**	**1**	**0**
	Enquires after a history of poor nutritional intake		**1**	**0**
	Establishes medications taken during (1) and prior to pregnancy (1)	**2**	**1**	**0**
	Establishes history of known drug allergies		**1**	**0**
	Smoking, alcohol and history of substance abuse (2=done well, 1=adequate)	**2**	**1**	**0**
	Relevant social history (e.g. housing circumstances, dependents, occupation etc.)		**1**	**0**
	Appropriate closure (e.g. explains next step, thanks patient and summarises) (2=does well, 1=adequately, 0=poorly or not done)	**2**	**1**	**0**
	Communication Skills			
	Appropriate questioning style (mix of open and closed questions) (2=does well, 1=adequately, 0=poorly or not done)	**2**	**1**	**0**
	Invites questions (1). Listens actively (1).	**2**	**1**	**0**
	Organised approach to history-taking (e.g. systematic, summarises, signposts change in focus of question)		**1**	**0**
	Simulated patient score (2=very good, 1=satisfactory, 0=poor)	**2**	**1**	**0**
	Total Score			

Global Rating	**1** Clear Fail	**2** Borderline	**3** Clear Pass	**4** Very Good	**5** Outstanding

Candidate Number:		University:	
Date:		Year of Study:	

STATION 12 – ABDOMINAL PAIN IN PREGNANCY

	Appropriate introduction (1=full name and role), checks patient's name, age and number of weeks in current pregnancy (1)	**2**	**1**	**0**
	Explains purpose of interview and checks consent (2=does well, 1=adequately, 0=poorly or not done)	**2**	**1**	**0**
	Establishes Presenting Complaint:			
	Establishes length of time of presenting complaint		**1**	**0**
	Takes a detailed history of abdominal pain (2=does well, 1=adequate)	**2**	**1**	**0**
	Asks about associated decrease in foetal movements		**1**	**0**
	Establishes any associated vaginal bleeding (e.g. volume, number of pads being soaked, passage of clots, number of episodes, any associated spontaneous rupture of membranes) (2=does well, 1=adequate)	**2**	**1**	**0**
	Enquires about history of urinary symptoms: dysuria (1) and urinary frequency (1)	**2**	**1**	**0**
	Enquires about bowel symptoms: vomiting (1), change in bowel habits (1)	**2**	**1**	**0**
	Asks after other systemic features: weight change, appetite, fever, rigors, seizures (2=three items; 1=two items; 0=one only or none)	**2**	**1**	**0**
	Current pregnancy:			
	Current pregnancy-related complications to date (1) and their management (1)	**2**	**1**	**0**
	Establishes time of last anomaly scan (1) and the findings of the scan, in particular of intra-uterine growth retardation and placenta position (1)	**2**	**1**	**0**
	Previous obstetric and gynaecology history:			
	Establishes history of previous pregnancies (1), pregnancy-related complications (1)	**2**	**1**	**0**
	Establishes history of previous miscarriages (1) or terminations (1)	**2**	**1**	**0**
	Establishes history of cervical smears: previous abnormal smears (1) and when last smear was taken (1)	**2**	**1**	**0**
	Previous general medical history:			
	Relevant past medical (1) and surgical history (1) specifically of hypertension or pre-eclampsia	**2**	**1**	**0**
	Establishes medications taken during (1) and prior to pregnancy (1)	**2**	**1**	**0**
	Establishes history of known drug allergies (1) and how they manifest (1)	**2**	**1**	**0**
	Smoking, alcohol and history of substance abuse (2=done well, 1=adequate)	**2**	**1**	**0**
	Enquires after social circumstance (e.g. housing, occupation, partner relationship)		**1**	**0**
	Appropriate closure (e.g. explains next step, thanks patient and summarises) (2=does well, 1=adequately, 0=poorly or not done)	**2**	**1**	**0**
	Communication Skills			
	Appropriate questioning style (mix of open and closed questions) (2=does well, 1=adequately, 0=poorly or not done)	**2**	**1**	**0**
	Invites questions (1). Listens actively (1).	**2**	**1**	**0**
	Organised approach to history-taking (e.g. systematic, summarises, signposts change in focus of question)		**1**	**0**
	Simulated patient score (2=very good, 1=satisfactory, 0=poor)	**2**	**1**	**0**
	Examiner to ask: 'What do you think the diagnosis is?'			
	Candidate suggests the diagnosis of concealed (1) placental abruption (1)	**2**	**1**	**0**
	Total Score			

Global Rating	**1** Clear Fail	**2** Borderline	**3** Clear Pass	**4** Very Good	**5** Outstanding

CHAPTER 6: MEDICAL ETHICS

Written by Dr. S. Shelmerdine

- Mental Health Act
- Capacity to Consent
- Maintaining Patient Confidentiality
- Do Not Attempt Resuscitation (DNAR) Order
- Advance Directives
- Breaking Patient Confidentiality
- Euthanasia
- Refusal of Medical Treatment

THE STATIONS

STATION 1
Time allowed: 10 minutes

You are a junior doctor working in psychiatry.

Mr Christopher Duffy is a 25 year old patient with a two year history of schizophrenia. He is non-compliant on treatment and occasionally suffers from acute paranoid delusions. Earlier this afternoon he was convinced that his best friend was stealing his car and was voicing intents of setting his friend's house on fire. He was refusing to come to hospital and his family were not contactable. As a result he was detained under Section 2 of the Mental Health Act 1983.

His mother has come to hospital this evening to visit him and has a few questions regarding why her son is detained in hospital. Please speak to her and address any questions she has.

STATION 2
Time allowed: 10 minutes

You are a junior doctor working in orthopaedics.

Mr Clancy is an elderly woman who was admitted with a fractured neck of femur. She was booked to undergo surgery to have a hemiarthroplasty this morning. However, the nurses call you to the ward to speak to the patient as she appears rather confused.

Please assess her capacity to consent for the operation.

STATION 3
Time allowed: 10 minutes

You are a junior doctor working in general surgery.

Miss Allan is a 16 year old patient who was admitted last night with appendicitis. Her father has come to the ward to visit her this morning and wants a quiet word with you. He is suspicious that his daughter is sexually active and would like to ask you whether his daughter disclosed this to you when you were taking her medical history.

Please speak to Mr Allan and address his concerns.

STATION 4
Time allowed: 10 minutes

You are a junior doctor working in genito-urinary medicine.

Miss Sally Vanstone has recently had a STI screening test which was negative for any infections but is suspicious that her boyfriend may be cheating on her. She knows that he is also a patient of yours in the clinic and has come to visit you today to ask you a few questions.

Please speak to Miss Vanstone and address her concerns appropriately.

STATION 5
Time allowed: 10 minutes

You are a junior doctor working in general medical.

Mr Kite is an elderly patient on the ward who has had multiple admissions in the last month with worsening COPD. He does not appear to be improving on his regular inhalers or nebulisers and is dependent on the BiPAP machine on the ward to maintain his oxygenation.

Your consultant would like to sign a DNAR (Do Not Attempt Resuscitation) form for the patient and mentioned this briefly to his daughter on the ward round. She is confused and doesn't really understand what is meant by a DNAR form. Please speak to Mr Kite's daughter and answer any questions she has.

STATION 6
Time allowed: 10 minutes

You are a junior doctor working in a general practice.

Mr Jones is an elderly man who has recently been diagnosed with brain cancer. He is aware that he does not have very long to live and that his health may deteriorate to such an extent that he will not be able to make his own decisions regarding his medical care.

Your colleague mentioned to him at his last visit to consider making an 'advanced directive'. He has spoken to some of his friends and family and would like more information about this.

Please speak to Mr Jones and address his questions.

STATION 7
Time allowed: 10 minutes

You are a junior doctor working in general medical.

Mr Zane is a middle-aged gentleman who has recently been admitted following a seizure. He is a known epileptic and his seizures are not particularly well controlled. A nurse on the ward informs you that he works as a bus driver and has overheard him speaking to his colleagues on the phone, saying that he'll be 'out driving again and back to work soon'. She is concerned that he is driving at all and would like you to speak to him with a view to stopping driving.

A colleague of yours has already spoken to him about his epileptic management.

Please speak to Mr Zane regarding his driving with a view to convincing him to inform the DVLA.

STATION 8
Time allowed: 10 minutes

You are a junior doctor working in general medical.

Mrs Potter is a middle-aged woman with motor neurone disease. She is bed-bound and entirely dependent on her husband for all aspects of care. She has been admitted to hospital with a severe chest infection and has stated on several occasions that she does not wish to be treated, and only to be 'kept comfortable'. She is still able to hold a conversation and speak in short sentences.

Please speak to Mr Potter with a view to assessing her capacity to refuse medical treatment.

STATION 9

Time allowed: 10 minutes

You are a junior doctor working in obstetrics.

Mrs Diamond is 39 weeks pregnant and has been admitted to hospital with the diagnosis of pre-eclampsia. The obstetricians have explained to her that in order to resolve this disorder and give both herself and her unborn child the best chance of survival, a caesarean section would be the next course of action. Mrs Diamond is extremely unhappy with this decision and is refusing to sign any consent forms.

Please speak to Mrs Diamond with a view to assessing her capacity to refuse medical treatment.

SIMULATED PATIENT BRIEFINGS

STATION 1 – Mental Health Act

Name: Mrs Glena Duffy

Age: 57 years old

Your 25 year old son, Chris, has been diagnosed with schizophrenia for the last two years. During this time he has not been compliant on his medication and has had frequent episodes of hallucinations mixed with episodes of being withdrawn. You have been quite distressed by his behaviour and are also concerned about his long-term future as he is currently unable to hold down any form of steady employment.

All the psychiatrists you have visited have, in your opinion, not offered him proper treatment. You feel that the mental health services have let your son down. You feel that sectioning your son is the physician's way of forcing him into doing what they want and that the doctors only do it because they are lazy, impatient and don't have time to sort out your son's health problems properly.

You specifically have a few questions you want the doctor to answer:
- How long is this Section 2 for?
- If you want to appeal against this Section how is it done? Is it possible?
- What happens when the section runs out? Can I take him home when it's over? Will it be automatically renewed?
- What will you do with my son whilst he is in hospital? What if he refuses your treatment and medicines? Will you force him into taking it or tranquilise him like an animal and inject him with it?

If the doctor tells you they do not know and refuse to give you a proper answer, you get quite upset and angry and feel that they do not take you seriously. You are very keen to get your son out of hospital if possible because you do not feel this is the best place for someone in his condition to be 'locked up'.

STATION 2 – Capacity

Name: Mr Dorothy Clancy

Age: 84 years old

You are an elderly woman who is rather happily confused and muddled. This is your normal state and you are not orientated in time, place or person. You can remember falling down some stairs in your nursing home yesterday and all you know is that your hip hurts a lot.

When the doctor tries to explain that you are in hospital and require an operation you say 'Yes, dear' and nod your head. When you are asked to explain and repeat what you have understood about your current condition, you stare at the doctor blankly and repeat 'Yes, dear'. You have a daughter who visits the nursing home regularly called Sally and if the doctors start to ask you any other questions that you don't feel you can answer you tell them to speak to Sally. If the doctors pressurise you further you end up saying 'Do what you think is best, dear. I don't really mind'.

You have fond memories of your cat, Felix, and summer holidays in the south of France. You occasionally try to engage the doctors in conversations about these two topics when you don't know what else to talk about.

STATION 3 – Confidentiality

Name: Mr Tom Allan

Age: 57 years old

Your daughter, Rachel, was admitted to the acute surgical unit this afternoon with suspected appendicitis. You love your daughter very much but are having problems with your relationship with her at home now that she is a teenager and wanting more independence. You suspect that she is sexually active and feel that this is inappropriate at her age as she should be concentrating on her GCSEs instead of boys. You have tried to speak to her about this subject at home but she doesn't seem willing to engage in a conversation about it.

You feel it is your duty as a parent to know what your daughter is up to and whether this is having any detrimental effect on her health. You wonder whether her abdominal pain may be due to pregnancy instead. You have asked to speak to the junior doctor in charge of this case to see if they can disclose your daughter's medical records to you. You specifically want to know if she has disclosed the fact she is sexually active, and whether or not a pregnancy test has been done and if it was, whether it is positive or not.

You get quite angry if the doctors refuse and keep saying 'This is ridiculous! I am her father! How can you not tell me?!' If the doctor suggests you speak to your daughter personally you tell them you have tried that and it hasn't worked.

STATION 4 – Confidentiality

Name: Miss Sally Vanstone

Age: 34 years old

You have been dating your boyfriend, Mike, for the last six months but lately find his behaviour rather odd and secretive. He keeps refusing to meet up with you for dates without giving any reason and he doesn't always reply to your text messages or telephone calls anymore. You suspect he is cheating on you and this has made you rather upset and suspicious about him.

You have visited the genito-urinary medicine clinic this week to check that he has not passed on any infections to you and was very relieved when this came back negative, including a negative HIV test. However, you do know that Mike has regularly attended the same clinic in the past and you want to find out if he has attended recently, and if so whether he disclosed any information about a new partner he is seeing or whether he was diagnosed with any infections.

You tell the doctors that this is important because you do not want to put your own health at risk if you sleep with him again. You also feel that this is the only way you can tell if he is being a 'good boyfriend' to you and feel that if you know that there is nothing going on it will stop you worrying at work and be a big weight off your shoulders.

If the doctors tell you to ask Mike yourself you tell them that you don't feel this is something you can chat about and don't think he will answer your questions honestly. If they refuse to give you any information then you start crying and begging for information. You keep saying you promise he will never find out and you won't tell anyone that the doctors told you. You keep repeating yourself and saying that you 'just have to know'!

STATION 5 – Do Not Resuscitate Order

Name: Miss Amanda Kite

Age: 28 years old

Your father has been suffering from chronic emphysema and COPD for as long as you can remember. He has recently taken a turn for the worse and is dependent on oxygen and some fancy new breathing equipment on the ward. You realise that his quality of life is not great but you love him dearly and only want him to have the best possible care. You still believe that he will be able to pull through this episode and return home to lead a reasonable quality of life.

He lives with his wife who helps to care for him at home. Although he is predominantly house-bound because he is on long-term oxygen therapy he was until recently able to dress and feed himself.

This morning the consultant on the medical team mentioned he was going to sign a DNAR form and muttered something about not needing to bother with CPR for your father because it probably wouldn't work. You are confused about this and want more information on what a 'DNAR' form involves.

You ask to speak to the junior doctor. Your specific questions are:
- What is a DNAR form?
- Why is it necessary for your father's case?
- Does this mean the doctors are no longer interested in keeping him alive?
- Is it possible to refuse to have the DNAR form written or to appeal against it?
- Can anyone just sign one of these forms?

You are not a difficult relative and if the junior doctor is able to adequately answer your concerns and questions you are happy for the DNAR form to remain. If you think the junior doctor does not take your concerns seriously and is not able to fully explain to you the details regarding a DNAR order you become quite anxious and upset and demand to speak to the consultant.

STATION 6 – Advance Directives

Name: Mr Alistair Jones

Age: 74 years old

You were recently diagnosed with brain cancer and have had this disease fully explained to you by your doctors. You are aware that you may not have very long to live and that your health may deteriorate to such an extent that you will not be able to make your own decisions regarding medical care. You have heard of something called an 'advanced will' or 'advanced directive' and would like some more information about this.

Your specific questions are:
- What are an advanced directive, living will and power of attorney? Are they the same thing?
- Are you allowed to ask for any sort of medical care?
- Are you allowed to state that you would like to refuse certain forms of medical treatment?
- How is an advanced directive drawn up?
- Once an advance directive is written, does this mean it is fixed and can't be changed?
- What happens if I decide later that I don't agree with my advance directive and get admitted to hospital before I have had the chance to change it?
- Are there situations where the advance directive doesn't hold?

You currently live at home with your wife, who is your main carer. You have not had a chance to discuss such matters with your wife yet and still have a lot to think about.

STATION 7 – Confidentiality

Name: Mr Bob Zane

Age: 45 years old

Job: Bus driver (for the last 10 years)

You were diagnosed as an epileptic since you were in your twenties. No intracranial cause has ever been found. You have never found your epileptic medication to be all that effective so as a consequence are not particularly compliant on it. Although you have been told that you should not drive by your GP, you still continue to drive because the pay as a bus driver is relatively good and you enjoy your job. Whenever you go back to your GP for other health problems you lie to him and say you no longer drive 'to get him off your back'.

You have a seizure about two times a year but this has never occurred whilst driving. You do not feel there is any reason to give up your job because no harm has ever come from doing what you do.

When the doctor confronts you about this you explain your situation and get quite cross and ask which nurse was eavesdropping on your phone call. When the doctor urges you to quit your job you say 'How else am I going to earn a living?' You have four children to feed and your wife doesn't work. No matter how much the doctor pleads with you, you say that you will refuse to tell the DVLA of your diagnosis.

If the doctor threatens to breach confidentiality and contact the DVLA against your wishes, you threaten him with legal action and say 'I am going to sue you for breaching confidentiality!' You tell him that he has no right and that 'you're onto him/her!'

If they tell you that they are legally allowed to breach confidentiality you say 'We'll see about that – my solicitors will be in touch'. You ask to take down their name, GMC number and job title and refuse to discuss the matter any further.

STATION 8 – Euthanasia

Name: Mrs Betty Potter

Age: 58 years old

You have been living with motor neurone disease for the last year and have had a steep decline in your ability to perform activities of daily living. You are totally dependent on your husband for all your care and have been in and out of hospital several times in the last month with infections, bed sores and DVTs. You are only just able to hold a meaningful conversation with someone and can speak in short slow sentences.

You do not feel it is fair to go on living. You have a poor quality of life and ideally would like the doctors to help you with medically-assisted suicide. Although you know that this is illegal in the UK you still ask in the hope that someone may take pity and help you.

If the doctor refuses to do so, you tell them that the next best thing is for them to stop treating you and feeding you so you can end all the torture. You understand that you cannot be cured from the motor neurone disease, that it is progressive and that refusing treatment will end in your death. You do not see what other alternatives exist and you are willing to die peacefully now rather than continue burdening your family. You have tried to speak to your husband several times about this but he refuses to comment and gets very tearful whenever the topic is brought up.

STATION 9 – Capacity

Name: Mrs Petula Diamond

Age: 23 years old

You are 39 weeks pregnant with your first baby and very excited. You have been planning your pregnancy for ages and have drawn up a birth plan with your midwife where you are absolutely determined that everything should be done in the most natural way possible. You ideally would like a home water birth and want your baby to be delivered vaginally with all your closest family members present.

In the last week you have started to develop high blood pressure and you have been told there is protein in your urine. The obstetricians have mentioned the diagnosis of 'pre-eclampsia' and explained to you in detail the risk of intra-uterine death and dangers to your own health in terms of liver damage, seizures and blood disorders if the baby is not delivered promptly by caesarean section and you do not take the appropriate medication. This has upset you very much because it was not the way you had hoped your pregnancy to go.

You do not want to have any operations at all and do not want any medication to be given to you or your baby. You understand the risks and possible consequences but still feel 'natural is best'. You state that 'mothers have been giving birth naturally for years and have been fine' and don't see why everyone is pressurising you into doing, something you really don't want to do. You have spoken to your husband who feels you should follow doctor's orders but you disagree and adamantly refuse any intervention, even if this may result in death to yourself or the baby. You have no history of any mental health disorders and no previous medical history of note.

MEDICAL ETHICS

Candidate Number:	University:
Date:	Year of Study:

STATION 1 – THE MENTAL HEALTH ACT

		2	1	0
	Appropriate introduction (1=full name and role), checks patient's name (1)	2	1	0
	Establishes rapport with the patient (1) and starts with an open question (1)	2	1	0
	Clarifies what the relative understands about her son's current situation		1	0
	Explains what the Mental Health Act is: The Mental Health Act 1983 is the law under which a person can be admitted, detained and treated for a mental health condition in hospital against their wishes (1). It comprises of different sections which involve admittance for treatment and for assessment of mental health disorder (1).	2	1	0
	Explains the duration of the detention powers: Under Section 2 of the Mental Health Act a patient can be detained for up to 28 days for assessment +/- subsequent treatment		1	0
	Knowledge of how the Section is made: The application for the Section is made by a relative or approved mental health professional (1) along with recommendations from two doctors, one of which has special experience in managing mental health disorders (1)	2	1	0
	Correct knowledge of rights to appeal under emergency detention powers: Appeal can be made to the 'Mental Health Tribunal' within the first 14 days of Section 2 (1). The patient may ask for a list of mental health solicitors who may represent them and are entitled to free legal representation at tribunals under the 'Legal Aid' scheme (1)	2	1	0
	Able to explain what happens when the Section expires: Section 2 of the mental health act cannot be renewed but a Section 3 Act may be enforced where the patient may be detained for treatment (1) which the doctors deem to be either necessary for the patient's health or the safety of others (1)	2	1	0
	Explain what is involved in Section 3: The duration of Section 3 is for 6 months (1) This Section may be renewed after a further 6 months, then annually thereafter if required (1)	2	1	0
	Explains that the patient has no right to refuse treatment for their mental health disorder (1) however there are some treatments that cannot be given e.g. ECT without the patient's direct consent (1)	2	1	0
	Clarifies that the Act only deals with mental health disorders and the patient will not be treated against their will for medical problems (1) unless their medical disorder is life-threatening and they are not deemed to have capacity (1)	2	1	0
	Demonstrates appropriate understanding of Mrs Duffy's fears and anxieties		1	0
	Explores Mrs Duffy's ideas, concerns and expectations		1	0
	Invites questions from the relative (1). Candidate was non-patronising (1).	2	1	0
	Avoids medical jargon		1	0
	Summarises the main points from the consultation		1	0
	Checks understanding of what has been explained		1	0
	Simulated patient score (2=very good, 1=satisfactory, 0=poor)	2	1	0
	Total Score			

Global Rating	1 Clear Fail	2 Borderline	3 Clear Pass	4 Very Good	5 Outstanding

Candidate Number:	University:
Date:	Year of Study:

STATION 2 – CAPACITY TO ACCEPT TREATMENT

	Appropriate introduction (1=full name and role), checks patient's name (1)	**2**	**1**	**0**
	Establishes rapport with the patient (1) and starts with an open question (1)	**2**	**1**	**0**
	Assesses patient's ability to:			
	Understand current situation		**1**	**0**
	Understand the risk of refusing current treatment		**1**	**0**
	Understand the alternative choices for treatment		**1**	**0**
	Sustain this information for long enough to weigh up the implications of treatment versus no treatment or alternative choices of treatment		**1**	**0**
	Communicate a decision about treatment		**1**	**0**
	Rationalise reason for this decision		**1**	**0**
	Communication Skills			
	Acknowledges the patient's right to refuse their treatment		**1**	**0**
	Expresses a wish to test the patient's mental state (examiner to state this is not required for this station)		**1**	**0**
	Avoids medical jargon		**1**	**0**
	Checks patient understanding		**1**	**0**
	Candidate was non-patronising, not prejudiced and patient		**1**	**0**
	Summarises current situation and decision regarding treatment		**1**	**0**
	Simulated patient score (2=very good, 1=satisfactory, 0=poor)	**2**	**1**	**0**
	Examiner to ask: 'In your opinion does this patient have capacity to refuse or make a decision regarding their medical management?'			
	Candidate states that the patient does not capacity (1) and states reasons (1) (i.e. patient is confused and unable to weigh up the risks and benefits of treatment/patient is unable to understand the proposed medical management)	**2**	**1**	**0**
	Total Score			

Global Rating	**1** Clear Fail	**2** Borderline	**3** Clear Pass	**4** Very Good	**5** Outstanding

Candidate Number:		University:
Date:		Year of Study:

STATION 3 – CONFIDENTIALITY

	Appropriate introduction (1=full name and role), checks patient's father's name (1)	**2**	**1**	**0**
	Establishes rapport (1) and starts with an open question (1)	**2**	**1**	**0**
	Establishes reason for discussion			
	Establishes reason for relative's discussion with doctor		**1**	**0**
	Enquires about circumstances leading to relative's queries		**1**	**0**
	Acknowledges relative's feelings and concerns		**1**	**0**
	Establishes that all patient information is confidential (1) and as the doctor you are not allowed to give out personal information about the patient without the patient's consent (1)	**2**	**1**	**0**
	Establishes that patient confidentiality also applies to divulging information to relatives, no matter how close their relationship		**1**	**0**
	Explains that to do so would undermine patient-doctor relationship		**1**	**0**
	Apologises for not being able to divulge any confidential information		**1**	**0**
	Suggests relative discusses the situation with the patient		**1**	**0**
	Offers to set up a meeting with the patient, doctors and relatives together to discuss the current medical management and treatment (1) if patient is happy for this to go ahead (1), but any personal information would not be for the doctors to disclose	**2**	**1**	**0**
	Acknowledges the difficult relationship that the patient and relative are going through (1) and offers assistance to help (e.g. counselling if this might be helpful) (1)	**2**	**1**	**0**
	Negotiates and agrees a course of action		**1**	**0**
	Communication Skills			
	Candidate avoids dismissive, threatening body language or interrupting the patient. Good use of eye contact and does not raise their voice.		**1**	**0**
	Candidate uses verbal and non-verbal clues to demonstrate active listening		**1**	**0**
	Demonstrates empathy (verbally and non-verbally)		**1**	**0**
	Simulated patient score (2=very good, 1=satisfactory, 0=poor)	**2**	**1**	**0**
	Total Score			

Global Rating	**1** Clear Fail	**2** Borderline	**3** Clear Pass	**4** Very Good	**5** Outstanding

Candidate Number:	University:
Date:	Year of Study:

STATION 4 – CONFIDENTIALITY

	Appropriate introduction (1=full name and role), checks patient's name (1)	2	1	0
	Establishes rapport (1) and starts with an open question (1)	2	1	0
	Establishes reason for discussion			
	Establishes reason for the patient's discussion with doctor		1	0
	Enquires about circumstances leading to patient's queries		1	0
	Acknowledges patient's feelings and concerns		1	0
	Establishes that all patient information is confidential (1) and as the doctor personal information about another patient cannot be discussed without their consent (1)	2	1	0
	Establishes that patient confidentiality also applies to divulging information to relatives/sexual partners no matter how close their relationship		1	0
	Explains that to do so would undermine patient-doctor relationship		1	0
	Apologises for not being able to divulge any confidential information		1	0
	Suggests patient discusses the situation with their partner instead		1	0
	Tells patient that confidentiality can only be broken in this circumstance if public health is put at risk (1), however, this is not the situation in this case (1)	2	1	0
	Explains that if the other patient was diagnosed with an infection then the doctor who was treating him would contact/encourage them to contact their partner to be treated (1), however, the candidate cannot just go and check the other patient's files and disclose this information (1)	2	1	0
	Refuses to divulge information despite patient's pleas not to tell anyone		1	0
	Establishes the relationship with the other patient (1) and offers any assistance to help (e.g. counselling if relative feels this might be helpful) (1)	2	1	0
	Negotiates and agrees a course of action	2	1	0
	Communication Skills			
	Candidate avoids dismissive, threatening body language or interrupting the patient. Good use of eye contact and does not raise their voice.		1	0
	Candidate uses verbal and non-verbal clues to demonstrate active listening		1	0
	Demonstrates empathy (verbally and non-verbally)		1	0
	Simulated patient score (2=very good, 1=satisfactory, 0=poor)	2	1	0
	Total Score			

Global Rating	**1** Clear Fail	**2** Borderline	**3** Clear Pass	**4** Very Good	**5** Outstanding

Candidate Number:	University:
Date:	Year of Study:

STATION 5 – DNAR

Appropriate introduction (1=full name and role), checks patient's father's name (1)	**2**	**1**	**0**
Establishes rapport with the patient's daughter (1) and asks an open question (1)	**2**	**1**	**0**
Establishes Current Clinical Circumstances			
Establishes what patient's daughter understands regarding current situation (1) and clarifies any misinterpretation (1)	**2**	**1**	**0**
DNAR orders			
Explores what daughter already knows regarding 'DNAR' orders		**1**	**0**
Explains that it only applies to CPR (1) not about medical treatment		**1**	**0**
Patient will still receive current medical management and therapy		**1**	**0**
Explains that CPR is a very distressing thing to put a patient through (1) and not usually successful especially in very frail patients (1)	**2**	**1**	**0**
Candidate explains that it is in the patient's best interest to be kept comfortable with dignity and self-esteem		**1**	**0**
Explains that a DNAR order is a medical decision (1) and made by the consultant or most senior doctor in charge (1)	**2**	**1**	**0**
It is not possible to appeal against it or refuse (1), however, if there are strong objections then they should be relayed to the consultant (1)	**2**	**1**	**0**
Offers to pass on the message to the consultant regarding father's DNAR status if relative is unhappy about it (1) and states patient and daughter may be present to discuss further issues (1)	**2**	**1**	**0**
Reassures relative that the medical team are still very much involved in her father's care (1) and this DNAR order does not stem from a lack of interest in him as a patient (1)	**2**	**1**	**0**
Communication Skills			
Listens actively (e.g. picks up cues/ responds appropriately to information)		**1**	**0**
Empathy (both nonverbally and verbally)		**1**	**0**
Avoids medical jargon (1) and repetition of questions/statements (1)	**2**	**1**	**0**
Professionalism and calm manner throughout consultation		**1**	**0**
Closing remarks			
Invites questions (1) and responds appropriately (1)	**2**	**1**	**0**
Summarises situation (1). Checks understanding (1).	**2**	**1**	**0**
Simulated patient score (2=very good, 1=satisfactory, 0=poor)	**2**	**1**	**0**
Total Score			

Global Rating	**1** Clear Fail	**2** Borderline	**3** Clear Pass	**4** Very Good	**5** Outstanding

Candidate Number:	University:
Date:	Year of Study:

STATION 6 – ADVANCE DIRECTIVES

		2	1	0
	Appropriate introduction (1=full name and role), checks patient's name (1)	2	1	0
	Establishes rapport with the patient (1) and starts with an open question (1)	2	1	0
	Elicits what patient understands regarding advance directives		1	0
	States that an advance directive is a set of instructions that a patient wishes to be carried out regarding their future medical treatment (1) and is put into action only when the patient can no longer provide these instructions themselves (1)	2	1	0
	A living will is a type of advance directive where these wishes are stated on paper (1) but does not involve decisions regarding money or property (1)	2	1	0
	Another type of advance directive is known as a power of attorney (1) where the patient appoints a person they trust to make decisions on their behalf (1)	2	1	0
	Explains that patients are allowed to make wishes both on treatment they would prefer (1) or prefer to refuse (1) within reason	2	1	0
	Advance directives are useful for stating wishes regarding decisions such as the use of life-saving treatment, CPR, administration of IV fluids or parenteral nutrition at the end of life (2=three examples, 1=two examples, 0=one or none)	2	1	0
	Advance directives cannot be used to ask for something that is illegal (i.e. assisted suicide), the use of a specific drug, refusal of treatment for a mental health condition (2=two examples, 1=one example, 0=not mentioned, no examples)	2	1	0
	It is not necessary to seek legal advice to draw up an advance directive (1), however, it is recommended in order to prevent a failure for wishes to be carried out (1)	2	1	0
	Advises on discussion with family members prior to drawing one up (1) and advises that this is made available to clinicians and kept within all medical notes (1)	2	1	0
	Even once an advance directive is drawn up it is possible to change your mind and alter the advance directive (1) providing patient capacity is maintained (1)	2	1	0
	Clarifies that even if the patient asks/refuses treatment that differs from what is stated in their advanced directive, and doesn't have a chance to change it before admitting to hospital, it can be over-ridden (1) if the patient still has capacity (1)	2	1	0
	Advance directives may be deemed invalid if it is felt the patient created the document under duress (1) or the document is not signed or witnessed (1)	2	1	0
	Communication Skills			
	Delivers information in manageable chunks		1	0
	Use of non-medical jargon		1	0
	Closing Remarks			
	Invites patients questions (1) and responds appropriately (1)	2	1	0
	Summarises situation (1) and checks patient understanding/offers leaflet (1)	2	1	0
	Organised (e.g. systematic, signposts change in focus of questions and topics)		1	0
	Total Score			

Global Rating	1 Clear Fail	2 Borderline	3 Clear Pass	4 Very Good	5 Outstanding

Candidate Number:		University:	
Date:		Year of Study:	

STATION 7 – BREAKING CONFIDENTIALITY

Appropriate introduction (1=full name and role), checks patient's name (1)	2	1	0
Establishes rapport with the patient (1) and starts with an open question (1)	2	1	0
Establishes reason for consultation			
Establishes how much patient understands about his current diagnosis		1	0
Confirms patient's current occupation as a bus driver (1) and confirms the information that patient is still driving and will continue to do so after discharge (1)	2	1	0
Explains to the patient that it is illegal to continue driving (1) and that the patient can be prosecuted if caught doing so (1)	2	1	0
Establishes that current driving license may not be valid (1) and having a seizure during driving could endanger the patient as well as others (1)	2	1	0
In the situation of an accident, the car insurance may not cover damages		1	0
Explains that patient can only drive cars if they have been seizure-free for one year (1) or only having seizures during the night for three years (1)	2	1	0
Explains that in order to drive buses the patient must be seizure-free for 10 years (1) off medication (1)	2	1	0
Explores reasons why patient continues to drive (1) and acknowledges the patient's difficult social circumstances (1)	2	1	0
Elicits whether patient has discussed the situation with his family and friends (1) and what their opinions on the matter are (1)	2	1	0
Encourages patient to disclose his health condition to the DVLA		1	0
Explains that if the patient is not willing to do this then the medical team are obliged to alert the DVLA		1	0
Explains that where public safety may be put at risk then patient confidentiality can be broken		1	0
Encourages patient to comply with medication in order to become seizure-free		1	0
Explores reasons why patient is not taking medication as prescribed		1	0
Encourages patient to discuss his health matters at work (1) and suggests that an alternative role within the same company may be possible (1)	2	1	0
Communication Skills			
Avoids ridiculing patient or being patronizing (1), demonstrates empathy (1)	2	1	0
Candidate remains calm and professional throughout consultation		1	0
Summarises situation (1) and checks patient understanding of action plan (1)	2	1	0
Total Score			

Global Rating	1 Clear Fail	2 Borderline	3 Clear Pass	4 Very Good	5 Outstanding

Candidate Number:	University:
Date:	Year of Study:

STATION 8 – CAPACITY TO REFUSE TREATMENT

	Appropriate introduction (1=full name and role), checks patient's name (1)	2	1	0
	Establishes rapport with the patient (1) and starts with an open question (1)	2	1	0
	Establishes what the patient understands about current clinical situation (1) and reasons for the discussion with doctors (1)	2	1	0
	Enquires about patient's social circumstances and home life		1	0
	Explores social support therapies to help patient's current situation such as counselling for depression (1) or perhaps living in a care home to alleviate stress on the family life (1)	2	1	0
	Explains that euthanasia in the UK is illegal (1) and refuses to carry out the patient's wishes relating to assisted suicide (1)	2	1	0
	Explains that refusal of medical treatment would slowly result in the patient's death		1	0
	Establishes rationale behind patient's decision (1) and that the patient has weighed up the risks of no treatment with the benefits of continued supportive therapy (1)	2	1	0
	Enquires after patient's mental health (1) and establishes they are not emotionally or mentally ill (1)	2	1	0
	Explores whether patient has discussed her feelings with her husband (1) and encourages discussion with husband and other family relatives before making decision (1)	2	1	0
	Expresses a wish to test the patient's mental state (examiner to state this is not required for this station)		1	0
	Communication Skills			
	Avoids medical jargon (1) and demonstrates empathy (1)	2	1	0
	Checks patient understanding		1	0
	Candidate was non-patronising, not prejudiced and patient		1	0
	Summarises current situation and decision regarding treatment		1	0
	Simulated patient score (2=very good, 1=satisfactory, 0=poor)	2	1	0
	Examiner to ask: 'In your opinion does this patient have capacity to refuse their recommended medical management?'			
	Candidate states that patient does have capacity (1) and states reasons (1) (i.e. patient is not confused, understands the information and risks, is able to weigh up the risks and benefits of treatment and communicate a rational decision)	2	1	0
	Total Score			

Global Rating	1 Clear Fail	2 Borderline	3 Clear Pass	4 Very Good	5 Outstanding

Candidate Number:		University:
Date:		Year of Study:

STATION 9 – CAPACITY TO REFUSE MEDICAL TREATMENT

Appropriate introduction (1=full name and role), checks patient's name (1)	2	1	0
Establishes rapport with the patient (1) and starts with an open question (1)	2	1	0
Establishes what patient understands about current clinical situation (1) and clarifies any misunderstandings (1)	2	1	0
Explains to patient the risks of not following medical advice to both herself (1) and her baby (1) (e.g. risk of maternal and foetal death)	2	1	0
Explains that this is the safest treatment given the circumstances (1) and there are no real safe alternative choices for treatment (1)	2	1	0
Explores patient's agenda for refusal of treatment (1) and responds appropriately (1)	2	1	0
Explores whether wife has discussed her feelings with her husband (1) and encourages further discussion with husband (1)	2	1	0
Acknowledges the patient's right to refuse their treatment (1) and establishes that patient is not under any duress and this decision is completely her own (1)	2	1	0
Establishes that a competent pregnant woman can refuse treatment, even if that refusal may result in harm to her unborn baby		1	0
Enquires after patient's mental health (1) and establishes they are not emotionally or mentally ill (1)	2	1	0
Acknowledges that sectioning under the Mental Health Act applies only to mental health conditions (1) and cannot be used to detain a patient for physical or medical therapy (1)	2	1	0
Expresses a wish to test the patient's mental state (examiner to state this is not required for this station)		1	0
Communication Skills			
Avoids medical jargon (1) and demonstrates empathy (1)	2	1	0
Checks patient understanding		1	0
Candidate was non-patronising, not prejudiced and patient		1	0
Summarises current situation and decision regarding treatment		1	0
Simulated patient score (2=very good, 1=satisfactory, 0=poor)	2	1	0
Examiner to ask: 'In your opinion does this patient have capacity to refuse their recommended medical management?'			
Candidate states that patient does have capacity (1) and states reasons (1) (i.e. patient is not confused, understands the information and risks, is able to weigh up the risks and benefits of treatment and communicate a rational decision)	2	1	0
Total Score			

Global Rating	1 Clear Fail	2 Borderline	3 Clear Pass	4 Very Good	5 Outstanding

CHAPTER 7: DIFFICULT COMMUNICATIONS
Written by Dr. S. Shelmerdine

- The Foreign Patient
- The Angry Patient
- The Difficult Relatives
- Negotiation Skills
- Jehovah's Witness
- Domestic Abuse
- Do Not Attempt Resuscitation (DNAR) Request
- Breaking Bad News
- Concerned Parent
- Difficult Colleague

THE STATIONS

STATION 1

Time allowed: 7 minutes

You are a junior doctor working in a general practice.

Mrs Gutierez is an elderly lady who has come into your surgery with a bad cough. She speaks very little English and you cannot speak any Portuguese.

Please take a brief focussed history from her and formulate a management plan.

Pen and paper is provided in the station.

STATION 2

Time allowed: 7 minutes

You are a junior doctor working in Accident and Emergency.

Mr Chong is a student visiting England from China. He speaks poor English and you cannot speak Chinese, but you notice him wincing in pain and holding his arm.

Please take a focussed history of his presenting complaint and formulate a management plan.

Pen and paper is provided in the station.

STATION 3

Time allowed: 7 minutes

You are a junior doctor working in a general practice.

One of your colleagues referred Mr Smith last week for a barium enema examination because he was complaining of a change in bowel habit. He had the procedure done yesterday and has come into your surgery this morning and is furious.

The nurse has asked that you see him first on your clinic. The results of the scan are not available yet. Please speak to him and address his concerns.

STATION 4

Time allowed: 7 minutes

You are a junior doctor working in obstetrics and gynaecology.

You are asked to see Mrs Jones on the ward who you prescribed Augmentin to earlier this morning for pyelonephritis. Unfortunately you failed to realise that she was allergic to this medication.

She did not develop a severe reaction when the nurses administered her medication but is now complaining of a rash and is very angry that she was given medication she is allergic to.

Please speak to her and address her concerns.

STATION 5

Time allowed: 7 minutes

You are a junior doctor working in general medicine.

Mr Catmin is an elderly man who was diagnosed with metastatic lung cancer last week during his current admission. He is not for active treatment and is under joint care with the palliative medicine team. He has asked that the doctors withhold the news of the diagnosis from his wife until he can find an appropriate time and place to discuss the issue with her. This morning when his wife was visiting hospital she saw the palliative care team speaking to her husband.

She has asked to speak to you urgently. Please speak to her and address her concerns.

STATION 6
Time allowed: 7 minutes

You are a junior doctor working in a general practice.

Miss Loong is a solicitor working in the city and has been complaining of a sore throat for the last two days. She is very upset about the pain and wants you to prescribe her antibiotics.

Please take a focussed history and negotiate a treatment plan.

STATION 7
Time allowed: 7 minutes

You are a junior doctor working in oncology.

Mrs Lee was recently diagnosed with Hodgkin's Lymphoma and is due to start her chemotherapy this week. She has a good prognosis and is expected to do well with this treatment. However, she has poor understanding of lymphoma and wants to speak to you about putting off her chemotherapy so she can go to China and give traditional herbal medicine a go.

Please address her concerns.

STATION 8
Time allowed: 7 minutes

You are a junior doctor working in general practice.

Mr Linkin has asked to see a doctor urgently. He appears very agitated and anxious. His usual GP, Dr. Rafi, is away and the surgery receptionist has asked you to speak to him instead.

Please take a brief history and formulate an appropriate management plan.

STATION 9
Time allowed: 7 minutes

You are a junior doctor working in general practice.

Sam Jenkins is a final year medical student who has come to see you this morning. He looks rather nervous and upset.

Please take a brief history and address his concerns.

STATION 10
Time allowed: 7 minutes

You are the junior doctor working on a busy surgical firm.

Mr Thompson, your patient, is a Jehovah's Witness and is due for a laparoscopic right hemicolectomy tomorrow morning. He has already had a discussion with your consultant regarding refusal of any blood products to be given to him and has signed a consent form accepting the risks of this procedure.

His wife, Mrs Thompson, has come to visit him on the ward this evening and asks to speak to you in private.

Please speak to her and address her concerns.

STATION 11
Time allowed: 7 minutes

You are a junior doctor working in general practice.

Mrs Scarlett has come in today to arrange a booking visit with the GP but you notice that she seems very anxious and feel there is something else going on. Your GP supervisor, Dr. Coombes, has asked you to talk to the patient and gain a clear picture of her social and personal circumstances.

Please speak to Mrs Scarlett and elicit her social circumstances. Offer any appropriate advice or support.

STATION 12
Time allowed: 7 minutes

You are a junior doctor working in general medicine.

You are asked by the nurses to see Miss Brown. Her 58 year old mother was admitted to hospital last week with a cardiac arrest due to ventricular fibrillation. After a brief admission to ITU and a successful resuscitation she is now on the ward, awake and alert. Miss Brown was horrified to see her mother on ITU and would like you to put a DNAR on her mother's chart so she will never have to go through the suffering again.

Please speak to Miss Brown and address her concerns.

STATION 13
Time allowed: 7 minutes

You are a junior doctor working in Accident and Emergency.

Mr Paterson is a young man who has just been involved in a road traffic accident where he was the driver. The car he was driving has been written off but other than a minor contusion and a fractured humerus he is medically stable.

Unfortunately for a young woman who was sitting in the passenger seat of his car, this was not the case. She was pronounced dead on arrival to hospital from severe head injuries. Mr Paterson is unaware of these events and wants to speak to a doctor.

Please explain the current events to him.

STATION 14
Time allowed: 7 minutes

You are a junior doctor working in Accident and Emergency.

Mrs Young is a 40 year old lady who is 6 weeks pregnant after having had her third course of IVF treatment. She has never had any children and this is the first time her IVF treatment has 'worked'.

Earlier this evening she came into the department complaining of vaginal bleeding. The triage nurse sent off a blood test. Beta hCG levels have come back as 'low' indicating a high chance of miscarriage. Two urine pregnancy tests performed in the department are both negative. She is in the waiting room with her husband.

Please explain the results and their significance to her.

STATION 15
Time allowed: 7 minutes

You are a junior doctor working in general surgery.

Mrs Tooke is a 40 year old lady with a history of breast cancer. She had a right mastectomy two years ago and has been well since this time. Last week she noticed a lump in her left breast and axilla, which was biopsied in clinic. The results show that the breast lump is malignant and there are metastatic cells within the enlarged axillary lymph node.

She is unaware of this and has returned to see you in clinic today for her results.

Please speak to her about the findings and address her concerns.

STATION 16
Time allowed: 7 minutes

You are a junior doctor in general surgery.

Mrs Lewis has asked to urgently speak to you. She is very distressed as her son, Greg, was admitted four days ago with appendicitis. Unfortunately, the surgery was delayed by five hours as another emergency surgery was being carried out. On operating, the surgeon found the appendix was perforated and Greg was suffering from early peritonitis. Greg was improving until this morning but now presents with a swinging pyrexia.

Mrs Lewis has little understanding of what has been going on and is very anxious.

Please explain the recent events to her and her son's likely outcome. Address any concerns she may have.

STATION 17
Time allowed: 7 minutes

You are a junior doctor working in your first medical job.

There is another junior doctor on your ward who is also working for your consultant. However, you have noticed that she is not doing her share of work on the firm. She arrives 30 minutes late to work every morning, leaves early and never completes all the jobs on her list. On several occasions you have had to stay behind to finish some tasks she was meant to have done.

You initially didn't want to make an issue of it, but last week your consultant was very angry because several of his patients (who the other junior doctor was meant to be looking after) did not have up-to-date blood results and you were blamed for this.

Please address your concerns with your junior doctor colleague.

SIMULATED PATIENT BRIEFINGS

STATION 1

Name: Mrs Juanita Gutierez

Age: 78 years old

Job: Retired shopkeeper

You speak very little English. You are Portuguese and have lived in England for the last five years with your son and daughter-in-law who speak fluent English but are both at work so could not come to the GP surgery with you today. For the last week you have been suffering with a sore throat and cough which is non-productive. You do not have a fever or any chest pain. You are not short of breath.

You want the doctor to check that everything is all right and that you don't need to go to hospital. You are generally fit and well. You only suffer from arthritis in your hips and back and take simple analgesia such as ibuprofen or paracetamol for this. You do not drink any alcohol and do not smoke.

STATION 2

Name: Mr Simon Chong

Age: 21 years old

Job: Computer sciences student

You speak very little English but are very keen to try to converse the best you know how. You are Chinese and have only been in England for a week on an English language course. Your only friends in England are the other students on your course who also speak very poor English and have left you to go to hospital on your own. This morning you were cycling into school when you fell off your bike and landed on your right elbow. There is a large bruise and it hurts for you to use that arm to write or lift objects. You are worried about a fracture.

You want the doctor to check that everything is all right and that you don't need an operation. You are generally fit and well. You do not take any medication and do not have any past medical history. You do not drink any alcohol but smoke 10 cigarettes a day.

STATION 3

Name: Mr John Smith

Age: 65 years old

Job: Retired postman

Last week you came to see a GP in the surgery because you have noticed that you have been unusually constipated over the last six months without changing your diet. He referred you for a barium enema and explained it would be an examination to look for evidence of bowel cancer. You had the procedure done yesterday and found it a most horrific experience. You did not feel the examination was explained to you properly and had not understood that you would have barium and air passed into the rectum. You feel this was an extremely degrading and undignified procedure and want to complain to someone.

You are also very worried about the results as your brother was recently diagnosed with bowel cancer and you desperately want to hear that everything is fine. You tell the doctor that you want to put in a formal complaint against their colleague for not counselling you properly before the barium enema but will drop the complaint if you can have your barium enema results immediately. You are furious when you find that the results are not available.

STATION 4

Name: Mrs Shelley Jones

Age: 46 years old

Job: Librarian

You are currently in hospital recovering from an operation you had to remove fibroids two days ago. Last night you developed dysuria and right flank pain. The consultant who saw you on ward round diagnosed you with pyelonephritis and you were started on a course of antibiotics. In the pre-operative assessment clinic you had told the junior doctor that you were allergic to Augmentin and had previously had an anaphylactic reaction. You made sure this was written in your clinical notes.

Unfortunately the doctor on the ward today carelessly prescribed this drug without checking your notes or the drug chart and it was administered to you by the nurses. You luckily did not develop an anaphylaxis reaction, only a severe rash which is now settling. Nevertheless you are extremely angry that this has happened. You are anxious and worried that other complications in your treatment will be made and want to make a formal complaint to ensure this does not happen again. You want a serious word with the doctor who made this mistake.

You have made up your mind before the doctor comes to see you that you will tell them you don't want them involved in your care and want to speak to their consultant about their negligent behaviour. However, if you feel that the mistake was a genuine oversight and that the doctor is apologetic you are willing to drop your complaint.

STATION 5

Name: Mrs Julia Catmin

Age: 80 years old

Job: Retired secretary

Your husband, James, was admitted to hospital last week with shortness of breath and chest pain. He has been telling you that the doctors were treating him for pneumonia and he was expected to make a full recovery so you wouldn't worry. However, this morning whilst visiting the hospital you bump into the palliative care team on the ward speaking to your husband. You confront him with this information and he ends up confessing his diagnosis of metastatic lung cancer.

You are deeply depressed and angry at the general medical doctors for not mentioning this to you sooner. You feel that you had a right to know and also feel betrayed by your husband and the team. You demand to know all the details of his treatment, previous scan results and future management plan. You want him to be for active management and do not want any palliative care involvement. You still believe that there is a chance of cure and do not want to accept that there is a high likelihood that your husband will die soon.

You have two daughters who are unaware of this diagnosis and five grandchildren who are very supportive. You live with your husband in a bungalow at the moment and your social support network is good.

STATION 6

Name: Miss Harriet Loong

Age: 29 years old

Job: Solicitor

You have a stressful job in the city and have been working late nights recently. For the last two days you have had a very sore throat which has prevented you from eating or drinking properly. You do not have a fever or cough. You are not short of breath and you haven't noticed any swellings in your throat.

You are quite upset about your symptoms because you hoped they would have got better by now and have come to see the GP because you want to be prescribed antibiotics to 'speed up the recovery process'. The sore throat has prevented you from going out to lunch with your clients and you have now 'had enough'.

STATION 7

Name: Mrs Sally Lee

Age: 50 years old

Job: Hairdresser

You have recently been diagnosed with Hodgkin's Lymphoma and have been told that you need chemotherapy to cure your illness. You have never heard of lymphoma and don't fancy the idea of chemotherapy. You have seen people on television who have been on chemotherapy and they all look miserable and bald.

You've spoken to your friends about your illness and none of them have ever heard of lymphoma either. However, they have told you that there is a renowned traditional herbal medical practitioner in China who has helped cure many patients with 'strange' diseases without the use of 'toxic' chemicals. You would like to give this treatment a try and have come to see your doctor today to cancel your chemotherapy treatment. You've already booked an airline ticket to China for next week.

STATION 8

Name: Mr Ashley Linkin

Age: 37 years old

Job: Unemployed

You used to be addicted to heroin but for the last two weeks have been enrolled onto a methadone replacement programme by your usual GP, Dr. Rafi. He is away on holiday and cannot see you. You ask to speak to another doctor because you claim you have 'lost your prescription for methadone' and want the junior doctor to give you a script for the week. You say that it was in your wallet and someone stole your wallet with the prescription in it, but in reality you have already used up all the methadone you picked up this week and want more.

You are agitated and craving the methadone. If the junior doctor does not oblige you start saying things like 'Do you want me to go back to the drugs? If I do it will all be on your head!' If they still refuse, you start to complain that you are being judged and that they are discriminating against you. You want your prescription now and walk out of the clinic if they continue to refuse.

STATION 9

Name: Mr Sam Jenkins

Age: 24 years old

Job: Final year medical student

You are a final year medical student and have your medical finals examination in three day's time. You have not slept well recently and have been studying very hard but still feel that you are not ready for the exams. You decide that the only hope you have is to see your GP and try to get them to write you a sick note explaining that you are unfit to sit the examination.

When you meet the GP you initially try to make up an excuse about why you are unwell but when questioned further about your illness you confess the truth and beg for a sick note. You have not spoken to your friends or family about this because you don't want to disappoint them. You have not spoken to your tutors either because you don't want to cause a fuss.

STATION 10

Name: Mrs Catherine Thompson

Age: 54 years old

Job: Shopkeeper

Your husband, Nathan, is due for a right hemicolectomy tomorrow to remove a tumour in his colon. He is a Jehovah's Witness and has already signed a consent form agreeing to the risks of the procedure and refusal of all blood products. You are very worried about the procedure and have tried to reason with him to change his mind and accept blood products in the event of an emergency. However, he is not willing to do so.

You have asked to speak to the doctor on the ward in private to see if there is any way you can ask them to just give him the blood if he needs it regardless of what he's agreed to on the consent form. You don't understand how the doctors can just 'let him die' if his life is at risk and urge them to 'pretend the consent form has gone missing' to make things less complicated. You tell the doctors that your husband will 'never know' as he will be anaesthetised during the operation and so long as his life is saved then 'everything will be OK'. You are very insistent on this and suggest the junior doctor brings this up with the consultant prior to the operation.

STATION 11

Name: Mrs Samantha Scarlett

Age: 29 years old

Job: Housewife

You are newly married to Mark, an officer in the army, and live in the army barracks with him. You are 12 weeks pregnant with your first child. Your pregnancy was not planned but you are both very happy about it. Mark was a very caring and loving husband until the last few months when you've noticed he has been having mood swings and occasionally comes home stressed and angry with you.

On one occasion you ended up having a shouting match where held you down firmly and caused you to have several bruises on your arms and thighs. He has never hit you or sexually abused you. You are worried about the violence but feel that things will be better once the baby arrives and that he's probably stressed that money is quite tight. You blame yourself for not being more supportive and feel that you aren't helping with matters as you are always feeling tired and nauseated from the pregnancy.

You do not have a job but occasionally volunteer at the local charity shop to get out of the house. You are close to your family but they do not live nearby and you don't have friends in the area. If the situation between you and Mark escalates you have no idea where to go for help. You don't want to tell the police or make a big deal about it and want the doctor to keep all these details completely confidential.

STATION 12

Name: Miss Jackie Brown

Age: 26 years old

Job: Receptionist

Your mother was recently admitted to hospital with a cardiac arrest. You saw her on ITU when she was intubated and felt sorry for her having to be 'put through so much'. You decide that it isn't right for someone of her age to go through this again and want the doctors to put a DNAR order in her notes without her knowledge. You don't understand the clinical indications for a DNAR order but just can't believe that further intervention can be appropriate for your mother.

You have not spoken to your mother about this and feel that after all she has been through, it is better not to bother her with these issues.

STATION 13

Name: Mr Ben Paterson

Age: 36 years old

Job: Sales manager

You were driving home tonight after having a lovely dinner out with your fiancée, Jane. You are due to get married in two month's time and have just put down a deposit on your first home together. On your way home you remember being hit by another car at high speed, which collided into the passenger side of your car. You have now just regained consciousness and find yourself in the Accident and Emergency department. You are very confused about the events of the evening and are desperate to find out what has happened to Jane.

STATION 14

Name: Mrs Judith Young

Age: 40 years old

Job: Beauty therapist

You have recently undergone your third course of IVF treatment. You have never had children and the previous two courses of IVF have not been successful. You are currently 6 weeks pregnant and recently had an ultrasound scan confirming an intra-uterine pregnancy. Your husband and you were utterly thrilled.

This evening you have noticed that there has been a bit of blood on your underwear. You also have been having severe pelvic pain similar to period pains. You are concerned that you may have miscarried but hope that this is not the case. You and your husband cannot afford another course of IVF and you feel that this is your last hope at having your own children.

If the doctor tells you that you have miscarried you ask them 'Is there anything you can do to save the baby?' and try to get them to admit that there is a possibility that they are wrong and you can still carry your pregnancy to term. You feel that if you cannot have children this will surely be the end of your marriage and you feel hopeless.

STATION 15

Name: Mrs Rachel Tooke

Age: 40 years old

Job: Healthcare assistant

Two years ago you had a mastectomy for a lump in your right breast that was found to be cancerous. You were told at the time that you did not have any other cancers elsewhere and that all the cancer was removed. Last week you arranged an emergency appointment with your doctor as you felt a new lump in your left breast. This was biopsied with another lump in your left armpit.

You are in clinic today for the results and are very nervous that it means the cancer has come back. When you are told that this is the case you break down crying and say 'But I thought all the cancer was removed, how can this happen?' and 'How long do I have?'

You are a single mother and work part-time as a healthcare assistant at your local GP surgery.

You are very upset because you think that you will surely die young whatever the doctors say and end up leaving your 8 year old daughter without a mother. Your ex-husband was abusive and you have not had any contact with him since the divorce three years ago. Your extended family lives abroad in Australia and your daughter has never met them.

STATION 16

Name: Mrs Laura Lewis

Age: 38 years old

Job: School teacher

You are a single mother to your son, Greg, who is 13 years old. He is a very active and energetic boy and generally fit and healthy. Four days ago he started complaining of right-sided abdominal pain and was taken to hospital. The casualty doctor who met Greg told you that it was highly likely Greg was suffering from appendicitis. The surgeons were not available to meet your son immediately as they were involved with a different emergency operation and Greg was kept waiting for five hours until he was finally taken to theatre.

He was initially doing well postoperatively but has developed a high temperature today and is complaining of worsening abdominal pains. No one spoke to you to tell you what was found at the initial operation, only that there was 'nothing to worry about'. You are worried that he needs another operation and don't want him to get forgotten about, which is why you want to speak to the doctor.

You feel angry at yourself because you think you should have taken Greg to a private hospital and that if he hadn't have been kept waiting for five hours he may not be this unwell.

Greg's father is on a business trip abroad and although you still keep in touch, he cannot come to be with the family at the moment. You have very little medical knowledge and need to have everything explained to you slowly and in non-medical jargon. You are very upset and blame yourself for Greg's situation. You keep repeating 'I'm a bad mother' when you speak to the doctors.

STATION 17

Name: Dr. Gillian Gall

Age: 25 years old

Job: F1 doctor

You have recently started your first medical job since graduating from medical school. You enjoy your job and feel that you are getting on well with your team. The other junior doctor on your ward is always very helpful and doesn't seem to mind doing your ward jobs for you when you feel overworked or stressed.

You are living with your parents at home as your mother has recently fractured her tibia in a skiing accident and you need to help care for her. It is a long drive away and due to the distance from work and the traffic, you are usually late but no one has minded so far. You are struggling with money and have a second part-time job working as a private tutor for A-level students and need to leave work early to make it on time to teach your classes.

You feel overstretched and tired all the time. You think you are working very hard and trying your best. When you find the other junior doctor doesn't appreciate you arriving late and leaving early, you are initially very upset because you thought that you were both good friends and you would help cover for them if they were in a similar predicament. If you believe that your feelings are being taken into consideration you eventually agree to pull more weight at work.

DIFFICULT COMMUNICATIONS

Candidate Number:	University:
Date:	Year of Study:

STATION 1 – THE FOREIGN PATIENT

	Appropriate introduction (1=full name and role), checks patient's name (1)	2	1	0
	Establishes rapport with the patient (1) and starts with an open question (1)	2	1	0
	Obtains a Clinical History			
	Establishes level patient can speak English		1	0
	Explores presenting complaint (2=in detail, 1=adequately, 0=not at all) Symptoms, time of onset, associated complaints, severity	2	1	0
	Explores patient's past medical history (2=in detail, 1=poorly, 0=not at all)	2	1	0
	Checks if patient is currently on any medication (1) or has allergies (1)	2	1	0
	Explores patient's social history – smoking, alcohol, social circumstances (2=all three, 1=any two, 0=one or none)	2	1	0
	Offers appropriate medical advice and follow-up • Clinical examination of respiratory system and throat • Investigation with chest X-ray and blood tests • Medication (e.g. antibiotics dependent on investigation results) (2=any two suggestions, 1=any one suggestion, 0=not mentioned)	2	1	0
	Suggests follow-up appointment (preferably with a translator)		1	0
	General Communication Skills			
	Uses non-verbal means of aiding communication (e.g. drawing or pointing at objects) (2=does well and creatively, 1=attempts, 0=does not attempt)	2	1	0
	Maintains eye contact with the patient (1) and persists in taking a good history (1)	2	1	0
	Avoids medical jargon	2	1	0
	Checks patient's understanding	2	1	0
	Rephrases questions to aid patient's understanding (2=attempts and persists in multiple methods, 1=rephrases only once and repeats self with failure to see that the patient is not understanding, 0=no attempt to rephrase any questions)	2	1	0
	Candidate was non-patronising and considerate with the patient		1	0
	Summarises presenting complaint and management plan	2	1	0
	Examiner to ask: 'What else could you do to improve communication?'			
	Explores whether patient is accompanied by anyone who speaks English		1	0
	Offers to find staff in the department who speak patient's language to translate or call 'Language Line'		1	0
	Offers to find if leaflet is provided within the department for patient's condition in their language		1	0
	Simulated patient score (2=very good, 1=satisfactory, 0=poor)	2	1	0
	Total Score			

Global Rating	1 Clear Fail	2 Borderline	3 Clear Pass	4 Very Good	5 Outstanding

Candidate Number:	University:
Date:	Year of Study:

STATION 2 – THE FOREIGN PATIENT

	Appropriate introduction (1=full name and role), checks patient's name (1)	2	1	0
	Establishes rapport with the patient (1) and starts with an open question (1)	2	1	0
	Obtains a Clinical History			
	Establishes level patient can speak English		1	0
	Explores presenting complaint (2=in detail, 1=adequately, 0=not at all) Symptoms, time of onset, severity of pain, range of movement	2	1	0
	Explores patient's past medical history (2=in detail, 1=poorly, 0=not at all)	2	1	0
	Checks if patient is currently on any medication (1) or has allergies (1)	2	1	0
	Explores patient's social history – smoking, alcohol, social circumstances (2=all three, 1=any two, 0=one or none)	2	1	0
	Offers appropriate medical advice and follow-up • Clinical examination of joint • Investigation with X-ray • Simple analgesia (e.g. ibuprofen with referral to orthopaedics depending on X-rays) (2=any two suggestions, 1=any one suggestion, 0=not mentioned)	2	1	0
	Suggests follow-up appointment (preferably with a translator)		1	0
	General Communication Skills			
	Uses non-verbal means of aiding communication (e.g. drawing or pointing at objects) (2=does well and creatively, 1=attempts, 0=does not attempt)	2	1	0
	Maintains eye contact with the patient (1) and persists in taking a good history (1)	2	1	0
	Avoids medical jargon		1	0
	Checks patient's understanding		1	0
	Rephrases questions to aid patient's understanding (2=attempts and persists in multiple methods, 1=rephrases only once and repeats self with failure to see that the patient is not understanding, 0=no attempt to rephrase any questions)	2	1	0
	Candidate was non-patronising and considerate with the patient		1	0
	Summarises presenting complaint (1) and management plan (1)	2	1	0
	Examiner to ask: 'What else could you do to improve communication?'			
	Explores whether patient is accompanied by anyone who speaks English		1	0
	Offers to find staff in the department who speak patient's language to translate or call 'Language Line'		1	0
	Offers to find if leaflet is provided within the department for patient's condition in their language		1	0
	Simulated patient score (2=very good, 1=satisfactory, 0=poor)	2	1	0
	Total Score			

Global Rating	1 Clear Fail	2 Borderline	3 Clear Pass	4 Very Good	5 Outstanding

Candidate Number:	University:
Date:	Year of Study:

STATION 3 – THE ANGRY PATIENT – MISCOMMUNICATION

	Appropriate introduction (1=full name and role), checks patient's name (1)	**2**	**1**	**0**
	Establishes rapport with the patient (1) and starts with an open question (1)	**2**	**1**	**0**
	Establishes Reason for GP Visit			
	Establishes current circumstance (1) and recent events (1)	**2**	**1**	**0**
	Enquires about circumstances leading to patient's dissatisfaction without prejudice		**1**	**0**
	Acknowledges patient's anger and validates their feelings		**1**	**0**
	Allows patient to vent their anger		**1**	**0**
	Explains how the situation leading to patient's anger may have arisen (1) without belittling the situation or creating excuses for the situation (1)	**2**	**1**	**0**
	Apologises (1) and offers to help (1) the patient or alleviate their dissatisfaction	**2**	**1**	**0**
	Apologises for absence of barium enema report (1) but offers to get the study reported soon by contacting the radiologist and the hospital (1)	**2**	**1**	**0**
	Candidate attempts to discover any other reason behind the anger such as frustration, fear or guilt (2=in detail and with patience, 1=briefly explored, 0=not explored)	**2**	**1**	**0**
	Negotiates and agrees a course of action (2=in detail and with agreement from both parties, 1=mentions a plan but not in detail or taking all patient's feelings into account, 0=not done)	**2**	**1**	**0**
	Offers to help patient with submission of a complaint if he wishes to proceed with this		**1**	**0**
	Communication Skills			
	Candidate avoids dismissive, threatening body language or interrupting the patient (1). Good use of eye contact and does not raise their voice (1).	**2**	**1**	**0**
	Avoids blaming colleagues, being judgmental or criticising the patient		**1**	**0**
	Candidate uses verbal and non-verbal clues to demonstrate active listening		**1**	**0**
	Demonstrates empathy (verbally and non-verbally)		**1**	**0**
	Candidate remains calm and professional throughout consultation		**1**	**0**
	Closing Remarks			
	Invites patient to offer suggestions for future improvement of service		**1**	**0**
	Invites patient's questions (1) and responds appropriately (1)	**2**	**1**	**0**
	Summarises situation (1) and checks patient understanding of action plan (1)	**2**	**1**	**0**
	Simulated patient score (2=very good, 1=satisfactory, 0=poor)	**2**	**1**	**0**
	Total Score			

Global Rating	**1** Clear Fail	**2** Borderline	**3** Clear Pass	**4** Very Good	**5** Outstanding

Candidate Number:		University:
Date:		Year of Study:

STATION 4 – THE ANGRY PATIENT – PRESCRIPTION ERROR

		2	1	0
	Appropriate introduction (1=full name and role), checks patient's name (1)	2	1	0
	Establishes rapport with the patient (1) and starts with an open question (1)	2	1	0
	Establishes Reason for Consultation			
	Enquires about the current circumstance leading to patient's dissatisfaction		1	0
	Acknowledges patient's anger and validates their feelings		1	0
	Allows patient to vent their anger		1	0
	Accepts responsibility for error and apologises for mistake	2	1	0
	Explains how the mistake may have arisen	2	1	0
	Corrective Action			
	Offers to do something to help the patient alleviate their dissatisfaction		1	0
	Suggests how situation may be sorted/prevented in future: • Highlighting allergy in red in the drug chart and clinical notes • Administration of antihistamines +/- steroids to alleviate rash • Discussion of situation with colleagues so team aware (2=all three of the above options, 1=any two of the above options, 0=only one or none)	2	1	0
	Advises patient on hospital complaints procedure with PALS should they wish to submit a letter of complaint		1	0
	Candidate explains they will submit a critical incident form		1	0
	Negotiates and agrees a course of action (2=a comprehensive plan performed in a sensitive manner, 1=vague plan or poorly done, 0=no clear decision on next course of action)	2	1	0
	Establishes whether patient has any other concerns or expectations of the situation (2=does well and sensitively, 1=asks but doesn't respond to patient's concerns, 0=not done)	2	1	0
	Communication Skills			
	Candidate avoids dismissive, threatening body language or interrupting the patient (1). Good use of eye contact and does not raise their voice (1).	2	1	0
	Avoids criticising the patient or blaming colleagues		1	0
	Candidate uses verbal and non-verbal clues to demonstrate active listening		1	0
	Demonstrates empathy (verbally and non-verbally)		1	0
	Candidate remains calm and professional throughout consultation	2	1	0
	Closing Remarks			
	Invites patients questions (1) and responds appropriately (1)	2	1	0
	Summarises situation (1) and checks patient understanding of action plan (1)	2	1	0
	Simulated patient score (2=very good, 1=satisfactory, 0=poor)	2	1	0
	Total Score			

Global Rating	1 Clear Fail	2 Borderline	3 Clear Pass	4 Very Good	5 Outstanding

Candidate Number:	University:
Date:	Year of Study:

STATION 5 – THE ANGRY FAMILY MEMBER

	Appropriate introduction (1=full name and role), checks patient's name (1)	2	1	0
	Establishes rapport with the patient (1) and starts with an open question (1)	2	1	0
	Establishes Reason for Consultation			
	Enquires about the current circumstance leading to patient's dissatisfaction		1	0
	Acknowledges patient's anger and validates their feelings		1	0
	Allows patient to vent their anger		1	0
	Candidate attempts to discover any other reason behind the anger such as frustration, fear or guilt (2=explores in detail, 1=explores briefly, 0=not done)	2	1	0
	Establishes Current Situation			
	Explains that patient has a right to privacy (1) and the fact the diagnosis was not discussed was due to the need to respect patient's wishes (1)	2	1	0
	Explains that to breach patient privacy would undermine the doctor-patient relationship		1	0
	Explores how much the wife already knows regarding husband's diagnosis		1	0
	Understands wife's reluctance for palliative care team involvement (1), however, curative treatment is not possible for the stage of the cancer (1)	2	1	0
	Encourages wife to have a frank conversation with her husband to resolve any misunderstandings		1	0
	Offers to do something to help the patient or alleviate their dissatisfaction		1	0
	Negotiates a course of action such as arranging to speak to wife regarding husband's situation with him present (if he agrees) or arranging a meeting with the consultant in charge of his care (2=performs well, 1=done poorly, 0=not done)	2	1	0
	Explores wife and patient's social circumstances and support network (2=in detail, 1=briefly touched upon, 0=not asked)	2	1	0
	Offers counselling for the current bad news if appropriate		1	0
	Communication Skills			
	Candidate avoids dismissive, threatening body language or interrupting the patient (1). Good use of eye contact and does not raise their voice (1).	2	1	0
	Avoids blaming colleagues or criticising the patient		1	0
	Candidate uses verbal and non-verbal clues to demonstrate active listening		1	0
	Demonstrates empathy (verbally and non-verbally)		1	0
	Candidate remains calm and professional throughout consultation	2	1	0
	Closing Remarks			
	Invites patients questions (1) and responds appropriately (1)	2	1	0
	Summarises situation (1) and checks patient's understanding of action plan (1)	2	1	0
	Simulated patient score (2=very good, 1=satisfactory, 0=poor)	2	1	0
	Total Score			

Global Rating	1 Clear Fail	2 Borderline	3 Clear Pass	4 Very Good	5 Outstanding

Candidate Number:	University:
Date:	Year of Study:

STATION 6 – NEGOTIATING SKILLS – ANTIBIOTIC PRESCRIPTION

	Appropriate introduction (1=full name and role), checks patient's name (1)	**2**	**1**	**0**
	Establishes rapport with the patient (1) and starts with an open question (1)	**2**	**1**	**0**
	Establishes Reason for GP Visit			
	Elicits details of presenting complaint		**1**	**0**
	Obtains a brief past medical history (1) and current medication including allergies (1)	**2**	**1**	**0**
	Acknowledges (1) and responds to patient's feelings appropriately (1)	**2**	**1**	**0**
	Establishes patient's agenda and desire for antibiotics		**1**	**0**
	Explores patient's ideas and concerns (1) and responds appropriately (1)	**2**	**1**	**0**
	Delivering Information			
	Empathises with patient's situation and work circumstances		**1**	**0**
	Explains that antibiotics are designed to kill bacteria (1) and have no effect on viruses (1)	**2**	**1**	**0**
	Explains that the patient's symptoms are likely to be viral in origin (1) and therefore it is unlikely that antibiotics would help (1)	**2**	**1**	**0**
	Outlines most appropriate medical plan would be to take simple analgesia (i.e. soluble aspirin or paracetamol) with plenty of fluids and rest (2=in detail, 1=briefly only mentions one of the points above, 0=no mention of medical plan)	**2**	**1**	**0**
	Negotiates prescription of antibiotics if no improvement of symptoms (1) and follow-up appointment in approximately one week's time (1)	**2**	**1**	**0**
	Outlines the danger of overprescribing of antibiotics (i.e. resistance to infection (1) and side effects from medication (1))	**2**	**1**	**0**
	Communication Skills			
	Candidate uses verbal and non-verbal clues to demonstrate active listening		**1**	**0**
	Candidate remains calm and professional throughout consultation		**1**	**0**
	Avoids intimidating or patronizing the patient (1). Use of non-medical jargon (1).	**2**	**1**	**0**
	Closing Remarks			
	Invites patients questions (1) and responds appropriately (1)	**2**	**1**	**0**
	Summarises situation (1) and checks patient's understanding of action plan (1)	**2**	**1**	**0**
	Organised (e.g. systematic, signposts change in focus of questions and topics)	**2**	**1**	**0**
	Simulated patient score (2=very good, 1=satisfactory, 0=poor)	**2**	**1**	**0**
	Total Score			

Global Rating	**1** Clear Fail	**2** Borderline	**3** Clear Pass	**4** Very Good	**5** Outstanding

Candidate Number:	University:
Date:	Year of Study:

STATION 7 – NEGOTIATING SKILLS – ALTERNATIVE THERAPY

	Appropriate introduction (1=full name and role), checks patient's name (1)	2	1	0
	Establishes rapport with the patient (1) and starts with an open question (1)	2	1	0
	Establishes Reason for Consultation			
	Establishes how much patient understands about her current diagnosis		1	0
	Establishes that patient is refusing to undergo current chemotherapy treatment		1	0
	Explores reasons behind this decision (1) and establishes whether patient has been coerced or if this is her own choice (1)	2	1	0
	Elicits whether patient has discussed feelings with family and friends (1) and what their opinions on the matter are (1)	2	1	0
	Acknowledges (1) and responds to patient's feelings appropriately (1)	2	1	0
	Explains patient's diagnosis and potential for curative therapy in easy to understand manner (2=does well, 1=does poorly, 0=not done at all)	2	1	0
	Negotiates Compromise			
	Acknowledges patient's concerns regarding chemotherapy (1) but explains that she may not necessarily suffer all the side effects (1)	2	1	0
	Explains how and why chemotherapy works (1) and that there have been numerous clinical trials to prove a beneficial outcome (1)	2	1	0
	Alternative therapy may work in certain circumstances, however, evidence is anecdotal		1	0
	Side effects from alternative therapies can be unpredictable (1) and delaying conventional therapy may cause a deterioration in patient's clinical situation (1)	2	1	0
	Encourages patient to take time to weigh up options first		1	0
	Negotiates a compromise of perhaps starting chemotherapy and if response is poor then considering alternative methods at a later date if appropriate (2=does professionally and allows patient to make decision in their own time, 1=does in an aggressive manner or only does poorly, 0=not done)	2	1	0
	Communication Skills			
	Candidate uses verbal and non-verbal clues to demonstrate active listening		1	0
	Avoids ridiculing patient's beliefs or being patronizing		1	0
	Demonstrates empathy (verbally and non-verbally)		1	0
	Candidate remains calm and professional throughout consultation		1	0
	Avoids medical jargon		1	0
	Closing Remarks			
	Invites patients questions (1) and responds appropriately (1)	2	1	0
	Summarises situation (1) and checks patient's understanding of action plan (1)	2	1	0
	Simulated patient score (2=very good, 1=satisfactory, 0=poor)	2	1	0
	Total Score			

Global Rating	1 Clear Fail	2 Borderline	3 Clear Pass	4 Very Good	5 Outstanding

Candidate Number:	University:
Date:	Year of Study:

STATION 8 – NEGOTIATING SKILLS – METHADONE PRESCRIPTION

	2	1	0
Appropriate introduction (1=full name and role), checks patient's name (1)	2	1	0
Establishes rapport with the patient (1) and starts with an open question (1)	2	1	0
Establishes Reason for GP Visit			
Establishes that patient has had prescription stolen		1	0
Enquires whether the case was reported to the police already		1	0
Acknowledges (1) and responds (1) to patient's feelings appropriately	2	1	0
Establishes patient's need for repeat prescription for the week		1	0
Elicits details of past medical history		1	0
Elicits details of drug abuse		1	0
Elicits details of past treatment and current treatment (1) including which doctor is currently supervising his methadone management (1)	2	1	0
Issues Regarding Prescribing Controlled Drugs			
Candidate establishes that they are not allowed to prescribe controlled drugs		1	0
Attempts to offer patient alternative means of obtaining prescription: • Does the patient have a psychiatrist who is available to prescribe for him? • Does the patient attend a chemist where photo identification and details regarding daily prescriptions are recorded who may be able to dispense to him? (2=any two options from above, 1=any one option)	2	1	0
Candidate refuses to give the week's course of methadone prescription		1	0
Offers to discuss situation with a senior partner in the clinic		1	0
Negotiates compromise of one supervised dose in the clinic if another GP is willing to prescribe the dose		1	0
Offers to inform the patient's regular GP when they return from leave (1) and arrange an early appointment with him (1)	2	1	0
Communication Skills			
Candidate uses verbal and non-verbal clues to demonstrate active listening		1	0
Demonstrates empathy (verbally and non-verbally)		1	0
Candidate remains calm and professional throughout consultation		1	0
Avoids medical jargon		1	0
Closing Remarks			
Offers to help with any other medical problems patient has other than the methadone prescription		1	0
Invites patient's questions (1) and responds appropriately (1)	2	1	0
Summarises situation (1) and checks patient's understanding of action plan (1)	2	1	0
Simulated patient score (2=very good, 1=satisfactory, 0=poor)	2	1	0
Total Score			

Global Rating	1 Clear Fail	2 Borderline	3 Clear Pass	4 Very Good	5 Outstanding

Candidate Number:		University:
Date:		Year of Study:

STATION 9 – NEGOTIATING SKILLS – THE SICK NOTE

Appropriate introduction (1=full name and role), checks patient's name (1)	2	1	0
Establishes rapport with the patient (1) and starts with an open question (1)	2	1	0
Obtains a Clinical History			
Elicits details of current presenting complaint (2=does well)	2	1	0
Elicits details of past medical history (1) and current medication (1)	2	1	0
Establishes that patient is not physically ill		1	0
Enquires after patient's mental health (1) and establishes they are not emotionally or mentally ill (1)	2	1	0
Establishes Real Reason Behind GP Visit			
Explores why patient is not prepared for exam		1	0
Establishes whether patient has obtained similar sick notes in the past		1	0
States that it is unethical for a doctor to write a note saying patient is ill when it is untrue		1	0
Refuses to write the sick note for the patient		1	0
Encourages patient to discuss circumstances and options with educational supervisor		1	0
Suggests re-sitting or delay sitting examination if not adequately prepared		1	0
Offers to speak to supervisor if patient wishes		1	0
Offers to help patient with future medical problems		1	0
Closing Remarks			
Invites questions from patient		1	0
Summarises situation (1) and checks patient's understanding (1)	2	1	0
Professionalism and calm manner throughout consultation		1	0
Candidate was non-patronising and non-judgmental		1	0
Simulated patient score (2=very good, 1=satisfactory, 0=poor)	2	1	0
Total Score			

Global Rating	1 Clear Fail	2 Borderline	3 Clear Pass	4 Very Good	5 Outstanding

Candidate Number:	University:
Date:	Year of Study:

STATION 10 – THE JEHOVAH'S WITNESS

	Appropriate introduction (1=full name and role), establishes patient's wife's name (1)	**2**	**1**	**0**
	Establishes rapport with the patient's wife (1) and starts with an open question (1)	**2**	**1**	**0**
	Establishes Reason for Consultation			
	Establishes the wife's agenda		**1**	**0**
	Acknowledges (1) and responds (1) to patient's feelings appropriately	**2**	**1**	**0**
	Explains that husband is aware of risks from the operation (1) and has signed a consent form detailing this (1)	**2**	**1**	**0**
	Establishes that doctors cannot go against the patient's wishes (1) and there is the potential of undermining the patient-doctor relationship (1)	**2**	**1**	**0**
	Explores whether wife has discussed her feelings with her husband (1) and encourages further discussion with husband (1)	**2**	**1**	**0**
	Explores whether other family members have been involved (1) and whether they share her view (1)	**2**	**1**	**0**
	Delivering Information			
	Outlines other options for minimizing blood loss: • Potential for autologous blood transfusion • Cell Saver device intra-operatively • Intravenous fluids to improve output if there is fluid loss (2=any two options, 1=any one option above)	**2**	**1**	**0**
	Explains details regarding the operation: • Laparascopic procedure to minimise blood loss (1) • Immediate ligation of any bleeding vessels identified (1)	**2**	**1**	**0**
	Offers to hold a meeting with surgical consultant with patient present if necessary		**1**	**0**
	Reassures wife where possible (1) without giving false hope (1)	**2**	**1**	**0**
	Negotiates an action plan (2=does thoroughly, 1=does adequately, 0=not done)	**2**	**1**	**0**
	Communication Skills			
	Listens actively (e.g. picks up cues/responds appropriately to information)		**1**	**0**
	Empathy (both non-verbally and verbally)		**1**	**0**
	Avoids medical jargon (1) and repetition of questions (1)	**2**	**1**	**0**
	Professionalism and calm manner throughout consultation		**1**	**0**
	Closing Remarks			
	Invites questions from wife (1) and responds appropriately (1)	**2**	**1**	**0**
	Summarises situation (1) and checks wife's understanding (1)	**2**	**1**	**0**
	Organised (e.g. systematic, summarises, signposts change in focus of questions)	**2**	**1**	**0**
	Simulated patient score (2=very good, 1=satisfactory, 0=poor)	**2**	**1**	**0**
	Total Score			

Global Rating	**1** Clear Fail	**2** Borderline	**3** Clear Pass	**4** Very Good	**5** Outstanding

Candidate Number:	University:
Date:	Year of Study:

STATION 11 – DOMESTIC VIOLENCE

Appropriate introduction (1=full name and role), checks patient's name (1)	2	1	0
Explains what interview will be about and asks for consent (2=does it well)	2	1	0
Starts with an open question		1	0
Social History			
Home circumstances (2=in some detail e.g. lives with husband, husband in army, lives on base)	2	1	0
Whether patient has children		1	0
Patient's occupation (2=explores in some detail)	2	1	0
Explores patient's support network of family and friends (2=explores in some detail)	2	1	0
Alcohol (1), recreational drugs (1)	2	1	0
Elicits Information About Violence			
Whether any violence or intimidation (2=asks in sensitive manner)	2	1	0
Explores nature of violence	2	1	0
Finds out how long violence has been going on (1) frequency of episodes (1)	2	1	0
Whether any other form of abuse or control (e.g. sexual, emotional, financial)	2	1	0
Explores patient's explanation for husband's behaviour (2=in detail)	2	1	0
Reassures that she is not to blame (1) acknowledges importance of explaining what has happened (1)	2	1	0
Explores what she wants to have happen now (2=in some detail and addresses issue of confidentiality)	2	1	0
Gives Information			
Higher prevalence of domestic violence in pregnancy (1) Suggests patient has a bag packed in safe place or keeps mobile phone close by (1)	2	1	0
Offers information on support (e.g. GP helpline, phone numbers of organisations, information leaflets or other sensible suggestions) (2=thorough)	2	1	0
Offers information about photographic evidence of bruising or writing notes (1) can be used as evidence if police prosecute (1)	2	1	0
Questioning skills (e.g. appropriate blend of open and closed questions, clarity)	2	1	0
Avoids leading questions (0=uses leading questions)		1	0
Listens actively (e.g. picks up cues/responds appropriately to information)		1	0
Organised (e.g. systematic, summarises, signposts change in focus of questions)	2	1	0
Simulated patient score (2=very good, 1=satisfactory, 0=poor)	2	1	0
Total Score			

Global Rating	**1** Clear Fail	**2** Borderline	**3** Clear Pass	**4** Very Good	**5** Outstanding

Candidate Number:		University:	
Date:		Year of Study:	

STATION 12 – DO NOT RESUSCITATE ORDER

Appropriate introduction (1=full name and role), establishes patient's daughter's name (1)	2	1	0
Establishes rapport with the patient's daughter (1) and asks an open question (1)	2	1	0
Establishes Current Clinical Circumstances			
Establishes what patient's daughter understands regarding current situation		1	0
Clarifies any misinterpretation regarding patient's clinical circumstance		1	0
Acknowledges and responds to daughter's feelings appropriately		1	0
DNAR Orders			
Explores what daughter already knows regarding 'DNAR' orders		1	0
Explains that a DNAR order is a medical decision (1) and cannot be dictated by family members (1)	2	1	0
Explains that DNAR order needs to be made by the consultant in charge		1	0
Asks if daughter has discussed use of life-sustaining treatment with the patient or what the patient's preferences are (i.e. any advance directives) (2= in detail, 1=brief discussion, 0=not done)	2	1	0
States patient's preferences might be different to daughter's		1	0
Explains mother has been resuscitated successfully on this occasion (1) and that future resuscitation may also be successful and life saving (1)	2	1	0
Asks about mother's quality of life prior to admission (1) and points out that patient still has a good quality of life to return to (1)	2	1	0
Offers to arrange a meeting with consultant regarding mother's DNAR status (1) and states patient and daughter may be present to discuss issue further (1)	2	1	0
Explains that discussion can be done in a sensitive way (1) and patient may welcome the opportunity to discuss her own treatment (1)	2	1	0
Candidate refuses to write a DNAR order without team discussion and patient's knowledge		1	0
Communication Skills			
Listens actively (e.g. picks up cues/responds appropriately to information)		1	0
Empathy (both non-verbally and verbally)		1	0
Avoids medical jargon (1) and repetition of questions/statements (1)	2	1	0
Professionalism and calm manner throughout consultation		1	0
Closing Remarks			
Invites questions (1) and responds appropriately (1)	2	1	0
Summarises situation and action plan (1). Checks understanding (1).	2	1	0
Organised (e.g. systematic, summarises, signposts change in focus of questions)	2	1	0
Simulated patient score (2=very good, 1=satisfactory, 0=poor)	2	1	0
Total Score			

Global Rating	1 Clear Fail	2 Borderline	3 Clear Pass	4 Very Good	5 Outstanding

Candidate Number:	University:
Date:	Year of Study:

STATION 13 – BREAKING BAD NEWS – ROAD TRAFFIC ACCIDENT

	Appropriate introduction (1=full name and role), checks patient's name (1)	2	1	0
	Establishes rapport with the patient (1) and starts with an open question (1)	2	1	0
	Current Situation and Delivers News			
	Establishes patient's understanding of situation so far		1	0
	Ask if patient would like anyone else to be present (e.g. family member)		1	0
	Gives warning shot		1	0
	Delivers bad news regarding patient's fiancé (2=does well)	2	1	0
	Use of silence to give patient space to think and absorb information		1	0
	Communication Skills			
	Acknowledges patient's feelings and concerns (1) and responds appropriately (1)	2	1	0
	Checks what and how much information patient wants at this point		1	0
	Reassures where possible		1	0
	Empathy (both non-verbally and verbally)		1	0
	Avoids medical jargon		1	0
	Listens actively (e.g. picks up cues/responds appropriately)		1	0
	Delivering Information			
	Explains diagnosis (1) and probable prognosis of patient's situation (e.g. full recovery but with physiotherapy and surgery for his fracture) (1)	2	1	0
	Explains referral to specialist (e.g. orthopaedics) (1) and for further investigations (e.g. X-rays, CT scans) (1)	2	1	0
	Describes possible treatment options (2=in detail regarding surgery, time to recover, hospital stay and physiotherapy post-operatively, 1=briefly mentions this, 0=none)	2	1	0
	Encourages patient to discuss news with family and call them if appropriate		1	0
	Offers counselling		1	0
	Closing Remarks			
	Invites questions from patient (1) and offers patient contact details in case of emergency or questions they have at a later stage (1)	2	1	0
	Summarises situation (1) and checks patient's understanding (1)	2	1	0
	Organised (e.g. systematic, signposts change in focus of interview)	2	1	0
	Simulated patient score (2=very good, 1=satisfactory, 0=poor)	2	1	0
	Total Score			

Global Rating	**1** Clear Fail	**2** Borderline	**3** Clear Pass	**4** Very Good	**5** Outstanding

Candidate Number:	University:
Date:	Year of Study:

STATION 14 – BREAKING BAD NEWS – MISCARRIAGE

Appropriate introduction (1=full name and role), checks patient's name (1)	2	1	0
Establishes rapport with the patient (1) and starts with an open question (1)	2	1	0
Current Situation and Delivers News			
Establishes patient's understanding of situation so far		1	0
Obtains consent from patient for consultation (1) and summarises situation to date (1)	2	1	0
Asks if patient would like anyone else to be present (e.g. family member)		1	0
Gives warning shot		1	0
Delivers bad news and results of the investigations (2=does well)	2	1	0
Use of silence to give patient space to think and absorb information		1	0
Communication Skills			
Acknowledges patient's feelings concerns (1) and responds appropriately (1)	2	1	0
Checks what and how much information patient wants at this point		1	0
Reassures where possible (1) without giving false hope (1)	2	1	0
Empathy (both non-verbally and verbally)		1	0
Avoids medical jargon		1	0
Listens actively (e.g. picks up cues/responds appropriately)		1	0
Delivering Information			
Explains referral to specialist (1) and for further investigations (1)	2	1	0
Encourages patient to discuss news with family		1	0
Offers counselling		1	0
Arranges follow-up (1) and offers patient information leaflet (1)	2	1	0
Closing Remarks			
Invites questions from patient (1) and offers patient contact details in case of emergency or questions they have at a later stage (1)	2	1	0
Summarises situation (1) and checks patient's understanding (1)	2	1	0
Checks that patient is fit to leave after consultation and can safely return home		1	0
Organised (e.g. systematic, signposts change in focus of interview)	2	1	0
Simulated patient score (2=very good, 1=satisfactory, 0=poor)	2	1	0
Total Score			

Global Rating	1 Clear Fail	2 Borderline	3 Clear Pass	4 Very Good	5 Outstanding

Candidate Number:	University:
Date:	Year of Study:

STATION 15 – BREAKING BAD NEWS

Appropriate introduction (1=full name and role), checks patient's name (1)	2	1	0
Establishes rapport with the patient (1) and starts with an open question (1)	2	1	0
Current Situation and Delivers News			
Establishes patient's understanding of situation so far		1	0
Obtains consent from patient for consultation (1) and summarises situation to date (1)	2	1	0
Asks if patient would like anyone else to be present (e.g. family member)		1	0
Gives warning shot		1	0
Delivers bad news and results of the investigations (2=does well)	2	1	0
Use of silence to give patient space to think and absorb information		1	0
Communication Skills			
Acknowledges patient's feelings and concerns (1) and responds appropriately (1)	2	1	0
Checks what and how much information patient wants at this point		1	0
Reassures where possible (1) without giving false hope (1)	2	1	0
Empathy (both non-verbally and verbally)		1	0
Avoids medical jargon		1	0
Listens actively (e.g. picks up cues/responds appropriately)		1	0
Delivering Information			
Explains diagnosis (1) and probable prognosis (1)	2	1	0
Explains referral to specialist (1) and for further investigations (1)	2	1	0
Describes possible treatment options (2=does in detail)	2	1	0
Encourages patient to discuss news with family and if appropriate, to accompany patient at subsequent appointments		1	0
Offers counselling		1	0
Arranges follow-up (1) and offers patient information leaflet (1)	2	1	0
Closing Remarks			
Invites questions from patient (1) and offers patient contact details in case of emergency or questions they have at a later stage (1)	2	1	0
Summarises situation (1) and checks patient's understanding (1)	2	1	0
Checks that patient is fit to leave after consultation and can safely return home		1	0
Organised (e.g. systematic, signposts change in focus of interview)	2	1	0
Simulated patient score (2=very good, 1=satisfactory, 0=poor)	2	1	0
Total Score			

Global Rating	1 Clear Fail	2 Borderline	3 Clear Pass	4 Very Good	5 Outstanding

Candidate Number:	University:
Date:	Year of Study:

STATION 16 – GIVING MEDICAL INFORMATION

	Appropriate introduction (1=full name and role), checks patient's name (1)	2	1	0
	Establishes rapport with the patient (1) and starts with an open question (1)	2	1	0
	Gathers Information			
	Establishes what the parent already knows about the situation (1) and who they have spoken to (1)	2	1	0
	Explores parent's ideas (1) and concerns (1) regarding situation	2	1	0
	Delivers Information			
	Apologises for not clarifying situation sooner (2=does well)	2	1	0
	Explains the situation clearly and in an easy to understand manner (2=clear and precise, 1=adequately but not easy to understand, 0=poor or not done)	2	1	0
	Offers explanation of likely diagnosis (i.e. intra-abdominal abscess)		1	0
	Explains the need for further investigation (e.g. CT scan to confirm diagnosis)		1	0
	Discusses possible management plans (i.e. surgery vs. intra-abdominal drain insertion and need for intravenous antibiotics) (2=in detail, 1=mentions briefly, 0=not done)	2	1	0
	Explains possible complications from treatment (recurrence of abscess, bleeding, further infection, failure of antibiotics, prolonged hospital stay) (2=any three, 1=any two)	2	1	0
	Reassures parent that prognosis is generally good		1	0
	Avoids false hope and promising a 'guaranteed recovery'		1	0
	Explores parent's (1) and patient's (1) social circumstances	2	1	0
	Offers parent the opportunity to discuss situation with consultant		1	0
	Communication Skills			
	Avoids patronizing parent		1	0
	Listens actively (e.g. picks up cues/responds appropriately)		1	0
	Demonstrates empathy (both verbally and non-verbally)		1	0
	Acknowledges parent's feelings and concerns (1) and responds appropriately (1)	2	1	0
	Avoids medical jargon (1) and paces information (1)	2	1	0
	Closing Remarks			
	Invites questions from parent (1) and responds appropriately (1)	2	1	0
	Summarises situation (1) and checks understanding (1)	2	1	0
	Offers parent a means of contacting doctors in case of emergency or if they have any questions at a later stage		1	0
	Organised (e.g. systematic, signposts change in focus of interview)	2	1	0
	Simulated patient score (2=very good, 1=satisfactory, 0=poor)	2	1	0
	Total Score			

Global Rating	1 Clear Fail	2 Borderline	3 Clear Pass	4 Very Good	5 Outstanding

Candidate Number:	University:
Date:	Year of Study:

STATION 17 – INTERPROFESSIONAL RELATIONSHIPS

		2	1	0
	Appropriate introduction (1=full name and role), checks patient's name (1)	2	1	0
	Establishes rapport with colleague (1) and starts with an open question (1)	2	1	0
	Establishes Reason for Meeting			
	States current problem with situation at work factually (1) in a non-threatening manner (1)	2	1	0
	Elicits colleague's response and perception of incident		1	0
	Explains personal agenda (1) and why colleague's behaviour has become a problem (1)	2	1	0
	Elicits colleague's agenda (1) and possible reasons behind circumstances at work (1)	2	1	0
	Offers advice and support to colleague (2=gives supporting advice in an understanding but firm manner, 1=gives advice but in a glib manner, 0=not done)	2	1	0
	Advises seeking help from educational supervisor if further support required		1	0
	Establishes that current situation is not ideal and the need for change		1	0
	Negotiates and agrees a course of action with colleague (2=clear plan of action, 1=vague or poor action plan, 0=not done)	2	1	0
	Communication Skills			
	Avoids being judgmental, blaming or criticising colleague (2=done sensitively without upsetting or creating a bad working atmosphere, 1=some attempt at being sensitive, 0=not done)	2	1	0
	Listens actively (e.g. picks up cues/ responds appropriately)		1	0
	Demonstrates empathy (both verbally and non-verbally)		1	0
	Closing Remarks			
	Invites further questions and remarks from colleague		1	0
	Summarises plan of action (1) and checks colleague is in agreement (1)	2	1	0
	Maintains a calm and professional manner throughout consultation		1	0
	Organised (e.g. systematic, signposts change in focus of interview)	2	1	0
	Simulated patient score (2=very good, 1=satisfactory, 0=poor)	2	1	0
	Total Score			

Global Rating	1 Clear Fail	2 Borderline	3 Clear Pass	4 Very Good	5 Outstanding

CHAPTER 8: CONSENTING AND EXPLAINING PROCEDURES

Written by Mr. J. Lynch

- Oesophagoduodenoscopy (OGD)
- Ultrasound Scan
- Capacity to Consent
- Appendicectomy
- Colonoscopy
- Endoscopic Retrograde Cholangio-Pancreatography (ERCP)
- Transurethral Resection of Prostate (TURP)
- Amniocentesis
- Liver Biopsy
- Laparascopic Cholecystectomy
- Chest Drain
- Lumbar Puncture
- Catheter Insertion

THE STATIONS

STATION 1
Time allowed: 7 minutes

You are a junior doctor working in gastrointestinal medicine outpatient-procedures department.

Runa Singh is an 83 year old lady who has been suffering from gastrointestinal-sounding chest pain and reflux symptoms, and has come in for an elective oesophagogastroduodenoscopy (OGD). She has been consented a couple of weeks ago in clinic, but has a few more questions.

Please address any concerns that Mrs Singh has with her procedure and re-discuss what she should expect during the OGD.

STATION 2
Time allowed: 7 minutes

You are a junior doctor working in the surgical outpatient's department.

You are working with a surgical consultant in the clinic. He has just seen a patient, Mr Steven Lo, and booked him for an ultrasound for his abdominal pain. The consultant is running late and explains that Mr Lo still has quite a few questions about his scan. He asks if you could help.

Please address any concerns that Mr Lo has with his ultrasound scan and re-discuss what he should expect during the scan.

STATION 3
Time allowed: 7 minutes

You are a junior doctor working in the surgical department.

A 7 year old patient, Victoria Grecker, has been admitted to hospital with right iliac fossa pain. She has been reviewed by the surgical registrar, who has consented and listed her for appendicectomy later this day. Victoria lives with her mother, who has been accompanying her throughout this process. The nurse informs you that the mother has some more questions about the operation.

Please address any concerns Victoria's mother has about her daughter's appendicectomy.

STATION 4
Time allowed: 7 minutes

You are a junior doctor working in the colorectal surgery outpatient clinic.

Your consultant has booked and consented Miss Susan Bingham for a colonoscopy, which is due to happen within the next two weeks. The patient has a nervous disposition and your consultant has asked you to discuss the procedure with her to help allay her concerns.

Please address any concerns that Miss Bingham has about her colonoscopy and re-discuss what she should expect during the procedure.

STATION 5

Time allowed: 7 minutes

You are a junior doctor working in the gastrointestinal medicine ward.

Your patient, Peter Peabody, has been admitted with abdominal pain and jaundice and an ultrasound revealed gallstones and dilated common bile duct. On the ward round this morning the consultant consented the patient for an endoscopic retrograde cholangio-pancreatography (ERCP) to retrieve the gallstones. The nurse calls you after the ward round as Mr Peabody has a few more questions.

Please address any concerns that Mr Peabody has about his ERCP and re-discuss what he should expect during the procedure.

STATION 6

Time allowed: 7 minutes

You are a junior doctor working in a urology firm.

Your patient, John Writter, is a 75 year old gentleman with benign prostatic hypertrophy who has come this morning in for a transurethral resection of the prostate (TURP). He was consented several months ago in clinic. Your registrar asks you to see him again before his surgery to find out if he has any more questions today.

Please address any concerns that Mr Writter has about his TURP and re-discuss what he should expect during the surgery.

STATION 7

Time allowed: 7 minutes

You are a junior doctor working in the obstetrics outpatient department.

Your patient, Cheryl Jones, has arrived for her amniocentesis. Your consultant is running late and has briefly consented her, but asked you to talk to her a bit further about her procedure.

Please address any concerns that Mrs Jones has about her amniocentesis procedure and re-discuss what she should expect.

STATION 8

Time allowed: 7 minutes

You are a junior doctor working in the gastrointestinal outpatient department.

Your consultant is running a liver biopsy list. Miss Gherkin is a 27 year old who has arrived for her appointment. She was consented in clinic a few weeks ago but has a few more questions today.

Please address any concerns that Miss Gherkin has regarding her liver biopsy.

STATION 9

Time allowed: 7 minutes

You are a junior doctor working in the surgical department.

Your patient, Mr John Hartman, has arrived for an elective laparoscopic cholecystectomy. He was consented in clinic several months ago but has a few more questions.

Please address any concerns that Mr Hartman has regarding his laparoscopic cholecystectomy and re-discuss what he should expect during the surgery.

CONSENT

Candidate Number:	University:
Date:	Year of Study:

STATION 1 – OESOPHAGODUODENSOCOPY (OGD)

		2	1	0
	Appropriate introduction (1=full name and role), checks patient's name (1)	2	1	0
	Establishes reason for consultation		1	0
	Informs Patient and Addresses Concerns			
	Asks what patient knows and what has happened so far		1	0
	Able to elicit patient's concerns about procedure (1), concerns about possible diagnosis (1)	2	1	0
	Elicits that patient would like a sedative		1	0
	Explains procedure – what it is (a camera test where a long thin device is inserted down the throat into the food pipe and images are taken looked at on a television screen) (1), why it is being done (to investigate causes for abdominal pain/stomach ulcers) (1)	2	1	0
	Explains biopsies may be taken, but these are painless		1	0
	Explains post-procedure plan – any 2 of: may have drowsiness (1), can go home same day after a few hours (1), should have someone to pick her up (1)	2	1	0
	Explains side effects: sore throat, sleepy if sedative given, bleeding, infection, perforation, dental complications (2=any three suggestions, 1=any two suggestions, 0=one or no suggestions)	2	1	0
	Explains follow-up: reports will be sent to GP within next few weeks		1	0
	Invites the patient to ask questions		1	0
	General Communication Skills			
	Uses non-verbal means of aiding communication (e.g. drawing or pointing at objects)		1	0
	Maintains eye contact with the patient and persists in taking a good history		1	0
	Avoids medical jargon		1	0
	Closing Remarks			
	Summarises key points		1	0
	Checks the patient's understanding		1	0
	Examiner to ask:			
	'What is the differential for epigastric pain after eating?' gastritis/oesophagitis, peptic ulcer, gallstones, pancreatitis, obstruction, mesenteric ischaemia, non-gastrointestinal (e.g. cardiac) (2=any three suggestions, 1=any two suggestions, 0=one or no suggestions)	2	1	0
	'What *initial* investigations would you consider?' blood tests (FBC, LFTs, amylase), ultrasound scan, ECG, abdominal X-ray (2=any three suggestions, 1=any two suggestions, 0=one or no suggestions)	2	1	0
	Simulated patient score (2=very good, 1=satisfactory, 0=poor)	2	1	0
	Total Score			

Global Rating	1 Clear Fail	2 Borderline	3 Clear Pass	4 Very Good	5 Outstanding

Candidate Number:	University:
Date:	Year of Study:

STATION 2 – ULTRASOUND SCAN

	Appropriate introduction (1=full name and role), checks patient's name (1)	2	1	0
	Establishes reason for consultation		1	0
	Informs Patient and Addresses Concerns			
	Asks what patient knows and what has happened so far		1	0
	Able to elicit patient's concerns about procedure (1), concerns about diagnosis (1)	2	1	0
	Explains that patient needs to be nil-by-mouth for his scan (1), and that it will take 15–20 mins (1)	2	1	0
	Explains procedure – what it is (invisible and silent sound waves targeting the abdomen and reflecting off the internal organs and captured back by the transducer device thereby creating an image on a video screen of the internal organs) (1), why it is being done (to investigate cause of abdominal pain and to look for liver lesions and gallstones) (1)	2	1	0
	Explains nature of gallstones: • why they cause pain (1) • can be uncomplicated but potential for development of cholecystitis or pancreatitis (1)	2	1	0
	Explains treatment options: • avoiding fatty foods may reduce the likelihood of abdominal pain (1) • if confirmed there is a curative surgical procedure (gallbladder removal) (1)	2	1	0
	Explains follow-up – reports will be sent to GP within next few weeks		1	0
	Invites the patient to ask questions		1	0
	General Communication Skills			
	Uses non-verbal means of aiding communication (e.g. drawing or pointing at objects)		1	0
	Maintains eye contact with the patient and persists in taking a good history		1	0
	Avoids medical jargon		1	0
	Closing Remarks			
	Summarises key points		1	0
	Checks the patient's understanding		1	0
	Examiner to ask:			
	'What are the most common clinical features of cholangitis?' abdominal pain, fever, jaundice (2=all three symptoms, 1=any two symptoms, 0=one or none)	2	1	0
	'When should cholecystectomy be performed after an acute attack of cholecystitis?' either within the first 3 days, or after a 6 week hiatus		1	0
	'What are the risks of cholecystectomy?' Immediate – bleeding, damage to common bile duct, complications of general anaesthesia, conversion to open procedure, chyle leak Early – infection, retained stone Late – retained stone (1 mark for dividing into immediate/early/late, 1 mark for two or more complications)	2	1	0
	Simulated patient score (2=very good, 1=satisfactory, 0=poor)	2	1	0
	Total Score			

Global Rating	**1** Clear Fail	**2** Borderline	**3** Clear Pass	**4** Very Good	**5** Outstanding

Candidate Number:	University:
Date:	Year of Study:

STATION 3 – PARENTAL CONSENT

	Appropriate introduction (1=full name and role), checks parent's name/child's name and relationship (1)	**2**	**1**	**0**
	Establishes reason for consultation		**1**	**0**
	Informs Parent and Addresses Concerns			
	Asks what parent knows and what has happened so far		**1**	**0**
	Able to elicit parent's concerns about procedure (1), concerns about diagnosis (1)	**2**	**1**	**0**
	Explains benefits of operation: to prevent abdominal sepsis due to perforation		**1**	**0**
	Explains details of procedure: general anaesthesia will be used and what this means (1), a small incision will be made in the RIF and the appendix removed (1)	**2**	**1**	**0**
	Explains possible complications: bleeding, infection, damage to bowel (2=all three suggestions, 1=any two suggestions, 0=one or none)	**2**	**1**	**0**
	Explains post-procedure plan: will be admitted overnight and if improves may be able to go home following day		**1**	**0**
	Elicits that parent is a Jehovah's Witness and does not want transfusion for her child (1), enquires whether patient has any reason to have an increased bleeding tendency (1)	**2**	**1**	**0**
	If asked whether the child will need blood during the operation, answers that it is possible (although unlikely) (1), answers that consultant will need to be involved in this discussion (1)	**2**	**1**	**0**
	General Communication Skills			
	Uses non-verbal means of aiding communication (e.g. drawing or pointing at objects)		**1**	**0**
	Maintains eye contact with the patient and persists in taking a good history		**1**	**0**
	Avoids use of medical jargon		**1**	**0**
	Closing Remarks			
	Summarises key points		**1**	**0**
	Checks the parent's understanding		**1**	**0**
	Invites the parent to ask questions		**1**	**0**
	Examiner to ask:			
	'In an emergency can you give blood to an unconscious child without the parent's consent?' Yes		**1**	**0**
	'Can a child give consent to an operation without the parent's knowledge?' Yes (1), if they are deemed Gillick competent (1)	**2**	**1**	**0**
	'Can a competent child refuse treatment that their parents have accepted?' No		**1**	**0**
	Simulated patient score (2=very good, 1=satisfactory, 0=poor)	**2**	**1**	**0**
	Total Score			

Global Rating	1 Clear Fail	2 Borderline	3 Clear Pass	4 Very Good	5 Outstanding

Candidate Number:	University:
Date:	Year of Study:

STATION 4 – COLONOSCOPY

	Appropriate introduction (1=full name and role), checks patient's name (1)	**2**	**1**	**0**
	Establishes reason for consultation		**1**	**0**
	Informs Patients and Addresses Concerns			
	Asks what patient knows and what has happened so far		**1**	**0**
	Able to elicit patient's concerns about procedure (1), concerns about diagnosis (1)	**2**	**1**	**0**
	Explains preparation for procedure: bowel preparation will be given as 2 sachets of 'Fleet' which need to be mixed with water and taken the morning and night before (1), intravenous sedation and pain relief will be administered immediately prior to the study (1)	**2**	**1**	**0**
	Explains procedure: what it is (a test where a long thin tube with a small camera at the end of it is inserted via the back passage and images viewed on a television screen to see for the presence of polyps and lesions) (1), why it is being done (to look for causes of change in bowel habits, bleeding and in particular to screen for cancer) (1)	**2**	**1**	**0**
	Explains possible complications: bleeding (1), infection (1), discomfort (1), risk of perforation (1) (maximum 2 marks)	**2**	**1**	**0**
	Explains post-procedure: drowsiness (1), will be in recovery area (1)	**2**	**1**	**0**
	Explains biopsies may be taken		**1**	**0**
	Explains follow-up: will be seen in outpatient appointment (1), results of biopsy (1)	**2**	**1**	**0**
	Warns of red-flag symptoms that patient should note: abdominal pain, excessive PR bleeding, temperature (2=any three suggestions, 1=any two suggestions, 0=one or none)	**2**	**1**	**0**
	Provides a leaflet		**1**	**0**
	General Communication Skills			
	Summarises key points		**1**	**0**
	Invites patient to ask questions		**1**	**0**
	Checks patient understanding		**1**	**0**
	Examiner to ask:			
	'What are the possible complications of colonoscopy?' Discomfort, failure to complete procedure, bleeding, perforation of colon (requiring operation), drowsiness from sedative, infection (2=three suggestions, 1=for two suggestions)	**2**	**1**	**0**
	'How do patients with ascending colon cancer present compared to those with descending or rectal cancer?' They tend to present with anaemia rather than obstruction (1) as the bowel contents are still not solid in the ascending colon (1)	**2**	**1**	**0**
	'What tumour markers would you request if you suspected colorectal carcinoma?' CEA (1), AFP (1)	**2**	**1**	**0**
	Simulated patient score (2=very good, 1=satisfactory, 0=poor)	**2**	**1**	**0**
	Total Score			

Global Rating	**1** Clear Fail	**2** Borderline	**3** Clear Pass	**4** Very Good	**5** Outstanding

Candidate Number:	University:
Date:	Year of Study:

STATION 5 – ENDOSCOPIC RETROGRADE CHOLANGIO-PANCREATOGRAPHY (ERCP)

	Appropriate introduction (1=full name and role), checks patient's name (1)	**2**	**1**	**0**
	Establishes reason for consultation		**1**	**0**
	Informs Patient and Addresses Concerns			
	Asks what patient knows and what has happened so far		**1**	**0**
	Able to elicit patient's concerns about procedure (1), concerns about diagnosis (1)	**2**	**1**	**0**
	Checks that patient has been nil-by-mouth for at least 6 hours		**1**	**0**
	Explains procedure – what it is (a test where a long thin device with a camera at the end is inserted down the throat into the stomach and then the small intestine to the level of where the common bile duct opens into the intestine, this tube is engaged and X-ray contrast agent administered into the duct. X-rays are then taken to look at the patency of the duct, gallstones and biopsies can be taken) (1), why it is being done (to look for gallstones, removal of gallstones, to investigate for growths at the opening of the bile or pancreatic ducts) (1)	**2**	**1**	**0**
	Explains that stents might be inserted into the bile-ducts to keep them patent (1), and that these may need to be removed later (1)	**2**	**1**	**0**
	Explains possible complications – any 2 of: sore throat, bleeding, infection, perforation of gut, damage to bile/pancreatic ducts, pancreatitis	**2**	**1**	**0**
	Warns that the procedure is not always successful, and that further procedures may be necessary		**1**	**0**
	Explores alternatives: MRCP		**1**	**0**
	Explains post-procedure plan: may have drowsiness (1), will be in recovery area (1)	**2**	**1**	**0**
	Explains follow-up – if successful they will stay overnight and may be able to go home tomorrow, but this is dependent on the consultant's decision		**1**	**0**
	General Communication Skills			
	Uses non-verbal means of aiding communication e.g. drawing or pointing at objects		**1**	**0**
	Maintains eye contact with the patient and persists in taking a good history		**1**	**0**
	Avoids medical jargon		**1**	**0**
	Closing Remarks			
	Summarises key points		**1**	**0**
	Checks the patient's understanding		**1**	**0**
	Invites the patient to ask questions		**1**	**0**
	Examiner to ask:			
	'What are the complications of ERCP?' Immediate – perforation (requiring operation), failure of procedure Early – bleeding, infection (cholangitis), pancreatitis, death (2=any three suggestions, 1=any two suggestions)	**2**	**1**	**0**
	Simulated patient score (2=very good, 1=satisfactory, 0=poor)	**2**	**1**	**0**
	Total Score			

Global Rating	**1** Clear Fail	**2** Borderline	**3** Clear Pass	**4** Very Good	**5** Outstanding

Candidate Number:		University:
Date:		Year of Study:

STATION 6 – TRANSURETHRAL RESECTION OF THE PROSTATE (TURP)

		2	1	0
	Appropriate introduction (1=full name and role), checks patient's name (1)	2	1	0
	Establishes reason for consultation		1	0
	Informs Patient and Addresses Concerns			
	Asks what patient knows about what has happened so far		1	0
	Able to elicit patient's concerns about procedure (1), concerns about diagnosis (1)	2	1	0
	Explains that BPH means Benign Prostatic Hyperplasia		1	0
	Checks that patient has been nil-by-mouth for at least 6 hours		1	0
	Explains procedure – what it is (i.e. a urological procedure where a thin device with a camera at the end is inserted into the urethra. The prostate is visualized and the prostate tissue is then removed with electrocautery or dissection) (1), why it is being done (1).	2	1	0
	Explains that anaesthetic will be used, either spinal or general		1	0
	Explains that alternatives exist (such as medication and catheterization)		1	0
	Explains possible complications – haematuria, injury to urethra/bladder, urinary incontinence, erectile dysfunction, retrograde ejaculation, urine infection, TURP syndrome, urinary retention (2=any three complications, 1=any two complications, 0=one or no complications mentioned)	2	1	0
	Warns that the condition can recur even with surgery		1	0
	Explains post-procedure plan: need to stay in overnight (1), will be catheterised, but this is usually removed within 24 hours (1)	2	1	0
	Explains follow-up: will be seen in outpatient's clinic in a few week's time		1	0
	General Communication Skills			
	Uses non-verbal means of aiding communication (e.g. drawing or pointing at objects)		1	0
	Maintains eye contact with the patient and persists in taking a good history		1	0
	Avoids medical jargon		1	0
	Closing Remarks			
	Summarises key points		1	0
	Checks the patient's understanding		1	0
	Invites the patient to ask questions		1	0
	Examiner to ask:			
	'How do you investigate suspected benign prostatic hyperplasia?' Digital examination of prostate, PSA blood test, ultrasound prostate, prostate biopsy, urodynamic flow tests (2=any three suggestions, 1=any two suggestions, 0=one or none)	2	1	0
	'How does tamsulosin work?' Alpha-blocker (1), causing smooth muscle relaxation in the prostate and bladder neck (1)	2	1	0
	Simulated patient score (2=very good, 1=satisfactory, 0=poor)	2	1	0
	Total Score			

Global Rating	1 Clear Fail	2 Borderline	3 Clear Pass	4 Very Good	5 Outstanding

Candidate Number:		University:	
Date:		Year of Study:	

STATION 7 – AMNIOCENTESIS

	Appropriate introduction (1=full name and role), checks patient's name (1)	**2**	**1**	**0**
	Establishes reason for consultation		**1**	**0**
	Informs Patient and Addresses Concerns			
	Asks what patient knows about what has happened so far		**1**	**0**
	Enquires about stage of pregnancy and progress so far		**1**	**0**
	Explains why test is being offered (the patient has blood tests which indicate higher risk of Down's syndrome) (1), and that it is not mandatory to know if Down's syndrome is present but the test is offered to all mothers in case they want to make plans for termination of pregnancy, should they wish (1)	**2**	**1**	**0**
	Able to elicit patient's concerns about procedure (1), worries regarding possibility of Down's syndrome (1)	**2**	**1**	**0**
	Explains procedure: • that ultrasound is used to identify foetus (1) • a needle is inserted and fluid is drawn off (1)	**2**	**1**	**0**
	Explains possible complications – miscarriage, infection, injury to the baby, Rhesus disease in the newborn (2=any three suggestions, 1=any two suggestions)	**2**	**1**	**0**
	Explains risk of miscarriage is 0.5–1%		**1**	**0**
	Warns of red-flag post-procedural symptoms requiring emergency attention: severe abdominal pain, contractions, PV bleeding, watery loss from vagina, fever (2=any three suggestions, 1=any two suggestions, 0=one or none)	**2**	**1**	**0**
	Explains post-procedure plan: can go home later, no need to stay in hospital overnight unless presence of complications		**1**	**0**
	Explains follow-up: will be seen in outpatients clinic in a couple of week's time with the results		**1**	**0**
	General Communication Skills			
	Uses non-verbal means of aiding communication (e.g. drawing or pointing at objects)		**1**	**0**
	Maintains eye contact with the patient and persists in taking a good history		**1**	**0**
	Avoids medical jargon		**1**	**0**
	Closing Remarks			
	Summarises key points		**1**	**0**
	Checks the patient's understanding		**1**	**0**
	Invites the patient to ask questions		**1**	**0**
	Examiner to ask:			
	'What is the chromosomal abnormality present in Down's' Trisomy 21		**1**	**0**
	Simulated patient score (2=very good, 1=satisfactory, 0=poor)	**2**	**1**	**0**
	Total Score			

Global Rating	**1** Clear Fail	**2** Borderline	**3** Clear Pass	**4** Very Good	**5** Outstanding

Candidate Number:	University:
Date:	Year of Study:

STATION 8 – LIVER BIOPSY

	Appropriate introduction (1=full name and role), checks patient's name (1)	**2**	**1**	**0**
	Establishes reason for consultation		**1**	**0**
	Informs Patient and Addresses Concerns			
	Asks what patient knows about what has happened so far		**1**	**0**
	Able to elicit patient's concerns about procedure (1), concerns about diagnosis (1)	**2**	**1**	**0**
	Explains procedure: what it is (an ultrasound scan will be taken of your liver to identify the lesion to biopsy, local anaesthetic will be used and a biopsy needle will be inserted through the skin into the liver to obtain a tissue sample) (1), why it is being done (to identify the pathology of the liver lesion, determine whether it is malignant) (1)	**2**	**1**	**0**
	Explains that local anaesthetic will be used		**1**	**0**
	Explains possible complications: bleeding (1), wound infection (1)	**2**	**1**	**0**
	Explains post-procedure plan: will be observed for a few hours to ensure no internal bleeding (1), can go home later on the same day if no apparent complications (1)	**2**	**1**	**0**
	Gives post-procedural advice: no contact sports for next few days (1), seek help if site looks infected or develops abdominal pain (1)	**2**	**1**	**0**
	Explains follow-up: will be seen in outpatient's clinic in a few weeks time with biopsy results		**1**	**0**
	General Communication Skills			
	Uses non-verbal means of aiding communication (e.g. drawing or pointing at objects)		**1**	**0**
	Maintains eye contact with the patient and persists in taking a good history		**1**	**0**
	Ensures that patient understands terms used		**1**	**0**
	Closing Remarks			
	Summarises key points		**1**	**0**
	Checks the patient's understanding		**1**	**0**
	Invites the patient to ask questions		**1**	**0**
	Examiner to ask:			
	'What blood test other than LFTs is a necessity before performing this procedure?' INR/clotting/platelets (1). The INR should be less than 1.5 before the procedure (1).	**2**	**1**	**0**
	'Please give your differential diagnosis for this patient.' Hepatic adenoma, hepatocellular carcinoma, liver metastases (any two for 1 mark)		**1**	**0**
	Simulated patient score (2=very good, 1=satisfactory, 0=poor)	**2**	**1**	**0**
	Total Score			

Global Rating	**1** Clear Fail	**2** Borderline	**3** Clear Pass	**4** Very Good	**5** Outstanding

Candidate Number:	University:
Date:	Year of Study:

STATION 9 – LAPAROSCOPIC CHOLECYSTECTOMY

	Appropriate introduction (1=full name and role), checks patient's name (1)	2	1	0
	Establishes reason for consultation		1	0
	Informs Patient and Addresses Concerns			
	Asks what patient knows about what has happened so far		1	0
	Able to elicit patient's concerns about procedure		1	0
	Explains procedure – what it is (a keyhole surgical operation to remove the gallbladder) (1), why it is being done (to remove gallbladder, improve symptoms) (1)	2	1	0
	Explains details of procedure: • General anaesthesia will be used and what this means (1) • Small incisions will be made in the abdomen and cameras/other instruments inserted through them (1)	2	1	0
	Explains possible complications: bleeding, infection, bile leak, larger wound in right upper quadrant if converted to open procedure (2=any three suggestions, 1=any two suggestions)	2	1	0
	Explains that normally patient should take at least a week off work		1	0
	Explains post-procedure plan: patient will be observed for a few hours (1), can often go home later that day, but sometimes requires staying the night (1)	2	1	0
	Gives post-procedural advice: seek help if wound site looks infected or develops abdominal pain		1	0
	General Communication Skills			
	Uses non-verbal means of aiding communication (e.g. drawing or pointing at objects)		1	0
	Maintains eye contact with the patient and persists in taking a good history		1	0
	Ensures that patient understands terms used		1	0
	Closing Remarks			
	Summarises key points		1	0
	Checks the patient's understanding		1	0
	Invites the patient to ask questions		1	0
	Examiner to ask:			
	'What is Murphy's sign?' An inspiratory 'catch' is observed (not necessarily pain) during palpation of the right upper quadrant, after asking the patient to breathe in		1	0
	'What is Courvoisier's law?' Jaundice in the presence of an enlarged non-tender gallbladder is unlikely to be due to gallstones		1	0
	Simulated patient score (2=very good, 1=satisfactory, 0=poor)	2	1	0
	Total Score			

Global Rating	1 Clear Fail	2 Borderline	3 Clear Pass	4 Very Good	5 Outstanding

Candidate Number:		University:		
Date:		Year of Study:		

STATION 10 – CHEST DRAIN

Appropriate introduction (1=full name and role), checks patient's name (1)	**2**	**1**	**0**
Establishes reason for consultation		**1**	**0**
Informs Patient and Addresses Concerns			
Asks what patient knows and what has happened so far		**1**	**0**
Able to elicit patient's concerns about procedure (1), concerns about diagnosis (1)	**2**	**1**	**0**
Explains procedure will be under local anaesthesia and what this means		**1**	**0**
Explains procedure: what procedure involves (insertion of a plastic tube attached to a drain to collect contents of the fluid which will be drained off the chest)		**1**	**0**
Explains why procedure is being done: diagnostic (1) and therapeutic (1)	**2**	**1**	**0**
Explains that the drain bottle will need to be kept under the bed/below the level of the insertion site (1) so that the pleural fluid will drain out under gravity (1)	**2**	**1**	**0**
Explains possible complications: bleeding, infection, discomfort, risk of lung damage (2=any three suggestions, 1=any two suggestions)	**2**	**1**	**0**
Explains a sample of the fluid will be kept and analysed in the laboratory		**1**	**0**
Post-procedure plan: explains that the drain will stay in overnight and taken out when most of the fluid has stopped draining (1) or is starting to drain at a very slow rate (1)	**2**	**1**	**0**
General Communication Skills			
Invites patient to ask questions		**1**	**0**
Checks patient understanding		**1**	**0**
Avoids use of medical jargon		**1**	**0**
Examiner to ask:			
'How would you classify pleural effusion?' transudate/exudate		**1**	**0**
'What investigations would you ask for on the form?' Protein, LDH, pH, Gram stain, AFB stain, cytology, and microbiological culture (2=any four suggestions, 1=any three suggestions, 0=one or none)	**2**	**1**	**0**
'What are the two most common causes of exudative pleural effusion?' Pneumonia (1), malignancy (1)	**2**	**1**	**0**
Simulated patient score (2=very good, 1=satisfactory, 0=poor)	**2**	**1**	**0**
Total Score			

Global Rating	**1** Clear Fail	**2** Borderline	**3** Clear Pass	**4** Very Good	**5** Outstanding

Candidate Number:	University:
Date:	Year of Study:

STATION 11 – LUMBAR PUNCTURE

	Appropriate introduction (1=full name and role), checks patient's name (1)	**2**	**1**	**0**
	Establishes reason for consultation		**1**	**0**
	Informs Patient and Addresses Concerns			
	Asks what patient knows and what has happened so far		**1**	**0**
	Able to elicit patient's concerns about procedure (1), concerns about diagnosis (1)	**2**	**1**	**0**
	Explains that it will be under local anaesthesia (1) using lignocaine injected under the skin to numb the area (1)	**2**	**1**	**0**
	Explains procedure: what procedure involves (i.e. a needle is inserted in between the spaces of two intervertebral bodies for about 1-2 cms and fluid which surrounds the spinal cord is collected (1) and that the amount collected is only a very small amount of the total fluid that is contained within the space (1)	**2**	**1**	**0**
	Explains why procedure is being done: i.e. for diagnosis/exclusion of meningitis or subarachnoid haemorrhage		**1**	**0**
	Explains possible complications: bleeding, infection of site, meningitis, possibility of result being ambiguous and CSF leak (2=any three suggestions, 1=any two suggestions, 0=one or none)	**2**	**1**	**0**
	Explains a sample of the fluid will be kept and analysed in the laboratory		**1**	**0**
	Post-procedure plan: to stay in hospital overnight as results may not be back until tomorrow (1) and the need to lie flat for at least 4 hours post-procedure to prevent CSF leak/headache (1)	**2**	**1**	**0**
	General Communication Skills			
	Invites patient to ask questions		**1**	**0**
	Checks patient understanding		**1**	**0**
	Avoids use of medical jargon		**1**	**0**
	Examiner to ask:			
	'What investigations would you ask for on the form?' CSF culture and sensitivity, cell count, glucose, protein, PCR (maximum 2 marks)	**2**	**1**	**0**
	'What are the most likely potential diagnoses?' Migraine, meningitis, subarachnoid haemorrhage, temporal arteritis, raised CSF pressure (e.g. cancer) (2=any three conditions, 1=any two conditions, 0=one or none)	**2**	**1**	**0**
	Simulated patient score (2=very good, 1=satisfactory, 0=poor)	**2**	**1**	**0**
	Total Score			

Global Rating	**1** Clear Fail	**2** Borderline	**3** Clear Pass	**4** Very Good	**5** Outstanding

Candidate Number:	University:
Date:	Year of Study:

STATION 12 – CATHETERISATION

	Appropriate introduction (1=full name and role), checks patient's name (1)	2	1	0
	Establishes reason for consultation		1	0
	Informs Patient and Addresses Concerns			
	Asks what patient knows and what has happened so far		1	0
	Able to elicit patient's concerns about procedure (1), concerns about diagnosis (1)	2	1	0
	Explains that it will be under local anaesthesia (1) using 'Instillagel' which contains lignocaine (1)	2	1	0
	Explains procedure: insertion of tube into bladder through the penis (1), connected to bag which drains urine (1)	2	1	0
	Explains why procedure is being done: diagnosis		1	0
	Explains possible complications: bleeding, infection of site, meningitis, risk of bladder damage (2=any three suggestions, 1=any two suggestions)	2	1	0
	Explains a sample of the fluid will be kept and analysed in the laboratory for infection		1	0
	Post-procedure plan: to stay in hospital overnight, catheter will be removed tomorrow		1	0
	General Communication Skills			
	Invites patient to ask questions		1	0
	Checks patient understanding		1	0
	Avoids use of medical jargon		1	0
	Examiner to ask:			
	'What are the most common causes of urinary retention?' Obstructive – BPH, prostate cancer, calculi Drug related – anticholinergics, opioids, alpha-agonists Neurological – cauda equina, spinal stenosis (2=any three suggestions, 1=any two suggestions, 0=one or none)	2	1	0
	Simulated patient score (2=very good, 1=satisfactory, 0=poor)	2	1	0
	Total Score			

Global Rating	**1** Clear Fail	**2** Borderline	**3** Clear Pass	**4** Very Good	**5** Outstanding

CHAPTER 9: EXPLAINING MANAGEMENT AND TREATMENT

Written by Dr. S. Shelmerdine & Dr. T. North

- Explanation of Colonoscopy Results
- Blood Transfusion Reaction
- Smoking Cessation
- Alternatives to General Anaesthesia
- Down's Syndrome Screening
- Cervical Smear Test Results and Colposcopy
- Rhesus Status in Pregnancy
- Needlestick Injury Counselling
- Explaining Cognitive Behavioural Therapy
- Explaining the Usage of Spacer Device
- Dietary Advice in Renal Failure
- Diabetic Management
- Osteoporosis Management

THE STATIONS

STATION 1

Time allowed: 10 minutes

You are a junior doctor working in general medicine.

Mr Robert Filcroft is a middle-aged man who was admitted to hospital with severe epigastric pain. The consultant has performed an OGD (oesophagoduodenoscopy) and taken biopsies from his stomach for a 'CLO test'. The results of the CLO test are positive. Apart from a solitary gastric ulcer there was no other abnormality to note. Biopsies of the ulcer were also taken and sent to pathology but results will take a week to return.

You have been told by your consultant to start one of two regimes:

1)   Omeprazole 20mg po bd + Clarithromycin 500 mg po bd + Amoxicillin 1g bd po **OR**

2)   Omeprazole 20mg po bd + Clarithromycin 500 mg po bd + Metronidazole 500 mg bd po

Please explain the results of the test, his subsequent management and answer any concerns or queries he has. You are not required to take a history from the patient.

STATION 2

Time allowed: 10 minutes

You are a junior doctor working in general surgery.

Mrs Daisy Hampton is an elderly lady who was admitted to your ward after a diverticular bleed. On admission her haemoglobin level was low (Hb = 7) and the consultant prescribed her 2 units of blood. The nurses have just put up the blood transfusion, however, they quickly call you to come and see the patient as she spiked a temperature, complained of flank pain, chills and nausea straight after this was started.

The nurses immediately stopped the transfusion and have disconnected it from the patient.

Her observations before the transfusion were: Temp: 37°C, Pulse: 75bpm, BP 110/70

Her observations after the transfusion started were: Temp: 38.5°C, Pulse: 100bpm, BP 100/70

Please take a quick focussed history of the presenting complaint from Mrs Hampton, explain what you think is happening to her and formulate a management plan.

STATION 3

Time allowed: 10 minutes

You are a junior doctor working in general practice.

Mr Stanislav Makov is a middle-aged man who is a heavy smoker. He is determined to give up smoking but is not sure the best way to go about doing this and has come for some advice.

Please obtain a relevant history from Mr Makov and offer him advice on smoking cessation including any concerns he may have.

STATION 4

Time allowed: 10 minutes

You are a junior doctor working in general surgery.

Mr Max Bamford is an elderly man has come to the pre-operative clinic for an assessment prior to his elective right hemicolectomy to remove a tumour from his caecum in two week's time. He appears rather anxious and is particularly concerned about pain relief options after the surgery.

The anaesthetist who will be in theatre on the day of the operation has told you that it would be possible for him to offer Mr Bamford either the option of a PCA device or an epidural should he wish. Your surgical consultant has therefore asked you to see Mr Bamford to discuss these options prior to his anaesthetic assessment clinic so he can have time to think about what he would like.

Please speak to Mr Bamford regarding these two options and answer any questions he may have.

You are not required to take a history from the patient and you do not need them to give you an answer today if they need further time to decide.

STATION 5

Time allowed: 10 minutes

You are a junior doctor working in general practice.

Mrs Nadia Hergozi is a 45 year old lady who is pregnant with her first child. She is rather concerned about her risk of giving birth to a Down's syndrome baby as she understands her age is a big factor.

Please discuss with Mrs Hergozi the various options available for Down's syndrome screening in the antenatal period. You do not need to take an obstetric history from the patient.

STATION 6

Time allowed: 10 minutes

You are a junior doctor working in general practice.

Miss Christine Grassfield had a cervical smear test performed last week which has revealed 'moderate dyskaryosis'. She is rather concerned as the letter she received asked her to come into clinic to speak to a doctor and she does not understand what the results mean or what the next step in her management will be.

Please discuss the findings of the cervical smear test result with Miss Grassfield and the most appropriate subsequent management plan. Answer any questions or concerns the patient may have.

STATION 7

Time allowed: 10 minutes

You are a junior doctor working in obstetrics and gynaecology.

Mrs Geraldine Starr is early into her first pregnancy and screening blood tests have revealed that she is Rhesus negative. She understands from her friends and family (who are non-medical) that this makes her pregnancy 'very risky'. It has obviously upset her a lot and she has come to clinic today to see you to straighten out the facts about what this means for her and the baby.

Please discuss the implications of her Rhesus negative status and answer any concerns she has.

STATION 8

Time allowed: 10 minutes

You are a junior doctor working in Accident and Emergency.

A medical student who is attached to the department was sent to try to take blood from a patient; however, she returns having failed to do so and tells you that she has sustained a needlestick injury in the process. She seems very upset and worried about the prospect of catching HIV and doesn't know what to do!

Please obtain more information regarding the incident from the medical student, offer her advice on management and address any concerns she has.

STATION 9
Time allowed: 10 minutes

You are a junior doctor working in psychiatry.

Mr Woodstock is a young gentleman with anxiety issues and obsessive compulsive disorder. He has been seen by the consultant psychiatrist and referred for CBT (Cognitive Behavioural Therapy). He is rather perplexed about what this will involve and was hoping to speak to someone about it.

Please speak to Mr Woodstock regarding CBT and address any concerns or questions he has about the therapy. You are not required to take a psychiatric history from the patient.

STATION 10
Time allowed: 10 minutes

You are a junior doctor working in general practice.

Mrs Sandrine Heinz is an elderly lady with rheumatoid arthritis and asthma. Although she has always been good at controlling her asthma in the past, the GP has noticed that her control is decreasing and suspects it is because her arthritis is preventing her from using her inhaler correctly. He has therefore issued her with a spacer device.

Mrs Heinz currently takes two puffs of her Beclomethasone (brown) inhaler every morning and only uses her Salbutamol (blue) inhalers when required.

Please speak to Mrs Heinz instructing her on how to use the spacer device (using the multiple breath technique) and answer any questions she may have. You will not be required to take a full history on her asthma control.

STATION 11
Time allowed: 10 minutes

You are a junior doctor working in general medicine.

Mr Rajiv Rahman is an elderly man who suffers from chronic renal failure. He has been in and out of hospital several times in the last 6 months and, although he is compliant with his medication, your consultant feels Mr Rahman could make some lifestyle improvements, especially regarding his dietary choices. Mr Rahman is due to be discharged from hospital this afternoon.

Please speak to him before he leaves and offer him advice and tips on his diet and fluid management once at home. You are not required to take a medical history from him or discuss any of his other treatments for chronic renal failure.

STATION 12
Time allowed: 10 minutes

You are a junior doctor working in general practice.

Miss Bonn is a patient with known diabetes. The GP has asked you to speak to Miss Bonn after her general appointment with him to discuss how she is managing with her medication and diet.

Please speak to Miss Bonn taking a history of her diabetes and asking about her current management. Offer her any advice and support you think is necessary.

STATION 13
Time allowed: 10 minutes

You are a junior doctor working in general practice.

Mrs Samantha Aldringham is a lady who attended clinic two weeks ago with back pain and was seen by the GP in the surgery. He suspected she had osteoporosis so sent her for a DEXA scan and blood test. Mrs Aldringham has returned to clinic today for the results of these tests.

The DEXA scan confirmed the GP's suspicion of osteoporosis. Her blood tests were normal. He would like to start her on calcium and vitamin D supplements as well as prescribing her some bisphosphonates.

Please explain to Mrs Aldringham the results of her tests and what the diagnosis of osteoporosis means. Please also suggest lifestyle modifications which may help and explain in detail the reasons for starting her on medication.

CHAPTER 10: PHARMACOLOGY

Written by Miss A. Verma and Dr. S. Shelmerdine

- Statins
- Inhaler Usage
- Warfarin
- Hormone Replacement Therapy (HRT)
- Combined Oral Contraceptive Pill (COCP)
- Antibiotics
- Steroids
- Prescribing a Sliding Scale

THE STATIONS

STATION 1
Time allowed: 10 minutes

You are a junior doctor working in general practice.

Mr Murphy has just been diagnosed with high cholesterol after having a heart attack two months ago.

Please explain statin therapy to him and address any concerns he may have.

STATION 2
Time allowed: 10 minutes

You are a junior doctor working in general practice.

Miss Kingsly has just been diagnosed with mild asthma.

Please explain how to use a meter dosed inhaler (MDI) containing Salbutamol and answer any questions or concerns she may have.

STATION 3
Time allowed: 10 minutes

You are a junior doctor working in the Accident and Emergency department.

Mrs Jenkins has just been diagnosed with a deep vein thrombosis and will be started on warfarin.

Please explain to her about warfarin therapy and answer any questions she may have.

STATION 4
Time allowed: 10 minutes

You are a junior doctor working in general practice.

Mrs Matterson is complaining of symptoms of hot flushes, dizziness and irregular light periods. The GP suspects she is undergoing the menopause and has prescribed her hormone replacement therapy.

Please explain to Mrs Matterson what you understand about hormone replacement therapy and answer any concerns she may have.

The examiner will stop you at 7 minutes to ask you a few questions.

STATION 5
Time allowed: 10 minutes

You are a junior doctor working in general practice.

Mrs Olson has been diagnosed with a chest infection and you have prescribed her oral co-amoxiclav for 7 days.

Please speak to the patient about taking this medication and answer any questions she may have.

STATION 6
Time allowed: 10 minutes

You are a junior doctor working in general practice.

Miss Nattley wants to start on the combined oral contraceptive pill (21 day pill taking regimen) for contraception. She is rather confused about what it involves and has never taken something like this before.

Please speak to her about this and explain about the regimen for taking Microgynon 30. Address any concerns or preconceptions about the pill that she may also raise.

The examiner will stop you at 7 minutes to ask you a few questions.

STATION 7
Time allowed: 10 minutes

You are a junior doctor working in general practice.

Mrs Noorma Norse is an elderly woman who suffers from rheumatoid arthritis. She is finding her pain rather difficult to control just on simple analgesics and the GP wants to start Mrs Norse on some steroids called 'Prednisolone' at a starting dose of 20mg once a day.

Please speak to her about this medication and explain any side effects she may have and how these will be dealt with. Address any concerns she may have.

STATION 8
Time allowed: 10 minutes

You are a junior doctor working in general medicine.

Mr Kevin Bellago (Hospital No: 123456, DOB: 1/1/1937) is a rather large elderly man with diabetes who has been admitted to the ward with gastroenteritis. He is feeling rather poorly and not eating or drinking very much at all as he keeps vomiting. The consultant thinks that the best method to keep his glucose levels under control whilst still rehydrating him is to put him on a sliding scale. His observations and electrolytes are all within normal range.

Please prescribe the sliding scale and appropriate intravenous fluids for the next 24 hours in the fluid section of his drug card overleaf. You are given a table by the nurse for prescribing the sliding scale:

Blood sugar levels (BMs):	Insulin Infusion (units/hr):
0 – 3.9	0.5
4 – 6.9	1.0
7 – 10.9	2.0
11 – 14.9	3.0
15 – 19.9	4.0
> 20	6.0

Name of Patient: _____

DOB: _____

Hospital No: _____

Date:	Route:	Type of Fluid:	Volume of Fluid:	Drug added to infusion:	Dose of Drug:	Rate of Infusion:	Doctor's Signature:

SIMULATED PATIENT BRIEFINGS

STATION 1

Name: Mr Phil Murphy

Age: 69 years old

Job: Retired builder

PC:

You have recently been discharged from hospital about two months ago after a sudden heart attack. Whilst you were in hospital the doctors mentioned to you that you would need to keep a healthy lifestyle from now on and gave you lots of advice on diet and exercise. You were told that your GP would arrange for you do have extra tests in their surgery and that you may be started on further medications but you don't quite remember exactly which ones or what tests you are supposed to have. You have never heard of 'statins' but you do understand that high cholesterol is bad and you have tried to cut out dairy products and eggs in your diet, only using 'Benecol' products to lower your cholesterol levels.

Past Medical History:

Myocardial infarction two months ago

Hypertension

Hypercholesterolaemia

Drug History:

Aspirin

Atenolol

Lisinopril

Social History:

You gave up smoking 10 years ago and only occasionally drink alcohol.

Family History:

Your mother died of a heart attack when she was 54 years old.

Ideas/Concerns/Expectations:

You are keen to prevent having another heart attack and understand that you currently lead an unhealthy lifestyle. You do not want to end up dying 'young' like your mother.

STATION 2

Name: Miss Maisie Kingsly

Age: 14 years old

Job: In school

PC:

You have been diagnosed recently with mild asthma, which is not that bad and only really affects you when it is very cold outside or when you are doing lots of sports. You are a little anxious about the diagnosis because your grandmother died quite young from an asthma attack and you realise that this condition can be life-threatening if it is not controlled well. As a result you are keen to learn how to use the inhaler and want to know how it works.

Past Medical History:

Mild asthma – recent diagnosis

Drug History:

None regular and no drug allergies.

Social History:

You do not smoke or drink alcohol.

Family History:

Asthma runs in the family and your brother, auntie and father all suffer from asthma.

Ideas/Concerns/Expectations:

You want to learn about using an inhaler but are worried you will not be able to use the inhaler properly. Your older brother who has asthma has been telling you how tricky it is and teasing you that you aren't 'clever' enough to do it properly.

STATION 3

Name: Mrs Rachel Jenkins

Age: 29 years old

Job: Florist

PC:

For the past week you have noticed that your right leg is looking increasingly puffy compared to the left leg. In addition the back of your right calf was rather tender and when you press on your leg, the area where you press leaves an indentation in your skin. You find this rather odd and when you saw your GP, he sent you for a scan which confirmed the presence of a DVT. You have been told you need to start warfarin and would like to know a bit more about this drug.

Past Medical History:

None

Drug History:

No allergies.

Microgynon 30 oral contraceptive pill

Paracetamol 1g qds po for pain relief

Social History:

You do not smoke and occasionally drink alcohol.

You live with your husband and were recently married three weeks ago. You have both only recently returned from a lovely honeymoon in Sri Lanka but you thought the flight was very long and you are glad to be back in the UK again!

You are both keen to start a family in the near future and have just bought a lovely little cottage in the countryside.

Ideas/Concerns/Expectations:

You are concerned about the side effects of warfarin especially as you know it will increase your chances of bleeding. You have heard that it is an ingredient in rat poisoning and this scares you a little bit!

STATION 4

Name: Mrs Sophie Matterson

Age: 52 years old

Job: Homemaker

PC:

For the last two months you have been suffering with hot flushes, feeling a dryness 'down below', night sweats and are complaining of irregular and light periods. You were told by your GP that you were probably going through the menopause and that this was a completely natural process. You have, however, found some of the symptoms a bit too difficult to handle and the GP mentioned to you something about potentially starting hormone replacement therapy. You have therefore come to the surgery today to discuss this with someone and to find out more information.

Past Medical History:

Fit and well.

Laparascopic cholecystectomy for gallstones aged 40 years old.

Drug History:

None. NKDA.

Social History:

You do not smoke and occasionally drink alcohol.

Ideas/Concerns/Expectations:

You used to be on the pill when you were younger without any problems and you don't have any problems with taking hormone treatments. You would like to know whether this drug is something you need to be on for the long term or not.

STATION 5

Name: Mrs Stacey Olson

Age: 40 years old

Job: Bank manager

PC:

You have not taken oral co-amoxiclav before and want to know how to take it and all about its side effects.

Past Medical History:

None.

Drug History:

None and NKDA.

Social History:

You do not smoke and only drink occasionally.

Family History:

None significant.

Ideas/Concerns/Expectations:

You have none.

STATION 6

Name: Miss Rebecca Nattley

Age: 19 years old

Job: Drama student

PC:

You are fit and well with no previous medical history or problems. You have recently begun a new relationship and you would like to start the pill so that you don't need to rely on condoms or buy them all the time. You have recently had a sexually transmitted infection check up which was negative and so has your partner.

Past Medical History:

Nil

Drug History:

None. NKDA.

Social History:

You do not smoke and only occasionally drink alcohol.

You are currently a drama student at college and find your life really disorganised and hectic. You are always being sent to castings and have plays to rehearse for, and you don't seem to have any order or routine in your days.

Family History:

Your father suffers with severe liver disease secondary to his heavy drinking and your aunt did suffer from cervical cancer when she was 40 years old but after radiotherapy and surgery she was cured. You do not know of anyone in your family who suffers from blood clots, strokes or migraines.

Ideas/Concerns/Expectations:

You want to know how effective this form of contraception will be.

STATION 7

Name: Mrs Norma Norse

Age: 71 years old

Job: Retired librarian

PC:

You have suffered with rheumatoid arthritis for the last five years and have found that your usual painkillers of paracetamol and ibuprofen are just not helping with your pain anymore. You are worried because you know it will soon be winter and that is when your joint pain seems to be at its worst! You have come to see your GP to find out if there is anything he can prescribe for you to improve your symptoms and relieve pain. He mentioned something about steroids but said that you needed to return for a good proper chat about it before really starting the medicines as there are lots of side effects. That is why you have attended the surgery today. You are ready to hear about all the side effects but would appreciate some written information as well as your memory is not too good!

Past Medical History:

Left total hip replacement from osteoarthritis aged 65 years old.

Rheumatoid arthritis affecting mainly both hands and the small joints in both feet.

Poor vision and hearing.

Drug History:

NKDA

Paracetamol 1g po qds

Ibuprofen 400mg po prn

Social History:

You do not smoke or drink. You live alone in your bungalow and have a cleaner in once a week to help you with your chores around the house. Your son lives about 20 minutes away and helps you with your shopping regularly. You are otherwise independent of activities of daily living but just need to take extra time to get around as your vision and hearing are a little poorer than they used to be.

Ideas/Concerns/Expectations:

You are keen to try steroids to help with your joint pain but are rather anxious because you have heard that athletes and boxers take steroids to bulk up their muscles and you don't fancy the idea of that! You have also heard that it is illegal to take steroids and are a little confused why the GP would have suggested this for you.

STATION 8

This station does not require a patient. Please find the instructions on how to correctly complete the drug chart in the mark schemes section of this chapter.

PHARMACOLOGY

Candidate Number:	University:
Date:	Year of Study:

STATION 1 – STATIN THERAPY

		2	1	0
	Appropriate introduction (1=full name and role), checks patient's name (1)	2	1	0
	Explains purpose of interview and checks consent (2=does well, 1=adequately, 0=poorly or not done)	2	1	0
	Presenting Complaint:			
	Explores what patient understands regarding statin therapy (1) and high cholesterol (1)	2	1	0
	Explains the reason for starting treatment (i.e. high cholesterol increases the risk of a future heart attack)	2	1	0
	Explains the benefits of therapy: reduction of cardiovascular risk, regression of coronary plaques, may ameliorate peripheral vascular disease, slight reduction in the risk of a stroke (2= any three benefits, 1= any two benefits)	2	1	0
	Explains that dosing will be once daily (1), at night (1)	2	1	0
	Explains the major side effects: hepatocellular damage (1), myalgia/myositis (1)	2	1	0
	Explains the minor side effects: abdominal pain, nausea/vomiting, headache, slight increase in liver enzyme levels		1	0
	Explores patient's ideas and concerns regarding the treatment		1	0
	Explains the duration of therapy will likely be life-long		1	0
	Enquires whether the patient wants to proceed with therapy		1	0
	Gives the patient the opportunity to think about the choice and take time to seek out further information they want to		1	0
	Other Relevant History:			
	Relevant past medical and surgical history		1	0
	Medication history (1) including allergies (1)	2	1	0
	Relevant family history		1	0
	Smoking (1) and alcohol (1)	2	1	0
	Appropriate closure (e.g. explains next step, thanks patient and summarises) (2=does well, 1=adequately, 0=poorly or not done)	2	1	0
	Communication Skills			
	Invites questions (1). Listens actively (1).	2	1	0
	Organised approach (e.g. systematic, summarises)	2	1	0
	Simulated patient score (2=very good, 1=satisfactory, 0=poor)	2	1	0
	Total Score			

Global Rating	1 Clear Fail	2 Borderline	3 Clear Pass	4 Very Good	5 Outstanding

305

Candidate Number:	University:
Date:	Year of Study:

STATION 2 – INHALER TECHNIQUE

	Appropriate introduction (1=full name and role), checks patient's name (1)	**2**	**1**	**0**
	Explains purpose of interview and checks consent (2=does well, 1=adequately, 0=poorly or not done)	**2**	**1**	**0**
	Presenting Complaint:			
	Establishes what patient understands by inhalers (1) and any previous experience (1)	**2**	**1**	**0**
	Explains how bronchodilators work – they relax the air passages in the lungs		**1**	**0**
	Explains the need for the medicine to reach deep down into the lungs (1) and to stay there for as long as possible so that the medicine can be absorbed (1)	**2**	**1**	**0**
	Explain when to use the inhaler (1) and that 2 puffs are to be taken at a time (1)	**2**	**1**	**0**
	Demonstrates How to Use the Inhaler			
	Talks through the steps of using inhaler:		**1**	**0**
	• Remove mouthpiece cover		**1**	**0**
	• Shake cannister		**1**	**0**
	• Hold the inhaler vertically with the mouthpiece near your mouth and with your index finger on top of the inhaler		**1**	**0**
	• Breathe all the way out		**1**	**0**
	• Put the mouthpiece in your mouth with your lips forming a tight seal around the mouthpiece		**1**	**0**
	• Start taking a deep breath in and press firmly down on the top of the inhaler with your index finger as you take the breath		**1**	**0**
	• Breathe in for as long and hard as you can		**1**	**0**
	• Hold your breath for 10 seconds, then breathe out normally		**1**	**0**
	• Repeat the process once more		**1**	**0**
	Ask the patient to perform the procedure (1) and corrects any errors (1)	**2**	**1**	**0**
	Appropriate closure (e.g. explains next step, thanks patient and summarises) (2=does well, 1=adequately, 0=poorly or not done)	**2**	**1**	**0**
	Communication Skills			
	Invites questions (1). Listens actively (1).	**2**	**1**	**0**
	Organised approach (e.g. systematic, summarises) and checks understanding	**2**	**1**	**0**
	Simulated patient score (2=very good, 1=satisfactory, 0=poor)	**2**	**1**	**0**
	Total Score			

Global Rating	**1** Clear Fail	**2** Borderline	**3** Clear Pass	**4** Very Good	**5** Outstanding

Candidate Number:	University:
Date:	Year of Study:

STATION 3 – WARFARIN THERAPY

	Appropriate introduction (1=full name and role), checks patient's name (1)	2	1	0
	Explains purpose of interview and checks consent (2=does well, 1=adequately, 0=poorly or not done)	2	1	0
	Presenting Complaint:			
	Checks patient's prior understanding about warfarin therapy		1	0
	Explains to patient need for warfarin (i.e. why their medical condition requires taking this drug and what it does to help)	2	1	0
	Explains that the medicine is taken once a day (1) and that the dose required may vary on different days depending on control of INR (1)	2	1	0
	Explains that treatment will be monitored in an anticoagulation clinic by blood tests to check the INR level (a measure of clotting) as warfarin increases the INR	2	1	0
	Explains that the patient will receive a yellow book (1) and this is used to record their INR levels and their warfarin dosage (1)	2	1	0
	Explains that on the first few days a higher dose called a 'loading dose' is given		1	0
	Explains the INR will need to be 2–3 (1) and the dose of warfarin will be adjusted depending on the INR by the doctor or nurse (1)	2	1	0
	Explains the possible side effects of warfarin (e.g. bleeding, skin necrosis, alopecia, DNV, jaundice)		1	0
	Warns the patient about possibility of over anticoagulation and need to seek medical help (e.g. epistaxis, haematuria, bleeding gums, excessive bruising) (2=any three, 1=any two)	2	1	0
	Explains the below lifestyle changes: • Alcohol intake to decrease as causes increased anticoagulation • Diet – decrease in food with vitamin K (e.g. green vegetables) • Avoid contact sports (2=all three suggestions, 1=any two suggestions)	2	1	0
	Warns the patient about getting pregnancy while on warfarin – teratogenic		1	0
	Tells patient to alert any health professionals and read all drug instruction leaflets carefully before taking warfarin with other medicines (e.g. NSAIDs, antibiotics etc.)		1	0
	Gives advice regarding missing doses of warfarin (do not take double) (1) and also do not suddenly stop taking warfarin without consulting a doctor (1)	2	1	0
	Tells the patient about need to inform dentist/surgeons re: warfarin		1	0
	Suggests that a Medical Alert bracelet may be worn		1	0
	Appropriate closure (e.g. explains next step, thanks patient and summarises) (2=does well, 1=adequately, 0=poorly or not done)	2	1	0
	Communication Skills			
	Invites questions (1). Listens actively (1).	2	1	0
	Organised approach to (e.g. systematic, summarises)	2	1	0
	Simulated patient score (2=very good, 1=satisfactory, 0=poor)	2	1	0
	Total Score			

Global Rating	**1** Clear Fail	**2** Borderline	**3** Clear Pass	**4** Very Good	**5** Outstanding

Candidate Number:	University:
Date:	Year of Study:

STATION 4 – HORMONE REPLACEMENT THERAPY (HRT)

	Appropriate introduction (1=full name and role), checks patient's name (1)	**2**	**1**	**0**
	Explains purpose of interview and checks consent (2=does well, 1=adequately, 0=poorly or not done)	**2**	**1**	**0**
	Presenting Complaint:			
	Explores how much patient already knows about hormone replacement therapy		**1**	**0**
	Explains what hormone replacement therapy is e.g. it is a replacement of the normal oestrogen and progesterone which your body used to produce (1) but is now slowly reducing in output due to menopause (1)	**2**	**1**	**0**
	Explains the benefits of therapy: hot flushes and vaginal dryness respond to HRT. HRT postpones menopausal bone loss and protects against cardiovascular disease and ovarian carcinoma (2=any three, 1=any two).	**2**	**1**	**0**
	Explains that HRT comes in many different formulations (e.g. gel, cream, pills)		**1**	**0**
	Explains the contraindications to HRT: breast carcinoma, PV bleeding, breast-feeding, DVT/PE (2=any three, 1=any two)	**2**	**1**	**0**
	Explains that contraception should still be continued for 1 year after the last period		**1**	**0**
	Explores patient's ideas and concerns regarding the treatment		**1**	**0**
	Gives the patient the opportunity to think about the choice and take time to seek out further information if they want to		**1**	**0**
	Other Relevant History:			
	Relevant past medical and surgical history (in particular regarding contraindications)		**1**	**0**
	Medication history (1) including allergies (1)	**2**	**1**	**0**
	Appropriate closure (e.g. explains next step, thanks patient and summarises) (2=does well, 1=adequately, 0=poorly or not done)	**2**	**1**	**0**
	Communication Skills			
	Invites questions (1). Listens actively (1).	**2**	**1**	**0**
	Organised approach (e.g. systematic, summarises)	**2**	**1**	**0**
	Simulated patient score (2=very good, 1=satisfactory, 0=poor)	**2**	**1**	**0**
	Total Score			

Global Rating	**1** Clear Fail	**2** Borderline	**3** Clear Pass	**4** Very Good	**5** Outstanding

Candidate Number:	University:
Date:	Year of Study:

STATION 5 – CO-AMOXICLAV PRESCRIBING

	Appropriate introduction (1=full name and role), checks patient's name (1)	**2**	**1**	**0**
	Explains purpose of interview and checks consent (2=does well, 1=adequately, 0=poorly or not done)	**2**	**1**	**0**
	Presenting Complaint:			
	Explains the reason for starting treatment – chest infection		**1**	**0**
	Checks for any reactions to penicillin/penicillin allergy		**1**	**0**
	Explains that dose will be 625 mg (1) three times a day (i.e. every 8 hours) (1)	**2**	**1**	**0**
	Encourages patient to take the medicine with food		**1**	**0**
	Explains the side effects: upset stomach, diarrhoea, vomiting	**2**	**1**	**0**
	Advises patient to use additional forms of contraception if they usually take the hormonal contraception (pill) (1) or experience diarrhoea when taking co-amoxiclav (1)	**2**	**1**	**0**
	Advises patient to see doctor again if they develop severe side effects or blood in the stool (1) as this may signify patient is suffering from colitis (1)	**2**	**1**	**0**
	Advises patient to stop taking the medicine and to seek immediate medical attention if they develop: itchy rash, swollen face/mouth, having difficulty breathing		**1**	**0**
	Explains that the patient must complete the course of antibiotics even if they think their symptoms have improved (1) as failure to do so increases bacterial resistance (1)	**2**	**1**	**0**
	Explores patient's ideas and concerns regarding the treatment and answers any questions patient has		**1**	**0**
	Appropriate closure (e.g. explains next step, thanks patient and summarises) (2=does well, 1=adequately, 0=poorly or not done)	**2**	**1**	**0**
	Communication Skills			
	Invites questions (1). Listens actively (1).	**2**	**1**	**0**
	Organised approach (e.g. systematic, summarises) (1) and checks understanding (1)	**2**	**1**	**0**
	Simulated patient score (2=very good, 1=satisfactory, 0=poor)	**2**	**1**	**0**
	Total Score			

Global Rating	**1** Clear Fail	**2** Borderline	**3** Clear Pass	**4** Very Good	**5** Outstanding

Candidate Number:	University:
Date:	Year of Study:

STATION 6 – COMBINED ORAL CONTRACEPTIVE PILL PRESCRIBING

	Appropriate introduction (1=full name and role), checks patient's name (1)	2	1	0
	Explains purpose of interview and checks consent (2=does well, 1=adequately, 0=poorly or not done)	2	1	0
	Side Effects/Contraindications and Benefits of the Pill			
	Explores the reason for the patient wanting to start treatment		1	0
	Explains that the pill is 99% effective if taken correctly		1	0
	Explains the benefits: periods are often lighter, less painful and more regular, it may relieve premenstrual tension, it reduces the risk of developing cancers of the ovary, colon and uterus ((2=any four options, 1=any three options)	2	1	0
	Explains side effects: nausea, headaches, sore breasts, tiredness, change in sex drive, breakthrough bleeding, skin changes and mood changes, rise in blood pressure, blood clots (1=any three options), advises to see GP if experiences side effects (1)	2	1	0
	Checks patient does not suffer from any contraindications to starting the COCP: past history or family history of blood clots, patient pregnant, patient complaining of unexplained vaginal bleeding, severe liver disease, sickle cell etc. (2=any three, 1=any two)	2	1	0
	Advises the patient that the pill reduces the risk of ovarian and uterine cancer (1), however, it may slightly increase chances of cervical and breast cancer and patients with a past history of breast cancer should not use the pill (1)	2	1	0
	Warns patient that the pill can increase the risk of blood clots (1) and advises patient to seek help if they suffer from any symptoms of severe migraines, swollen legs, severe chest pains (1)	2	1	0
	Candidate ensures patient is aware that the pill only protects against pregnancy and not against sexually transmitted infections (1) for which patient will require barrier methods of contraception as well or instead (1)	2	1	0
	Advises patient to use additional contraception if they have diarrhoea/vomiting (1) or if taking antibiotics for infections (1) as the pill may not be effective	2	1	0
	Advises patient to tell doctors that they are on the pill if they are being prescribed any new medication (1) or if they are due for an operation as the patient may be required to stop the pill for 4–6 weeks beforehand (1)	2	1	0
	Taking the Pill			
	Explain regimen – take the first pill on the first day of your period. If you start the pill on any other day, you need an additional contraceptive for the first 7 days. (1) Take your pill at about the same time each day for the 21 days. Then do not take the pill for 7 days (withdrawal bleed). Restart and follow the same regimen even if you have not finished bleeding. (1)	2	1	0
	If misses a pill and it was <12 hours from usual time of taking pill then just take the missed pill and continue as normal (1) no extra contraception required and you may end up taking 2 pills in one day but this is OK (1)	2	1	0
	If the missed pill is >12 hours late or more than one pill missed: take one pill as soon as you remember (1) NOT all the missed pills (1)	2	1	0
	If there are less than 7 remaining pills in your pack before your withdrawal bleed then start the next month's pack of pills without a 7 day break (1) and use condoms for the next 7 days from the date of the missed pills (1)	2	1	0
	If there are over 7 remaining pills in your pack before your withdrawal bleed use condoms for extra protection in the next 7 days (1) and when you finish your packet of pills allow for a withdrawal bleed before next packet (1)	2	1	0
	Explores patient's ideas and concerns regarding the treatment and checks understanding (2=in detail, 1=adequately)	2	1	0
	Communication Skills			
	Appropriate closure (e.g. explains next step, thanks patient and summarises) (2=does well, 1=adequately, 0=poorly or not done)	2	1	0
	Invites questions (1). Listens actively (1).	2	1	0
	Organised approach (e.g. systematic, summarises)		1	0
	Simulated patient score (2=very good, 1=satisfactory, 0=poor)	2	1	0
	Total Score			

Global Rating	**1** Clear Fail	**2** Borderline	**3** Clear Pass	**4** Very Good	**5** Outstanding

Candidate Number:	University:
Date:	Year of Study:

STATION 7 – STEROIDS

	Appropriate introduction (1=full name and role), checks patient's name (1)	**2**	**1**	**0**
	Explains purpose of interview and checks consent (2=does well, 1=adequately, 0=poorly or not done)	**2**	**1**	**0**
	Presenting Complaint:			
	Establishes what patient already understands about steroids (1) and dispels any myths patient may have regarding the drug (i.e. that this drug is for medical reasons and not the same preparation or type of steroids used by bodybuilders) (1)	**2**	**1**	**0**
	Explains why patient is being prescribed steroids (i.e. to reduce inflammation and swelling) (1) and that this will be in tablet form taken once a day (1)	**2**	**1**	**0**
	Explains to patient that being on steroids for their condition is long-term		**1**	**0**
	Explains/describes to patient serious side effects from taking steroids: risk of peptic ulcers, gastritis, hypertension, diabetes, osteoporosis, increased risk of infection and decreased immune response (2=any three, 1=any two)	**2**	**1**	**0**
	Explains/describes to patient less serious side effects from taking steroids: mood change, weight gain, proximal myopathy, acne, skin thinning (2=any three, 1=any two)	**2**	**1**	**0**
	States that in order to prevent some of the more serious side effects from occurring vitamin D and calcium supplements may be given to prevent osteoporosis (1), and an anti-acid tablet (proton pump inhibitor) is also given to prevent peptic ulcer disease (1)	**2**	**1**	**0**
	Informs patient that if they start to feel thirsty and are passing increasing amounts of urine, then to see GP for testing for diabetes		**1**	**0**
	Informs patient that during their time on the medication they will need to have their blood pressure more closely monitored to ensure this does not get raised		**1**	**0**
	Warns patient not to suddenly stop steroid medication at any point without consulting a doctor (1) as this can precipitate a severe reaction which may require hospitalization (i.e. an 'Addisonian crisis') (1)	**2**	**1**	**0**
	Warns patient not to take any additional NSAIDs whilst on steroids (1) and to alert doctors if they start to develop severe stomach pains or vomit any blood (1)	**2**	**1**	**0**
	Explains that many side effects do occur but the patient will be started on a low dose of steroids first		**1**	**0**
	Other Relevant History:			
	Relevant past medical and surgical history (in particular of peptic ulcer disease, osteoporosis and hypertension)	**2**	**1**	**0**
	Medication history in particular if already on NSAIDs (1). Establishes any drug allergies including nature of allergy (1).	**2**	**1**	**0**
	Communication Skills			
	Appropriate closure (e.g. explains next step, thanks patient and summarises) (2=does well, 1=adequately, 0=poorly or not done)	**2**	**1**	**0**
	Invites questions (1). Listens actively (1).	**2**	**1**	**0**
	Organised approach (e.g. systematic, summarises) and checks understanding	**2**	**1**	**0**
	Simulated patient score (2=very good, 1=satisfactory, 0=poor)	**2**	**1**	**0**
	Total Score			

Global Rating	**1** Clear Fail	**2** Borderline	**3** Clear Pass	**4** Very Good	**5** Outstanding

Candidate Number:	University:
Date:	Year of Study:

STATION 8 – SLIDING SCALE & IV FLUIDS PRESCRIBING

	Writes correct patient name, DOB and hospital number on chart (1=all correct)		1	0
	States the appropriate amount and type of insulin (Actrapid or alternative short-acting insulin) (1) to 49.5 mls of Normal 0.9% Saline (1) for infusion	2	1	0
	Copies the sliding scale infusion instructions correctly onto drug chart	2	1	0
	Includes instructions to call doctor if BMs are very low or very high		1	0
	Date of prescription of intravenous fluid infusion correctly written		1	0
	Correct route for infusion of intravenous fluids		1	
	Prescribes N. Saline and 5% dextrose as intravenous fluids (1) and gives instructions on when to give the appropriate bag according to BMs (1)	2	1	0
	Correct volume of fluid per bag to be infused		1	0
	Addition of 20mmols of KCL in 2 of the 3 bags of fluids to be given over the next 24 hours		1	0
	Correct rate of infusion for all intravenous fluids (8 hourly or 10 hourly acceptable)		1	0
	Doctor signs signature in correct box and/or puts down their bleep number		1	0
	Doctor states not to infuse over > 40mmols of KCL to patient in any 24 hours		1	0
	Fluid chart written legibly and neatly		1	0
	Total Score			

Global Rating	1 Clear Fail	2 Borderline	3 Clear Pass	4 Very Good	5 Outstanding

Candidate Number:	University:
Date:	Year of Study:

STATION 8 – ANSWERS

Name: Mr. Kevin Bellago
DOB: 1/1/1937
Hosp No: 123456

Date:	Route:	Type of Fluid:	Volume:	Drug added to infusion:	Dose of Drug:	Rate of Infusion:	Dr. Sign:
50 units of ACTRAPID in 49.5mls of 0.9% Normal Saline (therefore 1unit/ml) to be infused according to the following regime:							

BMs: Infusion of Insulin (units/hour):

0 – 3.9   0.5 and CALL DOCTOR

4 – 6.9   1.0

7 – 10.9   2.0

11 – 14.9   3.0

15 – 19.9   4.0

> 20   6.0 and CALL DOCTOR

Date:	Route:	Type of Fluid:	Volume:	Drug added to infusion:	Dose of Drug:	Rate of Infusion:	Dr. Sign:
1/1/12	IV	N. Saline (if BM >15)	1L	KCL	20mmol	8 hourly	X
1/1/12	IV	N. Saline (if BM >15)	1L	KCL	20mmol	8 hourly	X
1/1/12	IV	N. Saline (if BM >15)	1L	-	-	8 hourly	X
1/1/12	IV	5% Dextrose (if BM <15)	1L	KCL	20mmol	8 hourly	X
1/1/12	IV	5% Dextrose (if BM <15)	1L	KCL	20mmol	8 hourly	X
1/1/12	IV	5% Dextrose (if BM <15)	1L	-	-	8 hourly	X
DO NOT ADMINISTER MORE THAN 40MMOL KCL TO PATIENT IN 24 HOURS							

Please note that although it looks as if 6 bags of fluids have been prescribed, not all 6 bags will be given to the patient if there are instructions on when to give these bags according to the patient's BMs. The reason for writing up the different bags of fluids is so that the nurses can adjust the fluids they give the patient throughout the next 24 hours depending on what they measure as the patient's BMs.

SECTION 2 – CLINICAL SKILLS

CHAPTER 11: EXAMINATION SKILLS

Written by Dr. S. Shelmerdine

- Chest and Cardiovascular
  - Respiratory examination
  - Cardiovascular examination
  - Blood pressure measurement
  - Ankle brachial pulse index measurement
  - Peripheral vascular examination (arterial and venous)
- Neurology
  - Cranial nerves assessment
  - Cerebellar function assessment
  - Fundoscopy
  - Speech assessment
  - Hearing and ear assessment
  - Upper limb neurology assessment
  - Lower limb neurology assessment
  - Radial nerve examination
  - Ulnar nerve examination
  - Median nerve examination
  - Assessment of an acromegalic patient
- General Surgical
  - Thyroid assessment
  - Dermatology assessment
  - Lymph node examination
  - Abdominal examination
  - Assessment of an alcoholic patient
  - Rectal examination
  - Breast lump examination
- Orthopaedics and Rheumatology
  - GALS assessment
  - Spine
  - Shoulder
  - Wrist
  - Hip
  - Knee
  - Ankle and Foot
- Paediatrics, Obstetrics and Gynaecology
  - Developmental assessment
  - Pregnant abdomen
  - Bimanual examination
  - Speculum examination and swab taking

THE STATIONS

CHEST & VASCULAR MEDICINE

RESPIRATORY EXAMINATION
Time allowed: 10 minutes

You are a junior doctor in general medicine.

Miss Victoria Tuck has attended your outpatient chest clinic with a bad cough.

Please perform a full respiratory examination on the patient with a view to making a diagnosis.

You will be stopped by the examiner after 8 minutes to give your differential diagnoses and opinions on further investigation and treatment.

CARDIOVASCULAR EXAMINATION
Time allowed: 10 minutes

You are a junior doctor working in general medicine.

Mr Arthur Brook has been admitted to hospital complaining of chest pain.

Please perform a full cardiovascular examination of this patient.

The examiner will stop you after 9 minutes to ask you to present your findings.

BLOOD PRESSURE MEASUREMENT
Time allowed: 8 minutes

You are a junior doctor working in general practice.

Mr Harper Magden is a middle-aged gentleman who is diabetic and overweight. Your colleagues suspect that he may have blood pressure problems and would like you to take his blood pressure manually to be certain.

Please measure Mr Magden's blood pressure using a manual sphygmomanometer.

After 7 minutes the examiner will stop you to ask a few questions.

ANKLE BRACHIAL PULSE INDEX MEASUREMENT
Time allowed: 10 minutes

You are a junior doctor working in vascular surgery.

One of your patients, Mr Trevor Yonas, has been complaining of long-standing bilateral leg pain on walking. Your consultant has asked you to perform an ankle-brachial pressure index (ABPI) to assess the severity of his claudication.

Please perform an ABPI on the patient.

After 8 minutes the examiner will stop you to ask you a few questions.

PERIPHERAL VASCULAR EXAMINATION – ARTERIAL
Time allowed: 8 minutes

You are a junior doctor working in general surgery.

Mr Raymond Chau is a middle-aged overweight diabetic man with high blood pressure. You have been asked by your consultant to perform a peripheral arterial examination on Mr Chau due to his risk factors for peripheral vascular disease.

The examiner will stop you after 7 minutes to ask you a few questions.

PERIPHERAL VASCULAR EXAMINATION – VENOUS
Time allowed: 8 minutes

You are a junior doctor in vascular surgery.

Miss Jane Thomas is a middle-aged lady who has recently noted some unsightly blue 'snake-like' lesions over both her lower legs.

Please perform a peripheral venous examination of both of Miss Thomas' legs.

After 7 minutes the examiner will stop you to ask you a few questions.

NEUROLOGY STATIONS

CRANIAL NERVES EXAMINATION
Time allowed: 8 minutes

You are a junior doctor working in Accident and Emergency.

Mrs Leona Lee has attended the department today with severe headaches.

Please perform an examination of her cranial nerves.

The examiner may stop you after 7 minutes to ask a few questions.

CEREBELLAR EXAMINATION
Time allowed: 5 minutes

You are a junior doctor in general medicine.

You notice one of your patients, Mr Pete Lewis, is looking unusually unsteady on his feet on the ward.

Please assess Mr Lewis' cerebellar function.

You will be stopped after 4 minutes when the examiner will ask you to present your findings.

FUNDOSCOPY EXAMINATION
Time allowed: 8 minutes

You are a junior doctor working in general medicine.

Mr Rahman Ahmed is a middle-aged diabetic man with high blood pressure who has attended the outpatient diabetes clinic today for an eye check.

You are provided with a fundoscope.

Please examine and perform fundoscopy of both of Mr Ahmed's eyes. The examiner will ask you what you are looking for as you inspect his retina and after 7 minutes the examiner will ask you a few questions.

SPEECH ASSESSMENT
Time allowed: 5 minutes

You are a junior doctor working in your first medical job.

Mr James Jackson is an elderly gentleman who has been brought in by his wife to the outpatient's clinic because of 'speech problems'. These have been going on for a week now and she is rather worried.

Your consultant has asked you to speak to Mr Jackson to assess his speech. The examiner will stop you after 4 minutes to ask you to present your findings and ask you a few questions.

HEARING AND EAR ASSESSMENT
Time allowed: 10 minutes

You are a junior doctor working in general practice.

Miss Stephanie Wright has attended clinic today complaining of difficulty hearing in her left ear. You have been asked to examine Miss Wright's ears with a view to making a diagnosis of her decreased hearing.

The equipment available to you includes a selection of tuning forks and an otoscope with clean replacement speculums. You will be stopped after 8 minutes and asked to present your findings.

UPPER LIMB NEUROLOGY EXAMINATION
Time allowed: 8 minutes

You are a junior doctor working in Accident and Emergency.

Miss Indigo Waterman has attended the department with odd pins and needle-like symptoms in both her arms.

Please perform a neurological examination of both her arms and present your findings to the examiner as you go along.

LOWER LIMB NEUROLOGY EXAMINATION
Time allowed: 8 minutes

You are a junior doctor working in Accident and Emergency.

Mr Rueben Smith has been referred to the department by his GP feeling 'off legs'.

Please perform a neurological examination of both his lower limbs and present your findings to the examiner as you go along.

RADIAL NERVE EXAMINATION
Time allowed: 5 minutes

You are a junior doctor working in Accident and Emergency.

You notice that Mr Henry Douglas has attended your department with what looks like a 'wrist drop'. You suspect he has a radial nerve palsy but will need to examine him to confirm your suspicions.

Please examine both of Mr Douglas' hands to assess whether he has a radial nerve palsy.

ULNAR NERVE EXAMINATION
Time allowed: 5 minutes

You are a junior doctor working in general practice.

Mrs Yoland Ingleby has attended your clinic because she has noticed that she is unable to grip hold of objects as tightly as she once could in her right hand.

Please examine both of Mrs Ingleby's hands with a particular focus on assessing the function of her ulnar nerve.

MEDIAN NERVE EXAMINATION

Time allowed: 5 minutes

You are a junior doctor working in general practice.

Mrs Greta Jerboa is 30 weeks pregnant and within the last week has noticed odd shooting pains in the middle of the night affecting her left hand in the thumb and first two fingers. She is rather concerned.

Please examine both of Mrs Jerboa's hands with a particular focus on assessing the function of her median nerve.

ACROMEGALY

Time allowed: 8 minutes

You are a junior doctor working in general practice.

One of the senior partners in the clinic has asked you to come and examine an 'interesting patient' with acromegaly.

Please comment upon the positive clinical signs that the patient displays and examine for complications of this condition.

The examiner will stop you after 7 minutes to ask you a few questions.

GENERAL SURGERY

THYROID EXAMINATION

Time allowed: 10 minutes

You are a junior doctor working in a general practice.

Mrs Gabrielle Luna has attended clinic today complaining of a lump in her neck and weight loss.

Please examine her thyroid status.

The examiner will stop you after 7 minutes to ask you a few questions.

DERMATOLOGICAL EXAMINATION

Time allowed: 5 minutes

You are a junior doctor working in Accident and Emergency.

Mrs Jennifer Alston has attended the minor's department with a rash.

Please examine her rash and present your findings to the examiner.

EXAMINATION OF LYMPH NODES

Time allowed: 8 minutes

You are a junior doctor working in general practice.

Miss Grace Kissock has attended your clinic complaining of 'swollen glands' in her neck and armpit. Please examine the lymph nodes within both her cervical chain and both axillae to determine whether any are enlarged.

You will be expected to name the groups of lymph nodes you are examining and after 7 minutes you will be stopped and the examiner will ask you a few questions.

ABDOMINAL EXAMINATION
Time allowed: 10 minutes

You are a junior doctor working in Accident and Emergency.

Miss Adriana Lemington has attended your department complaining of right iliac fossa pain.

Please perform a full abdominal examination of the patient with a view to making a diagnosis of her pain. You will be stopped by the examiner after 8 minutes to give your differential diagnoses and opinions on further investigation and treatment.

RECTAL EXAMINATION
Time allowed: 8 minutes

You are a junior doctor working in general surgery.

Mr Phillip Squires is an elderly lady who has been complaining of rectal bleeding and difficulty urinating.

Please perform a thorough per rectal examination and present your findings to the examiner.

THE ALCOHOLIC PATIENT
Time allowed: 8 minutes

You are a junior doctor working in general medicine.

Mr Ed Wothington is a chronic alcoholic patient on your ward. Please examine Mr Worthington for any signs and complications of chronic alcohol consumption.

You will be stopped by the examiner after 7 minutes and asked some questions.

BREAST LUMP EXAMINATION
Time allowed: 8 minutes

You are a junior doctor working in general surgery.

Mrs Theresa Tooke has attended the breast clinic today because she has recently noticed a small lump in her right breast. She is very anxious.

Please examine both of Mrs Tooke's breasts and present your findings to the examiner.

You will be stopped after 7 minutes and asked some questions.

ORTHOPAEDIC STATIONS

GALS EXAMINATION
Time allowed: 8 minutes

You are a junior doctor working in general practice.

Mr Germaine Reddick is a young gentleman who has come into your clinic complaining of 'pain all over'. He denies any trauma and says all his joints 'hurt the same'.

Please perform a quick screening GALS examination on Mr Reddick.

The examiner will ask you to present your findings after 7 minutes.

SPINE EXAMINATION
Time allowed: 8 minutes

You are a junior doctor working in general practice.

Mr Gregory Hilton has attended your clinic complaining of lower backache. He denies any neurology but is finding it difficult to continue with his daily activities.

Please perform a full spinal examination on Mr Hilton.

The examiner will ask you to present your findings after 7 minutes.

SHOULDER EXAMINATION
Time allowed: 8 minutes

You are a junior doctor working in general practice.

Mr Sebastian Green is a young gentleman who is complaining of left shoulder pain. He says he fell down some stairs last week and his shoulder has just 'not felt quite right' since the accident.

Please perform an examination of both his shoulders.

The examiner will ask you to present your findings after 7 minutes.

WRIST EXAMINATION
Time allowed: 5 minutes

You are a junior doctor working in a general practice.

Mr Samuel Lam has attended clinic with a painful right wrist.

Please examine both of his wrists and present your findings to the examiner.

The examiner will stop you after 4 minutes to ask you a few questions.

HIP EXAMINATION
Time allowed: 8 minutes

You are a junior doctor working in general practice.

Miss Katie Pollock has attended your clinic today complaining of pain in the right hip.

Please examine both of her hips and present your findings to the examiner.

KNEE EXAMINATION
Time allowed: 5 minutes

You are a junior doctor working in a general practice.

Mr Tom Russell has attended clinic with a painful right knee. Please examine both his knees and present your findings to the examiner.

The examiner will stop you after 4 minutes to ask you a few questions.

ANKLE AND FOOT EXAMINATION
Time allowed: 8 minutes

You are a junior doctor working in general practice.

Miss Letitia Barker is a keen tennis player and reports having fallen onto her ankle during a match last weekend. She is complaining of swelling and pain in her left ankle and would like you to take a look at it.

Please examine both of Miss Barker's ankles and feet.

The examiner will stop you after 7 minutes to ask you a few questions.

PAEDIATRICS, OBSTETRICS AND GYNAECOLOGY

DEVELOPMENTAL ASSESSMENT
Time allowed: 8 minutes

You are a junior doctor working in paediatrics.

Mrs Jasmine Khan has brought her one year old daughter, Alex, into your outpatient's clinic today because she is worried that Alex is not advancing as quickly as her friends' children in the playgroup. She is worried that her daughter may have developmental delay.

Please assess Alex's developmental milestones and determine whether you feel there is any developmental delay for her age or not.

PREGNANT ABDOMEN EXAMINATION
Time allowed: 8 minutes

You are a junior doctor working in a general practice.

Mrs Jacinda Lawry has attended your antenatal clinic today for a routine check-up. She is 30 weeks pregnant with her first child.

Please perform a general obstetric assessment of Mrs Lawry. You should present your findings to the examiner as you go along.

BIMANUAL EXAMINATION
Time allowed: 8 minutes

You are a junior doctor working in Accident and Emergency.

Miss Alice Green has attended the department with severe left pelvic pain. Abdominal examination was unremarkable. Please perform a bimanual pelvic examination on the patient and present your findings to the examiner.

After 7 minutes the examiner will stop you and ask you a few questions.

SPECULUM EXAMINATION AND SWAB TAKING
Time allowed: 8 minutes

You are a junior doctor working in gynaecology.

Miss Sharon Broadmoore has been complaining of foul-smelling vaginal discharge for the last week and is concerned that she may be suffering from a sexually transmitted infection such as chlamydia.

Please perform a speculum examination and take swabs for a chlamydia screen for Miss Broadmoore ensuring you explain the procedure carefully to her prior to starting.

COMMONLY EXAMINED SIGNS & CONDITIONS

CHEST AND VASCULAR EXAMINATIONS:

Respiratory Examination

It is not uncommon to get a patient who has undergone a previous lobectomy within the OSCE as these patients are usually stable and have large scars which examiners like to quiz candidates upon. (A lobectomy scar is from an incision where a thoracic surgeon has removed a lobe or part of a lobe of one lung. It looks like an oblique scar at the back of the patient which slopes downwards anteriorly following the contours of the ribs.)

An asthmatic/COPD patient with an expiratory wheeze, or a patient with pulmonary fibrosis (inspiratory crackles which don't clear on coughing) are other likely subjects. You will not get a patient with a pneumothorax and it is unlikely that you will be presented with a patient with a pleural effusion.

Cardiovascular Examination

In previous clinical examinations students have always worried about getting a cardiac murmur or a paediatric patient. This is often put in the exam by the examiners to throw off the less confident candidates even though there is nothing fancy expected from you.

Paediatric patients for the examination will normally be about 8–14 years old and healthy. The fact that they are younger than your normal patient should not deter you from performing exactly the same steps you would for an adult patient.

The commonest cardiac murmurs to hear in the medical OSCEs are those of aortic stenosis or mitral regurgitation. These murmurs are characterised in the table below:

Aortic Stenosis Murmur	Mitral Regurgitation Murmur
Ejection systolic murmur	Pansystolic murmur
Radiates to the carotid arteries	Radiates to the back
Loudest in expiration	Loudest in expiration and with patient lying on their left side
Heard best in the second intercostal space at the right upper sternal border	Heard best with the bell of the stethoscope at the apex within the fifth intercostal space, midclavicular line
In more severe cases the second heart sound becomes softer	The loudness of the murmur does not correlate to its severity
Associated with a narrow pulse pressure and precordial thrill	Commonly associated with atrial fibrillation, laterally displaced apex and occasionally a third heart sound

Other types of patient you may have are those with a previous CABG and midline sternotomy scar; valve replacement surgery with a midline sternotomy scar or a patient with atrial fibrillation.

Peripheral Arterial and Venous Examination

It is impossible to get a patient with an acutely ischaemic limb in your OSCE so don't worry about missing the 6 Ps of an ischaemic limb in the examination! However, it is very likely you could get a patient with diabetic foot ulcers or varicose veins, therefore ensure you are slick with your venous examination and that you can differentiate and describe the various forms of ulcers which you may see:

Arterial Ulcers	Venous Ulcers	Neuropathic Ulcers
Painful	Associated with other signs of venous disease (e.g. eczema, varicosities, haemosiderin deposits)	Poor healing
Deep	Painless	Painless
Usually on pressure areas (heels, base of big toe etc.)	Shallow	Occur on pressure sites as well as areas of repetitive damage (e.g. base of metatarsals, big toe)
Well defined 'punched out' lesions	Large	Commonly associated with diabetics and ill-fitted shoes
	Gaitor region (medial aspect of calf)	
	Poorly irregularly defined	

NEUROLOGICAL EXAMINATIONS:

Cranial Nerves Examination

Again, it is unlikely that you would get real signs for this examination, but if you do it may be a patient with a Bell's Palsy or alternatively someone with a third nerve palsy (ptosis, fixed dilated pupil which looks down and out). Other cranial nerve signs are difficult to find in patients and to simulate.

Cerebellar Examination

This is an easy examination and most of the time the patient will not have symptoms. If they do, it will be an actor pretending to simulate all the symptoms of the cerebellar signs. You are unlikely to get a mix match of a few signs and not others.

Speech

Although there are a huge variety of speech disorders, the most likely ones you will get in your examination will either be an expressive or receptive dysphasia. However, in the majority of cases the actor/patient will probably have no signs at all.

Fundoscopy

Again, it is unusual to get a patient willing to sit through several candidates shining a bright light from a fundoscope directly into their eye. This station, if it occurs, will most likely be with a plastic model of a head that you practice your technique upon. Revise the differences between hypertensive and diabetic retinopathies and make sure you have seen a few images of diabetic patients who have undergone macular oedema laser treatment.

Hearing

It is uncommon to have any significant pathology to see on otoscopy (if this is being tested in the medical OSCEs) and it will be unusual to have a real patient willing to be examined by several students with an otoscope!

However, when examining a patient's hearing, the actor or patient may simulate either a conductive or sensorineural hearing loss. Remember how to differentiate this with the Rinne's and Weber's tests:

Rinne's Test:

Louder transmission of sound through the air than the bone is normal.

If the patient reports that they can hear the tuning fork sound louder through the bone on the same side then this signifies conductive hearing loss and the test is said to be 'positive'.

PAEDIATRICS, OBSTETRICS & GYNAECOLOGY EXAMINATIONS:

Developmental Assessment

It is unusual to have a real paediatric patient with cerebral palsy to practice your development assessment skills upon and more common to be introduced to a short film of a child performing different tasks and either being questioned on your presumed developmental age for the child in question or to be given the age of the patient and then asked what tasks you witnessed them struggling with which you would expect them to have already mastered.

Bimanual and Cervical Swab Sampling

With the bimanual examination and cervical swab sampling (also rectal examination), you will be asked to perform these on a model. However, you may be asked to obtain consent and explain the procedure to a real actor/patient. Practice your opening gambit for these stations as it is important to appear confident and clear about what you propose to do, especially when it is an intimate examination. Always ensure you ask for a chaperone – this will earn you easy marks!

Pregnant Abdomen Examination

The same can be said about examination of a pregnant abdomen. You will be more likely asked to examine a model of the pregnant abdomen to ensure you understand the basic principles of what to look for. However, you may be asked to explain what you want to do to a real patient beforehand.

EXAMINATIONS

Candidate Number:	University:
Date:	Year of Study:

RESPIRATORY EXAMINATION

		2	1	0
	Appropriate introduction (1=full name and role), checks patient's name (1)	2	1	0
	Explains procedure appropriately and obtains consent (2=does well, 1=adequately, 0=poorly or not done)	2	1	0
	Ensures good exposure of patient's chest wall and neck		1	0
	Applies alcogel to hands before and after examination (1=both)		1	0
	General inspection of patient and around the bed (use of accessory muscles, scars, deformity, asymmetry, presence of respiratory paraphernalia) (2=three observations, 1=two observations, 0=one or none)	2	1	0
	Examines hands for peripheral stigmata of respiratory disease (clubbing, nicotine stains, peripheral cyanosis, hypercapnic flap, fine beta agonist tremor) (2=three observations, 1=two observations, 0=one or none)	2	1	0
	Comments on respiratory rate and pulse rate (1=both)		1	0
	Examines eyes for anaemia, Horner's syndrome		1	0
	Examines for central cyanosis		1	0
	Examines cervical lymph nodes from behind patient		1	0
	Checks central position of trachea		1	0
	Examines JVP (raised in cor pulmonale)		1	0
	Checks position of apex beat and comments on position		1	0
	Examines for chest expansion – both front (1) and back (1) in the upper and lower chest	2	1	0
	Percusses chest (correct technique and all areas) – front (1) and back (1)	2	1	0
	Assesses for vocal or tactile fremitus – front (1) and back (1)	2	1	0
	Auscultates chest (correct techniques and areas – bell at the apices and diaphragm in all other areas) – front (1) and back (1)	2	1	0
	Examines for sacral and pedal oedema		1	0
	Treats patient with consideration throughout (2=does well, 1=adequately, 0=poorly or not done)	2	1	0
	Gives clear instructions to patient during examination (2=does well, 1=adequately, 0=poorly or not done)	2	1	0
	Examiner to ask: 'What else would you like to do to complete your examination?'			
	Offers to perform a cardiovascular examination, inspect the observation charts with oxygen saturation, BP, pulse and respiratory rate, perform a PEFR, CXR, check sputum pot, look in patient notes for any ABG measurements. (2=any three suggestions, 1=any two suggestions, 0=one or none)	2	1	0
	Examiner to ask: 'Please present your findings and offer a diagnosis.'			
	Candidate presents findings (1) in a logical and structured manner (1)	2	1	0
	Candidate presents offers a suitable diagnosis (1) and differential (1)	2	1	0
	Total Score			

Global Rating	1 Clear Fail	2 Borderline	3 Clear Pass	4 Very Good	5 Outstanding

Candidate Number:	University:
Date:	Year of Study:

PERIPHERAL VASCULAR EXAMINATION – VENOUS

	Appropriate introduction (1=full name and role), checks patient's name (1)	**2**	**1**	**0**
	Explains procedure appropriately and obtains consent (2=does well, 1=adequately, 0=poorly or not done)	**2**	**1**	**0**
	Appropriately exposes patient (preferably down to underwear)		**1**	**0**
	Applies alcogel to hands before and after examination (1=both)		**1**	**0**
	Asks if patient in any pain prior to examination		**1**	**0**
	Inspection of lower limbs with patient standing looking for shape of legs (beer bottle), eczema, venous stars, haemosiderin deposition, scars, ankle swelling, lipodermatosclerosis (2=any three observations, 1=any two, 0=one or none)	**2**	**1**	**0**
	Palpates for any temperature change (1) along patient's legs and for pitting oedema (1)	**2**	**1**	**0**
	Establishes the location and distribution of varicose veins (inspects both in the path of the long (1) and short saphenous veins (1))	**2**	**1**	**0**
	Specific palpation and inspection of long saphenous vein for tenderness/thrombosis	**2**	**1**	**0**
	Specific palpation and inspection of short saphenous vein for tenderness/thrombosis	**2**	**1**	**0**
	Examine for saphena varix at sapheno-femoral junction (1) and feels for cough impulse here and at the sapheno-popliteal junction (1)	**2**	**1**	**0**
	Whilst patient remains standing, candidate performs the tap test by placing their finger at the bottom of a long varicosity and tapping above this site (1). Comments on the presence of an impulse (1).	**2**	**1**	**0**
	Candidate offers to perform the Trendelenberg's or Tourniquet test (examiner to state that only one test is necessary)		**1**	**0**
	Asks patient to lie supine and elevate leg until superficial veins are drained		**1**	**0**
	Either occludes the saphenofemoral junction with two fingers and asks patient to stand (Trendelenberg's test) or places a tourniquet tightly around the upper thigh and asks patient to stand (Tourniquet test)		**1**	**0**
	Observes for filling of superficial veins		**1**	**0**
	States that filling of the veins below the tourniquet/saphenofemoral junction indicates that the incompetent perforators originate below this level		**1**	**0**
	Suggests to repeat test and continue occluding vessels distally until no superficial filling (examiner to state this is not required)		**1**	**0**
	Offers to perform Perches' test (examiner to state this is not required)	**2**	**1**	**0**
	Auscultates over any obvious varicosities for bruits suggesting an arterio-venous malformation	**2**	**1**	**0**
	Treats patient with consideration throughout (2=does well, 1=adequately, 0=poorly or not done)	**2**	**1**	**0**
	Gives clear instructions to patient during examination (2=does well, 1=adequately, 0=poorly or not done)	**2**	**1**	**0**
	Examiner to ask: 'What else would you like to do to complete your examination?'			
	Examine the peripheral arterial system, the abdomen, rectum and pelvis for a low abdominal mass causing inferior vena caval obstruction, measurement of ankle brachial pulse index (ABPI) and a neurological assessment of the lower limbs (2=suggests all four options, 1=any three of the above options).	**2**	**1**	**0**
	Examiner to ask: 'Please present your findings and offer a diagnosis.'			
	Candidate presents findings (1) in a logical and structured manner (1)	**2**	**1**	**0**
	Candidate presents offers a suitable diagnosis		**1**	**0**

Global Rating	**1** Clear Fail	**2** Borderline	**3** Clear Pass	**4** Very Good	**5** Outstanding

Candidate Number:		University:
Date:		Year of Study:

CRANIAL NERVES EXAMINATION

		2	1	0
	Appropriate introduction (1=full name and role), checks patient's name (1)	2	1	0
	Explains procedure appropriately and obtains consent (2=does well, 1=adequately, 0=poorly or not done)	2	1	0
	Appropriately exposes patient (ensures patient face and neck not covered)		1	0
	Applies alcogel to hands before and after examination (1=both)		1	0
	I – Olfactory Nerve			
	Enquires whether patient has noticed a change in smell		1	0
	Offers to test with smelling salts (examiner to state this is not required)		1	0
	II – Optic Nerve			
	Test for visual acuity with Snellen chart (both eyes separately)		1	0
	States the correct visual acuity for each eye separately		1	0
	Tests visual fields for both eyes separately (1=both)		1	0
	Accommodation for both eyes separately (1=both)		1	0
	Direct and consensual light reflex (1=both, 0=partly done)		1	0
	The examiner is to state the following are not required if the candidate offers:			
	Offers to perform fundoscopy		1	0
	Offers to perform the corneal reflex		1	0
	Offers to test for colour vision with Ishihara plates		1	0
	III, IV, VI – Opthalmic, Trochlear, Abducens			
	Inspects for equal pupil sizes and ptosis		1	0
	Tests full range of eye movements (asking about diplopia) (2=full range, 1=limited, 0=does poorly or not at all)	2	1	0
	Pauses at extremities for nystagmus		1	0
	V – Trigeminal			
	States jaw jerk reflex (examiner to state this is not required)		1	0
	Tests sensation over face bilaterally in all 3 areas (2=well done, 1=partly done)	2	1	0
	Tests strength of masseter and temporalis muscles (clench teeth, move jaw side to side, open jaw against resistance) (1=both)		1	0
	VII – Facial			
	Inspects face and comments on any asymmetry		1	0
	Asks about taste (anterior 2/3rd of tongue)		1	0
	Examines muscles of facial expression (asks patient to raise eyebrows, scrunch up eyes, smile and puff out cheeks) (2=all four actions, 1=three actions, 0=two or less)	2	1	0
	VIII – Vestibulocochlear			
	Tests hearing using stimulus such as whisper in both ears (1=both)		1	0
	Offers to perform Rinne's and Weber's tests (examiner to state not required)		1	0
	IX – Glossopharyngeal and Vagus			
	Examines for uvula deviation		1	0
	States would check 'gag reflex' (examiner to state not required)		1	0
	XI – Accessory			
	Asks patient to shrug shoulders against resistance (1=both)		1	0
	Deviates head to left and right against resistance (1=both sides)		1	0
	XII – Hypoglossal			
	Examines for tongue deviation (1) and wasting or fasciculations (1)	2	1	0
	Tests tongue strength by pressing over cheek to test tongue movement		1	0
	Examiner to ask: 'Please present your findings.'			
	Candidate presents key findings (1) in a logical and fluent manner (1)	2	1	0
	Communicates with patient appropriately during examination		1	0
	Professional behaviour (gentle, watches for pain, maintains dignity)		1	0
	Total Score			

Global Rating	1 Clear Fail	2 Borderline	3 Clear Pass	4 Very Good	5 Outstanding

Candidate Number:	University:
Date:	Year of Study:

CEREBELLAR EXAMINATION

Appropriate introduction (1=full name and role), checks patient's name (1)	2	1	0
Explains procedure appropriately and obtains consent (2=does well, 1=adequately, 0=poorly or not done)	2	1	0
Appropriately exposes patient so face and limbs are clearly visible		1	0
Applies alcogel to hands before and after examination (1=both)		1	0
Assesses gait by asking patient to walk heel-to-toe in a straight line		1	0
Whilst patient is standing, candidate offers to perform the Romberg test (examiner to state that this is not necessary)		1	0
Asks patient to lie supine on the examining bed		1	0
Asks patient to place the heel of one foot to the knee of the other leg and run their heel down the shin of the other leg repeatedly		1	0
Repeats for the other leg		1	0
Tests the tone of upper and lower limbs for hypotonia		1	0
Asks patient to speak on a topic familiar to them (1) to assess for scanning/slurred speech (1) e.g. 'Can you describe in detail everything you did today?' or 'Can you tell me about your house and describe each room in detail?'	2	1	0
Asks patient to rapidly clap their hands and alternate between clapping the palm of one hand with the other palm, then with the back of the hand and so forth to test for dysdiadochokinesis (2=demonstrates action clearly and comments on presence of sign, 1=done poorly, 0=not done)	2	1	0
Swaps the hand that is alternating		1	0
Asks patient to use one finger and place it on their nose then to touch the candidate's finger repeatedly whilst the candidate changes the position of their own finger to check for intention tremor and past pointing (2=demonstrates action clearly and comments on presence of sign, 1=done poorly, 0=not done)	2	1	0
Checks for nystagmus at extremes of eye movements		1	0
Treats patient with consideration throughout (2=does well, 1=adequately, 0=poorly or not done)	2	1	0
Gives clear instructions to patient during examination (2=does well, 1=adequately, 0=poorly or not done)	2	1	0
Examiner to ask: 'Please present your findings.'			
Candidate presents findings (1) in a logical and structured manner (1)	2	1	0
Examiner to ask: 'If there was a right-sided cerebellar lesion, which side would the symptoms manifest themselves?'			
Candidate to state that the symptoms and signs would be right-sided		1	0
Examiner to ask: 'What sort of diseases affect cerebellar function?'			
Candidate to suggest stroke, hydrocephalus, posterior fossa tumours/abscesses, thiamine deficiency (Wernicke's encephalopathy) or excessive alcohol intake (2=any three suggestions, 1=any two, 0=one or none)	2	1	0
Total Score			

Global Rating	1 Clear Fail	2 Borderline	3 Clear Pass	4 Very Good	5 Outstanding

Candidate Number:	University:
Date:	Year of Study:

FUNDOSCOPY EXAMINATION

	Appropriate introduction (1=full name and role), checks patient's name (1)	**2**	**1**	**0**
	Explains procedure appropriately (warning the patient that the room will be darkened and the candidate may need to approach closely with a very bright light directed at the eye). Obtains consent (2=does well, 1=adequately, 0=poorly or not done).	**2**	**1**	**0**
	Checks patient is not driving home (1) or operating machinery (1)	**2**	**1**	**0**
	Appropriately exposes patient so face is clearly visible, asking patient to remove glasses if appropriate		**1**	**0**
	Applies alcogel to hands before and after examination (1=both)		**1**	**0**
	Candidate explains they would ideally like dilating eye drops prior to examination (e.g. Tropicamide)		**1**	**0**
	Inspects and comments on the exterior part of both eyes (e.g. conjunctivitis, proptosis, eyelid droop, scleritis, glass eye) (2=two observations, 1=one observations 0=none)	**2**	**1**	**0**
	Instructs patient to stare at point on the wall straight ahead and to keep head still		**1**	**0**
	Sets lens to power 0 or any appropriate setting if candidate wears glasses		**1**	**0**
	Switches the fundoscope on and checks that the light source is working		**1**	**0**
	Requests for room to be darkened		**1**	**0**
	Approaches patient from one side about an arm's length away and examines for red reflex		**1**	**0**
	Approaches patient more closely and inspects the retina		**1**	**0**
	Whilst candidate performing test, examiner to ask: 'Explain what you are looking for.'			
	Locate and examine the optic disc (1). Comments on presence of papilloedema (1).	**2**	**1**	**0**
	Checks for vessels in all 4 quadrants of each eye		**1**	**0**
	Look for additional features such as haemorrhages or exudates		**1**	**0**
	Repeats on contralateral side		**1**	**0**
	Candidate uses their right eye to examine patient's right eye and their own left eye to examine patient's left eye	**2**	**1**	**0**
	Treats patient with consideration throughout (2=does well, 1=adequately, 0=poorly or not done)	**2**	**1**	**0**
	Gives clear instructions to patient during examination (2=does well, 1=adequately, 0=poorly or not done)	**2**	**1**	**0**
	Examiner to ask: 'Please summarise your key findings.'			
	Candidate presents key findings (1) in a fluent and logical manner (1)	**2**	**1**	**0**
	Examiner to ask: 'What are the early signs of diabetic retinopathy in the eye?'			
	Candidate to suggest presence of microanuerysms, haemorrhages, venous beading and hard exudates (2=any three suggestions, 1=any two, 0=one or none)	**2**	**1**	**0**
	Examiner to ask: 'What are the complications with using Tropicamide eye drops?'			
	Candidate to suggest glaucoma, allergic reactions with reddening and itchiness of the eyes, blurred vision and inability to operate machinery or drive immediately after use (2=any three suggestions, 1=any two suggestions, 0=one or none)	**2**	**1**	**0**
	Total Score			

Global Rating	1 Clear Fail	2 Borderline	3 Clear Pass	4 Very Good	5 Outstanding

Candidate Number:	University:
Date:	Year of Study:

SPEECH ASSESSMENT

	Appropriate introduction (1=full name and role), checks patient's name (1)	2	1	0
	Explains procedure appropriately and obtains consent (2=does well, 1=adequately, 0=poorly or not done)	2	1	0
	Appropriately exposes patient so face and neck are clearly visible		1	0
	Applies alcogel to hands before and after examination (1=both)		1	0
	Asks patient to speak fluently and talk on a topic familiar to them such as describing their house, room, day or a hobby (1). Comments on the presence of dysphasia and dysphonia (1).	2	1	0
	Asks patient to repeat 'British Constitution' and 'Baby Hippopotamus' to assess for dysarthria		1	0
	Asks patient to repeat the sounds 'Pataka' repeatedly then to repeat 'Papapa', 'Tatata' and 'Kakaka' to assess for apraxia of speech (here the repetition rate of 'Pataka' will be much slower than for the single syllables) (2=does well and comments on apraxia of speech, 1=performs poorly and makes some comment on apraxia of speech)	2	1	0
	Asks patient to repeat the phrase 'No ifs, ands or buts'		1	0
	Asks patient to follow a three step command such as 'clap your hands, touch your nose then stick out your tongue' to test for receptive dysphasia (2=asks patient to perform all three commands and comments on receptive dysphasia, 1=performs poorly and makes some comment on receptive dysphasia)	2	1	0
	Examines for any uvula (1) and tongue (1) diversion	2	1	0
	Inspects tongue for any fasciculations or muscle wasting in a lower motor neurone lesion		1	0
	Asks patient to name objects that they point to such as a pen, name badge, watch, paper etc. (1) to check for expressive dysphasia (1)	2	1	0
	Offers to perform the mini mental state examination (examiner to state this is not required)		1	0
	Offers to assess the jaw jerk reflex to check for an upper motor neurone lesion if brisk (examiner to state that this is not required)		1	0
	Treats patient with consideration throughout (2=does well, 1=adequately, 0=poorly or not done)	2	1	0
	Gives clear instructions to patient during examination (2=does well, 1=adequately, 0=poorly or not done)	2	1	0
	Examiner to ask: 'Please summarise your key findings.'			
	Candidate presents key findings (1) in a fluent and logical manner (1)	2	1	0
	Examiner to ask: 'Can you describe the three main classes of dysphasia?'			
	Broca's (expressive) dysphasia (1): lesion in the inferior frontal gyrus on the language dominant hemisphere. Comprehension is intact but speech is slow and there is difficulty in description of objects (1).	2	1	0
	Wernicke's (receptive) dysphasia (1): lesion in the posterior part of the superior temporal gyrus on the language dominant hemisphere. Comprehension is impaired and speech is fluent but doesn't make sense (1).	2	1	0
	Conduction aphasia (1): lesion within the arcuate fasciculus in the inferior parietal lobe of the language dominant hemisphere that connects Wernicke's and Broca's areas. There is difficulty in repetition of speech (1).	2	1	0
	Total Score			

Global Rating	1 Clear Fail	2 Borderline	3 Clear Pass	4 Very Good	5 Outstanding

Candidate Number:	University:
Date:	Year of Study:

HEARING AND EAR ASSESSMENT

Appropriate introduction (1=full name and role), checks patient's name (1)	2	1	0
Explains procedure appropriately and obtains consent (2=does well, 1=adequately, 0=poorly or not done)	2	1	0
Appropriately exposes patient so face and ears are clearly visible		1	0
Applies alcogel to hands before and after examination (1=both)		1	0
Inspects both ears and behind ears for scars, skin pigmentation, deformity, presence of hearing aids and looking for any obvious discharge (2=any 3 observations, 1=any 2 observations, 0=one or none)	2	1	0
Gross assessment of hearing by whispering a number followed by a letter into one ear whilst covering the contralateral ear (1). Asks patient to repeat the number and letter whispered (1).	2	1	0
Repeats test for the other ear		1	0
Selects the correct tuning fork (512Hz)		1	0
Performs Weber's test by vibrating the tuning fork and placing in the centre of the patient's head (1). Asks patient to describe which side the sound is loudest (1).	2	1	0
Performs Rinne's test by vibrating the tuning fork and holding it behind the ear on the mastoid process until the sound disappears (1). Then immediately holding it in front of the same ear (1).	2	1	0
Asks patient to state which position could they hear the sound louder		1	0
Repeats test for the other ear		1	0
Correct interpretation of Rinne's and Weber's tests to confirm sensorineural or conductive hearing loss		1	0
Performs Otoscopy:			
Checks the light source is working for the otoscope		1	0
Places a clean speculum on the end of the otoscope		1	0
Gently pulls the pinna of the patient's ear backwards to straighten the auditory canal and places tip of the speculum into the external acoustic canal (1) under direct vision (1) not whilst looking through the otoscope	2	1	0
Correctly holds the otoscope as if it was a pen or pencil (1) in the same hand of the side of the patient they are examining (1) (i.e. candidate holds otoscope in right hand when examining patient's right ear)	2	1	0
Comments on the skin of the auditory canal for wax, infection, foreign bodies		1	0
Comments on the tympanic membrane for light reflex, perforation, bulging drum, discharge, middle ear mass (2=comments on at least three aspects, 1=any two aspects)	2	1	0
Slowly withdraws the otoscope (1), disposes of the speculum and replaces with a new one (1)	2	1	0
Repeats the examination with the contralateral ear (2=does well, 1=does adequately but not slick enough to score full marks)	2	1	0
Treats patient with consideration throughout (2=does well, 1=adequately, 0=poorly or not done)	2	1	0
Gives clear instructions to patient during examination (2=does well, 1=adequately, 0=poorly or not done)	2	1	0
Examiner to ask: 'Please summarise your key findings.'			
Candidate presents key findings (1) in a fluent and logical manner (1)	2	1	0
Total Score			

Global Rating	1 Clear Fail	2 Borderline	3 Clear Pass	4 Very Good	5 Outstanding

Candidate Number:	University:
Date:	Year of Study:

RADIAL NERVE EXAMINATION

	Appropriate introduction (1=full name and role), checks patient's name (1)	**2**	**1**	**0**
	Explains procedure appropriately and obtains consent (2=does well, 1=adequately, 0=poorly or not done)	**2**	**1**	**0**
	Appropriately exposes patient (sleeves above the elbow and without any jewellery)		**1**	**0**
	Applies alcogel to hands before and after examination (1=both)		**1**	**0**
	Inspection (with patient's hands on a table):			
	Inspects for any asymmetry of the hands, swelling, pallor, cyanosis, bruising or blistering to suggest recent trauma (inspects both palmar and dorsal surfaces) (2=three observations, 1=two observations, 0=one or none)	**2**	**1**	**0**
	Assesses for vascular compromise by palpating for radial pulse (1) and checking capillary refill (1)	**2**	**1**	**0**
	Sensation:			
	Checks for sensation using light touch/cotton wool tip over the little finger, index finger and first web space on dorsal aspect of hand (2=checks sensation over all three peripheral nerve areas and confirms that it is only the radial nerve sensation that is lacking, 1=only checks in area supplied by radial nerve)	**2**	**1**	**0**
	Candidate to comment on area supplied by radial nerve (1) and whether this is intact or not (1)	**2**	**1**	**0**
	Movement (examines the muscles supplied by radial nerve):			
	Asks patient to extend elbows against resistance (triceps)	**2**	**1**	**0**
	Asks patient to flex elbow (1) against resistance (1) with hand held halfway between supination and pronation (Brachioradialis)	**2**	**1**	**0**
	Asks patient to extend wrist (1) with fingers extended against resistance (1) (extensor carpi radialis/ulnaris)	**2**	**1**	**0**
	Asks patient to turn wrist so palm facing ceiling (1) whilst resisting pronation (1) (supinator)	**2**	**1**	**0**
	Asks patient to extend fingers at metacarpophalangeal joint (1) against resistance (1) (extensor digitorum)	**2**	**1**	**0**
	Asks patient to extend thumb (1) against resistance (1) (extensor pollicis)	**2**	**1**	**0**
	Examines all the above actions bilaterally		**1**	**0**
	Treats patient with consideration throughout (2=does well, 1=adequately, 0=poorly or not done)	**2**	**1**	**0**
	Gives clear instructions to patient during examination (2=does well, 1=adequately, 0=poorly or not done)	**2**	**1**	**0**
	Examiner to ask: 'Please summarise your key findings.'			
	Candidate presents key findings (1) in a fluent and logical manner (1)	**2**	**1**	**0**
	Total Score			

Global Rating	**1** Clear Fail	**2** Borderline	**3** Clear Pass	**4** Very Good	**5** Outstanding

Candidate Number:	University:
Date:	Year of Study:

ULNAR NERVE EXAMINATION

	Appropriate introduction (1=full name and role), checks patient's name (1)	2	1	0
	Explains procedure appropriately and obtains consent (2=does well, 1=adequately, 0=poorly or not done)	2	1	0
	Appropriately exposes patient so face and limbs are clearly visible		1	0
	Applies alcogel to hands before and after examination (1=both)		1	0
	Inspection (with patient's hands on a table):			
	Inspects for any asymmetry of the hands, swelling, pallor, cyanosis, bruising or blistering to suggest recent trauma (inspects both palmar and dorsal surfaces) (2=three observations, 1=two observations, 0=one or none)	2	1	0
	Assesses for vascular compromise by palpating for radial pulse and checking capillary refill	2	1	0
	Inspect for 'clawing of the hand' flexion of the ring and little finger		1	0
	Wasting of the hypothenar muscles		1	0
	Sensation:			
	Checks for sensation using light touch/cotton wool tip over the little finger, index finger and first web space on dorsal aspect of hand (2=checks sensation over all three peripheral nerve areas and confirms that it is only the radial nerve sensation that is lacking, 1=only checks in area supplied by radial nerve)	2	1	0
	Candidate to comment on area supplied by ulnar nerve (1) and whether this is intact or not (1)	2	1	0
	Movement:			
	Assesses for power grip		1	0
	Asks patient to spread out fingers as wide as possible. Candidate to attempt to adduct the fingers (dorsal interossei) (2=all spaces between fingers tested, 1=only partly tested, 0=not at all).	2	1	0
	Asks patient to hold a piece of paper between each of the finger spaces whilst candidate attempts to pull paper out between the spaces (palmar interossei) (2=all spaces between fingers tested, 1=only partly tested, 0=not at all).	2	1	0
	Asks patient to adduct thumb (1) against resistance (1) (adductor pollicis)	2	1	0
	Assesses integrity of the lumbrical muscles by resisting flexion of the metacarpophalangeal joint (1) and resisting extension of the interphalangeal joints (1) (NB only the ulnar two lumbricals are innervated by the ulnar nerve)	2	1	0
	Performs all actions above bilaterally		1	0
	Special Tests:			
	Performs Froment's sign by asking patient to clutch a piece of paper between thumb and index finger, then attempting to pull paper away from the clasp of the patient (1). If this is not possible, candidate to suggest that there is ulnar nerve compromise (1).	2	1	0
	Treats patient with consideration throughout (2=does well, 1=adequately, 0=poorly or not done)	2	1	0
	Gives clear instructions to patient during examination (2=does well, 1=adequately, 0=poorly or not done)	2	1	0
	Examiner to ask: 'Please summarise your key findings.'			
	Candidate presents key findings (1) in a fluent and logical manner (1)	2	1	0
	Total Score			

Global Rating	1 Clear Fail	2 Borderline	3 Clear Pass	4 Very Good	5 Outstanding

Candidate Number:	University:
Date:	Year of Study:

MEDIAN NERVE EXAMINATION

Appropriate introduction (1=full name and role), checks patient's name (1)	2	1	0
Explains procedure appropriately and obtains consent (2=does well, 1=adequately, 0=poorly or not done)	2	1	0
Appropriately exposes patient so face and limbs are clearly visible		1	0
Applies alcogel to hands before and after examination (1=both)		1	0
Inspection:			
Inspects for any asymmetry of the hands, swelling, pallor, cyanosis, bruising or blistering to suggest recent trauma (inspects both palmar and dorsal surfaces) (2=three observations, 1=two observations, 0=one or none)	2	1	0
Assesses for vascular compromise by palpating for radial pulse (1) and checking capillary refill (1)	2	1	0
Comments upon any wasting of the thenar eminence		1	0
Sensation:			
Checks for sensation using light touch/cotton wool tip over the little finger, index finger and first web space on dorsal aspect of hand (2=checks sensation over all three peripheral nerve areas and confirms that it is only the radial nerve sensation that is lacking, 1=only checks in area supplied by radial nerve)	2	1	0
Candidate to comment on area supplied by median nerve (1) and whether this is intact or not (1)	2	1	0
Movement:			
Asks patient to abduct their thumb (1) against resistance (1) (abductor pollicis brevis) – the most important muscle to assess	2	1	0
Asks patient to touch their little finger with their thumb of the same hand and form a circle (1). Candidate to copy this action and intertwine their circle with patient in an attempt to pull and break the circle (1) (opponens pollicis).	2	1	0
Asks patient to flex thumb (1) against resistance (1) (flexor pollicis)	2	1	0
Assesses integrity of the lumbrical muscles by resisting flexion of the metacarpophalangeal joint (1) and resisting extension of the interphalangeal joints (1) (NB only the radial two lumbricals are innervated by the median nerve)	2	1	0
Examines all the above actions bilaterally		1	0
Special Tests:			
Performs Phalen's test by holding the wrists fully hyperflexed (1) for 1-2 minutes to reproduce symptoms of pain or tingling (1)	2	1	0
Performs Tinel's test by tapping over the carpal tunnel (1) and asks patient whether there is reproduction of symptoms of pain or tingling (1)	2	1	0
Treats patient with consideration throughout (2=does well, 1=adequately, 0=poorly or not done)	2	1	0
Gives clear instructions to patient during examination (2=does well, 1=adequately, 0=poorly or not done)	2	1	0
Examiner to ask: 'Please summarise your key findings.'			
Candidate presents key findings (1) in a fluent and logical manner (1)	2	1	0
Total Score			

Global Rating	1 Clear Fail	2 Borderline	3 Clear Pass	4 Very Good	5 Outstanding

Candidate Number:		University:	
Date:		Year of Study:	

ACROMEGALY

	Appropriate introduction (1=full name and role), checks patient's name (1)	**2**	**1**	**0**
	Explains procedure appropriately and obtains consent (2=does well, 1=adequately, 0=poorly or not done)	**2**	**1**	**0**
	Appropriately exposes patient (down to shorts or underwear)		**1**	**0**
	Applies alcogel to hands before and after examination (1=both)		**1**	**0**
	General inspection commenting on the prominence of the lower jaw (prognathism), supraorbital ridges, large nose, ears and tongue (2=any three aspects, 1=any two)	**2**	**1**	**0**
	Examines and comments on large hands (spade-like), thickened skin and prominent superficial veins (if present)		**1**	**0**
	Performs examination of visual fields (1) and comments on findings (1)	**2**	**1**	**0**
	Candidate asks for previous photographs of patient		**1**	**0**
	Candidate enquires after change in clothes/shoe/hat size		**1**	**0**
	Offers to perform a blood pressure measurement (examiner to state this is not required)		**1**	**0**
	Candidate to offer to perform a cardiovascular examination to determine whether the apex beat is displaced due to cardiomegaly (examiner to state this is not required)		**1**	**0**
	Candidate to offer to examine for median nerve palsy secondary to carpal tunnel syndrome (examiner to state this is not required)		**1**	**0**
	Treats patient with consideration throughout (2=does well, 1=adequately, 0=poorly or not done)	**2**	**1**	**0**
	Examiner to ask: 'What do you think is the most likely diagnosis?'			
	Candidate offers an appropriate diagnosis (1) and differential (1)	**2**	**1**	**0**
	Examiner to ask: 'How would you support your diagnosis?'			
	Candidate suggests to perform an oral glucose tolerance test (OGTT) with demonstrated elevated levels of insulin-like growth factor 1 (IGF-1) (1) in combination with a failure of growth hormone to suppress after an intake of oral glucose (1)	**2**	**1**	**0**
	Examiner to ask: 'What complications do you know of this condition?'			
	Candidate to suggest: blindness from an enlarged pituitary adenoma, hypertension, diabetes, sleep apnoea, carpal tunnel syndrome (2=three complications, 1=any two, 0=one or none)	**2**	**1**	**0**
	Examiner to ask: 'What further investigations could you suggest to rule out these complications?'			
	Candidate to suggest MRI pituitary gland, fasting glucose level, monitor blood pressure, overnight sleep test for PaCO2 levels (2= any three options, 1 = any two)	**2**	**1**	**0**
	Examiner to ask: 'What sort of treatment(s) would this patient require for his primary condition?'			
	Candidate to suggest referral to endocrinologist (1) and, if appropriate, neurosurgical referral for pituitary gland surgery (1)	**2**	**1**	**0**
	Total Score			

Global Rating	1 Clear Fail	2 Borderline	3 Clear Pass	4 Very Good	5 Outstanding

Candidate Number:	University:
Date:	Year of Study:

THYROID EXAMINATION

	Appropriate introduction (1=full name and role), checks patient's name (1)	2	1	0
	Explains procedure appropriately (1) and obtains consent (1)	2	1	0
	Applies alcogel to hands before and after examination (1=both)		1	0
	Ensures patient seated with access to examine from behind (1) and exposure of the neck (1)	2	1	0
	Observes patient from front commenting on any lumps/scars/swellings/general appearance e.g. dress, hair distribution etc. (2=comments on any three aspects, 1=any two)	2	1	0
	Asks patient to swallow (1) and also stick tongue out (1) whilst commenting on any lumps/swelling with ascend of thyroid	2	1	0
	Palpates thyroid gland from behind commenting on size (1) and symmetry (1)	2	1	0
	Palpates thyroid (+/- lump) on movement on swallowing (1) and protrusion of tongue (1)	2	1	0
	Palpates neck for cervical lymphadenopathy (2=does well, 1=adequately)	2	1	0
	Check for central located trachea		1	0
	Percusses for retrosternal extension over the upper sternum		1	0
	Auscultates over thyroid gland for bruit		1	0
	Examines eyes for lid retraction, lid lag, exophthalmus, ophthalmoplegia, periorbital odema, chemosis (2=comments on any three aspects, 1=any two)	2	1	0
	Examines hands to look for tremor and sweating, palmar erythema, vitiligo, onycolysis, thyroid acropachy (2=comments on any three aspects, 1=any two)	2	1	0
	Checks radial pulse and comments on rhythm and rate (1=both)		1	0
	Checks for pretibial myxoedema		1	0
	Checks for slow relaxation of reflexes (1) and proximal myopathy (1)	2	1	0
	Communicates with patient appropriately during examination		1	0
	Professional behaviour (gentle, watches for pain, maintains dignity)		1	0
	Thanks patient and allows patient to redress		1	0
	Examiner to ask: 'Please summarise your key findings.'			
	Candidate presents key findings (1) in a fluent and logical manner (1)	2	1	0
	Examiner to ask: 'What is your likely diagnosis?'			
	Candidate gives a reasonable diagnosis (1) and offers a differential (1)	2	1	0
	Examiner to ask: 'What further management would you suggest?'			
	Candidate offers biochemical investigations (1) and radiological examination (ultrasound scan) with or without FNA of lump (1)	2	1	0
	Examiner to ask: 'If the FNA reveals follicular cells, what would be the management and why?'			
	Candidate to suggest thyroid lobectomy (1) because unable to differentiate follicular adenoma from carcinoma on FNA results alone (1)	2	1	0
	Total Score			

Global Rating	**1** Clear Fail	**2** Borderline	**3** Clear Pass	**4** Very Good	**5** Outstanding

Candidate Number:	University:
Date:	Year of Study:

DERMATOLOGICAL EXAMINATION

		2	1	0
	Appropriate introduction (1=full name and role), checks patient's name (1)	2	1	0
	Explains procedure appropriately and obtains consent (2=does well, 1=adequately, 0=poorly or not done)	2	1	0
	Appropriately exposes patient whilst maintaining dignity		1	0
	Applies alcogel to hands before and after examination (1=both)		1	0
	Inspection of lesion commenting on site, size (using ruler), colour and shape (offer only 1 mark for any two and 2 marks for three or more observations)	2	1	0
	Palpates lesion commenting on consistency, surface, fixation, raised, tenderness (offer 1 mark for any two and 2 marks for three or more observations)	2	1	0
	Enquires whether patient has similar lesions elsewhere		1	0
	Examines local lymph nodes (2=does well, 1=adequately)	2	1	0
	Communicates with patient appropriately during examination		1	0
	Examines patient in a professional manner (gentle, maintains dignity, watches for pain)		1	0
	Thanks patient and leaves patient comfortable and covered		1	0
	Examiner to ask: 'Please summarise your key findings.'			
	Candidate presents key findings (2=key findings given comprehensively, 1=only some of the findings mentioned, 0=not given)	2	1	0
	Candidate presents findings in a fluent, logical manner		1	0
	Examiner to ask: 'What is your likely diagnosis?'			
	Candidate offers reasonable diagnosis (offer 1 mark for one diagnosis, 2 marks for giving reasonable differential)	2	1	0
	Examiner to ask: 'What further management do you recommend?'			
	Candidate offers further investigations (2= in detail, 1=poorly, 0=no suggestions)	2	1	0
	Candidate suggests possible treatment options (2=in detail, 1=poorly, 0=no suggestions)	2	1	0
	Total Score			

Global Rating	**1** Clear Fail	**2** Borderline	**3** Clear Pass	**4** Very Good	**5** Outstanding

Candidate Number:	University:
Date:	Year of Study:

RECTAL EXAMINATION

	Appropriate introduction (1=full name and role), checks patient's name (1)	2	1	0
	Explains procedure appropriately (2=does well, 1=adequately, 0=poorly or not done)	2	1	0
	Checks that patient consents to examination (1) and indicates that chaperone is required (1)	2	1	0
	Washes hands before and after examination (1=both)		1	0
	Prepares equipment – gloves, lubricating jelly and tissue		1	0
	Appropriately exposes patient (asks patient to remove underwear and trousers and offers blanket/gown to maintain dignity)		1	0
	Positions patient appropriately on the bed (in the left lateral decubitus with knees drawn to chest)		1	0
	Puts on gloves (1=both hands)		1	0
	Examines perianal region for skin tags, warts, fistulae, excoriation, prolapsed piles (2=any three signs, 1=two signs, 0=one or none)	2	1	0
	Applies lubricating gel to index finger		1	0
	Inserts index finger and performs a 360 degree sweep of the internal anal canal (1) examining the anterior, posterior and lateral walls (1)	2	1	0
	Palpates the prostate gland by identifying central sulcus and both lobes (1). Candidate to comment appropriately on size and shape of the gland (1).	2	1	0
	Asks patient to 'squeeze finger' (1) and comments on anal tone (1)	2	1	0
	After examination, thanks patient (1) and offers tissues, privacy to get dressed (1)	2	1	0
	Disposes of gloves in rubbish bag		1	0
	Candidate presents findings (1) in a logical and structured manner (1)	2	1	0
	Systematic and organised approach to examination		1	0
	Clear explanations to patient throughout procedure		1	0
	Maintains dignity throughout		1	0
	Simulated patient score (full marks if patient felt comfortable with candidate)	2	1	0
	Total Score			

Global Rating	1 Clear Fail	2 Borderline	3 Clear Pass	4 Very Good	5 Outstanding

Candidate		University:
Date:		Year of Study:

	Candidate Number:
	Date:

THE ALCOHOLIC PATIENT

		2	1	0
	Appropriate introduction (1=full name and role), checks patient's name (1)	2	1	0
	Explains procedure appropriately and obtains consent (2=does well, 1=adequately, 0=poorly or not done)	2	1	0
	Applies alcogel to hands before and after examination (1=both)		1	0
	Appropriately exposes patient		1	0
	Inspects from the end of the bed for jaundice, abdominal distension, spider naevi, caput medusa, resting tremor from acute withdrawal (2=three observations, 1=any two, 0=one or none)	2	1	0
	Examines hands for leuconychia, palmar erythema or Dupuytren's contracture		1	0
	Asks patient to bend both hands back to check for asterixis		1	0
	Examines eyes and comments on presence of anaemia, icterus, nystagmus, ophthalamoplegia (2=any two, 1=any one, 0=none)	2	1	0
	Cardiovascular			
	Offers to measure blood pressure (raised in heavy alcohol usage)		1	0
	Palpates for apex beat to determine presence of cardiomegaly		1	0
	Abdominal Examination			
	Palpates abdomen for hepatomegaly		1	0
	Assesses for fluid thrill (1) or shifting dullness (1) to determine presence of ascites	2	1	0
	Neurological Examination			
	Gross examination of power in upper (1) and lower limbs (1) (lost in central pontine myelinolysis)	2	1	0
	Gross examination of upper (1) and lower limb (1) sensation (lost in central pontine myelinolysis)	2	1	0
	Examines for loss of upper (1) and lower limb reflexes (1)	2	1	0
	Co-ordination – checks for heel-to-shin co-ordination in lower limbs and finger-to-nose test within the upper limbs bilaterally. (Ataxia is seen with cerebellar damage and Wernicke's encephalopathy.)	2	1	0
	Asks patient questions regarding orientation in time, place, person (2=all three aspects, 1=two aspects)	2	1	0
	Treats patient with consideration throughout (2=does well, 1=adequately, 0=poorly or not done)	2	1	0
	Gives clear instructions to patient during examination (2=does well, 1=adequately, 0=poorly or not done)	2	1	0
	Examiner to ask: 'Please summarise your key findings.'			
	Candidate presents key findings (1) in a fluent and logical manner (1)	2	1	0
	Examiner to ask: 'What health complications would you expect in a patient with chronic alcoholism?'			
	Candidate suggests hypertension, pancreatitis, Wernicke's encephalopathy, alcoholic dementia, liver cirrhosis, pernicious anaemia, malnutrition, vitamin B deficiency, hepatic carcinoma (2=any three, 1=any two, 0=one or none)	2	1	0
	Total Score			

Global Rating	1 Clear Fail	2 Borderline	3 Clear Pass	4 Very Good	5 Outstanding

Candidate Number:	University:
Date:	Year of Study:

BIMANUAL EXAMINATION

		2	1	0
	Appropriate introduction (1=full name and role), checks patient's name (1)	**2**	**1**	**0**
	Applies alcogel to hands before and after examination (1=both)		**1**	**0**
	Explains what bimanual examination will involve: One hand on abdomen (1) Will insert two fingers in vagina (1)	**2**	**1**	**0**
	Checks that patient consents to examination (1) and indicates that chaperone is required (1)	**2**	**1**	**0**
	Appropriately exposes patient (patient to remove underwear and trousers) and offers a gown or blanket to maintain dignity		**1**	**0**
	Positions patient on bed correctly (supine with a pillow) and instructs them to draw knees up, feet together and open legs		**1**	**0**
	Puts on gloves (1=on both hands)		**1**	**0**
	Inspects vulva: comments on presence/absence of e.g. warts, ulcers, inflammation, rashes, swelling, discharge (2=three or more, 1=two, 0=one or none)	**2**	**1**	**0**
	Lubricates fingers (examiner to stop candidate from using lubricant)		**1**	**0**
	Separates labia and inserts 2 fingers into vagina (1). Places other hand in correct position on abdomen (1).	**2**	**1**	**0**
	Comments correctly on position (1) and size (1) of uterus	**2**	**1**	**0**
	Comments on mobility of uterus		**1**	**0**
	Specifically checks with patient whether any tenderness/pain		**1**	**0**
	After examination, thanks patient (1) and offers tissues, privacy to get dressed (1)	**2**	**1**	**0**
	Disposes of gloves in rubbish bag		**1**	**0**
	Systematic and organised approach to examination	**2**	**1**	**0**
	Clear explanations to patient throughout procedure (2=does well, 1=vague instructions or mumbling to patient, 0=not done)	**2**	**1**	**0**
	Maintains dignity throughout		**1**	**0**
	Simulated patient score (full marks if patient felt comfortable with candidate)	**2**	**1**	**0**
	Total Score			

Global Rating	**1** Clear Fail	**2** Borderline	**3** Clear Pass	**4** Very Good	**5** Outstanding

Candidate Number:		University:	
Date:		Year of Study:	

SPECULUM EXAMINATION AND SWAB TAKING

	Appropriate introduction (1=full name and role), checks patient's name (1)	**2**	**1**	**0**
	Explains what a speculum examination will involve: passing a speculum into the vagina (1) and obtaining a sample of cells by insertion of a swab into the cervix (1)	**2**	**1**	**0**
	Checks that patient consents to examination (1) and indicates that chaperone is required (1)	**2**	**1**	**0**
	Appropriately exposes patient (patient to remove underwear and trousers) and offers a gown or blanket to maintain dignity		**1**	**0**
	Positions patient on bed correctly (supine with a pillow) and instructs them to draw knees up, feet together and open legs		**1**	**0**
	Washes hands (1) and wears appropriately sized gloves (1)	**2**	**1**	**0**
	Mentions need to warm speculum		**1**	**0**
	Checks speculum is clean and not damaged (1) and assembles parts together correctly (1)	**2**	**1**	**0**
	Inspects vulva: comments on presence/absence of e.g. warts, ulcers, inflammation, rashes, swelling, discharge (2=three or more, 1=two, 0=one or none)	**2**	**1**	**0**
	Lubricates speculum (examiner to stop candidate from using lubricant)		**1**	**0**
	Parts labia with left hand		**1**	**0**
	Inserts speculum (1) and opens correctly (open with handles then tighten screw) (1)	**2**	**1**	**0**
	Locates cervix (examiner to check cervix visible)		**1**	**0**
	Comments on normal appearance of cervix		**1**	**0**
	Removes swab from packet, maintaining sterility		**1**	**0**
	Correctly inserts endocervical swab		**1**	**0**
	Examiner to ask: 'Where have you taken swab from?'			
	1=Swab taken from endocervix, 0=any other answer		**1**	**0**
	Correctly puts swab into transport medium (puts in medium tube and puts cap back on)		**1**	**0**
	Removes speculum correctly (1) disposes into correct disposal box (1)	**2**	**1**	**0**
	Labels swab tube with patient's name, d.o.b, date of collection, type of swab taken (2=all, 0=less than all)	**2**	**1**	**0**
	After examination, thanks patient (1) and offers tissues, privacy to get dressed (1)	**2**	**1**	**0**
	Disposes of gloves in rubbish bag (1). Washes hands (1).	**2**	**1**	**0**
	Systematic and organised approach to examination	**2**	**1**	**0**
	Clear explanations to patient throughout procedure (2=does well, 1=vague instructions or mumbling to patient, 0 = not done)	**2**	**1**	**0**
	Maintains dignity throughout		**1**	**0**
	Simulated patient score (2=I felt comfortable with this candidate)	**2**	**1**	**0**
	Total Score			

Global Rating	**1** Clear Fail	**2** Borderline	**3** Clear Pass	**4** Very Good	**5** Outstanding

CHAPTER 12: PRACTICAL SKILLS

Written by Dr. S. Shelmerdine

- Phlebotomy
- Intravenous Cannulation
- Intravenous Injection
- Blood Transfusion
- Setting up an Intravenous Infusion of Normal Saline
- Nasogastric Tube Insertion
- Male Catheterisation

THE STATIONS

STATION 1
Time allowed: 5 minutes

You are a junior doctor working in the Accident and Emergency department.

Miss Ursula James (DOB: 2/12/1981, Hosp No: 213415) is a young patient who has attended the department with abdominal pain. You suspect the patient has got either gallstones or pancreatitis and need to send off a set of bloods.

Please decide which blood tests you should send for, obtain consent from the patient and perform phlebotomy on the patient using the 'Vacutainer' device. The following blood form is provided for you to complete.

ST. NOSUCH HOSPITAL – BLOOD REQUEST FORM

Patient Forename: _____

Patient Surname: _____

DOB: _____

Hospital Number: _____

Blood Tests Required: _____

Clinical Indication:

Doctor Signature: _____

Doctor Bleep: _____

STATION 2
Time allowed: 5 minutes

You are a junior doctor working in the Accident and Emergency department.

Mr Jack Brewer, a policeman, has been in a road traffic accident after a high speed car chase and is in the resuscitation area of the department. He is responsive but complaining of back and chest pains. There are many doctors and nurses around him who are examining him and attaching him to monitors. You have been asked to get intravenous access so that the nurse can start fluids.

Please choose the most appropriate sized cannula for this situation, obtain consent and perform intravenous cannulation on the patient.

STATION 3
Time allowed: 5 minutes

You are a junior doctor working in the surgical department.

Mrs Chewy Long is two days post right hemicolectomy and has been feeling nauseated and dizzy as a result of her pain medication. You have decided to administer her some intravenous cyclizine to help alleviate these symptoms. She already has a cannula in situ.

Please administer the correct dose of cyclizine prescribed below for Mrs Long.

CHAPTER 13: DATA INTERPRETATION

Written by Mr. J. Lynch

- Chest X-rays
- Abdominal X-rays
- Electrocardiograms (ECGs)
- Arterial Blood Gas interpretation (ABGs)
- Pathology Reports
- Blood Test Results
- Urine Dipstick Results

THE STATIONS

STATION 1
Time allowed: 7 minutes

Scenario 1

You are a junior doctor working in A&E. A 34 year old man presents with sudden onset shortness of breath. His CXR reveals:

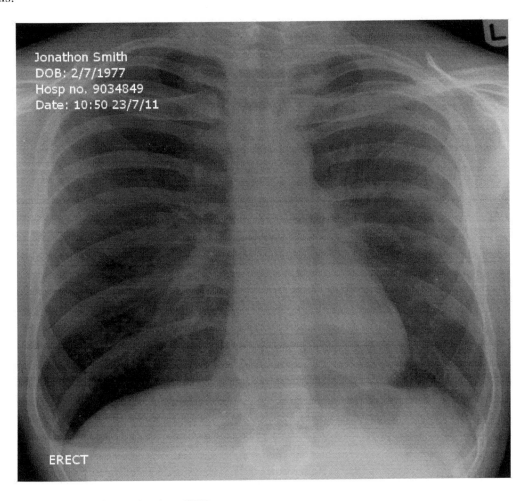

1. Describe your system for reviewing CXRs.
2. Comment on the abnormalities found on this CXR.
3. What is the usual aetiology, and what risk factors predispose?
4. What management plan would you suggest?
5. Under what circumstances would you treat this condition conservatively?

DATA INTERPRETATION

Candidate Number:	University:
Date:	Year of Study:

STATION 1 – INTERPRETATION OF A CHEST X-RAY

Scenario 1 – Examiner to ask: 'Describe your system for reviewing CXRs.'				
Checks name and age of patient			1	0
Notes date of X-ray (1) and type of film i.e. chest X-ray (1)		2	1	0
Identifies X-ray as PA (1), identifies X-ray is erect (1)		2	1	0
Comments on penetration, rotation and inspiration			1	0
Inspects the lungs (1) and comments on trachea (1)		2	1	0
Inspects the cardiac silhouette (1) and comments on cardiothoracic ratio (1)		2	1	0
Inspects the soft tissue (1) and skeleton (1)		2	1	0
Inspects the hila			1	0
Inspects the diaphragm, costophrenic angles (1) and comments on any free air below the diaphragm (1)		2	1	0
Examiner to ask: 'Comment on the abnormalities present in this CXR.' No tracheal/mediastinal shift (1), lack of lung markings in the right peripheral lung field (1) consistent with a spontaneous pneumothorax		2	1	0
Examiner to ask: 'What are the usual aetiologies and what risk factors predispose to pneumothoraces?' Congenital bleb/idiopathic spontaneous (1) Risk factors: asthma/COPD, tall thin habitus, male, connective tissue disorders, smoking (states at least two risk factors for one mark)		2	1	0
Examiner to ask: 'What management plan would you suggest?' Oxygen and saturation monitoring; needle decompression of pneumothorax; chest drain (2=all three suggestions, 1=any two suggestions, 0=one or none)		2	1	0
Examiner to ask: 'Under what circumstances would you treat this condition conservatively?' (see the British Thoracic Guidelines for comprehensive management) If patient is breathless and/or > 2 cm rim of air on CXR then treat (1), otherwise consider discharge and follow-up CXR of patient (1)		2	1	0
Scenario 2 – Examiner to ask:				
'What does the CXR show?' Right middle zone opacification (1) consistent with consolidation/infection (1)		2	1	0
'Give 3 necessary investigations.' Blood tests (FBC, U&E, CRP), ABG, blood cultures, sputum culture (2=any three suggestions, 1=any two suggestions, 0=one or none)		2	1	0
'What parameters might help you decide the severity of this illness?' CURB-65 – confusion < 8 AMT, urea > 7, respiratory rate > 30, blood pressure < 90, age >=65 (offer 1 mark for stating the criteria and 2 marks for criteria including values)		2	1	0
'If he is to be admitted, what 3 treatments will he have?' Oxygen, intravenous antibiotics, IV fluids (2=three suggestions, 1=two suggestions, 0=one or none)		2	1	0
Total Score				

Global Rating	1 Clear Fail	2 Borderline	3 Clear Pass	4 Very Good	5 Outstanding

Candidate Number:		University:	
Date:		Year of Study:	

STATION 2 – INTERPRETATION OF AN ABDOMINAL X-RAY

	Scenario 1 – Examiner to ask:			
	'What condition does this AXR show?' Small bowel (1) obstruction (1)	**2**	**1**	**0**
	'Give 3 features that support your diagnosis.' Centrally placed loops of bowel, diameter of bowel is > 3 cm, presence of valvulae conniventes (2=all three features, 1=two features, 0=one or none)	**2**	**1**	**0**
	'What is the typical presentation?' Colicky abdominal pain, early vomiting, bloating, absolute constipation in later stages (2=any three features, 1=two features, 0=one or none)	**2**	**1**	**0**
	'What features would you expect to find on examination?' Distended abdomen; high pitched tinkling bowel sounds; empty rectum; possible hernia or abdominal mass (2=any three suggestions, 1=any two suggestions, 0=one or none)	**2**	**1**	**0**
	'Give 3 of the commonest causes.' Adhesions secondary to intra-abdominal surgery, hernias, tumours and Crohn's disease secondary to strictures (2=any three suggestions, 1=any two suggestions, 0=one or none)	**2**	**1**	**0**
	'What conservative treatment would you initiate?' Intravenous fluids and NG tube		**1**	**0**
	'What radiographic sign describes air visible on both sides of the bowel wall after perforation or surgery?' Rigler's sign		**1**	**0**
	Scenario 2 – Examiner to ask:			
	'What evidence on this radiograph is there that this patient has had surgery?' Surgical staples (1), right hip replacement (1)	**2**	**1**	**0**
	'Describe the other abnormalities present.' Large and small bowel dilatation		**1**	**0**
	'What is the likely cause?' Postoperative paralytic ileus		**1**	**0**
	'What would you expect to hear on auscultation of the abdomen?' Absent or sluggish bowel sounds		**1**	**0**
	'What factors predispose to this condition?' Increased surgical operating time; electrolyte imbalance (especially hypokalaemia), hypothyroidism; medications such as opiates (2=any three suggestions, 1=any two suggestions, 0=one or none)	**2**	**1**	**0**
	Total Score			

Global Rating	**1** Clear Fail	**2** Borderline	**3** Clear Pass	**4** Very Good	**5** Outstanding

Candidate Number:		University:	
Date:		Year of Study:	

STATION 3 – ECG INTERPRETATION

	Part 1 – Examiner to ask: 'Please describe your system for interpreting ECGs.'			
	Confirms patient's name and date of birth (1), date and time of investigation (1)	**2**	**1**	**0**
	Notes patient symptoms		**1**	**0**
	Checks calibration of the ECG – strip recorded at a setting of 25 mm/s		**1**	**0**
	Comments on rate, rhythm and axis		**1**	**0**
	Comments on morphology of the QRS complex: ST elevation		**1**	**0**
	Comments on ST segment (elevation anterior leads), PR interval (normal), QT interval (normal), T waves (inverted in III, aVR, aVF)		**1**	**0**
	'Please calculate the rate, rhythm and axis.'			
	Calculates rate: 100 bpm		**1**	**0**
	Comments of rhythm: sinus rhythm		**1**	**0**
	Determines axis: left deviated		**1**	**0**
	'Please give a diagnosis.' Candidate suggests ST-elevation myocardial infarction (1) of anterioseptal leads (1)	**2**	**1**	**0**
	'How would you investigate this patient?' 12 hour troponin (1), serial ECGs (1)	**2**	**1**	**0**
	'Outline the management of this patient.' Requires thrombolysis or angioplasty, anticoagulation (clopidogrel, aspirin), nitroglycerins, morphine, oxygen (2=any three suggestions, 1=any two suggestions, 0=one or none)	**2**	**1**	**0**
	Part 2 – Examiner to ask:			
	'Please describe this rhythm and give a diagnosis.' Irregularly, irregular rhythm (1), atrial fibrillation (1)	**2**	**1**	**0**
	'How would you treat this patient?' Chemical cardioversion (using amiodarone) or rate control (using digoxin or beta-blocker medication), anticoagulation (using warfarin) (2=all three suggestions, 1=any two suggestions, 0=one or none)	**2**	**1**	**0**
	Part 3 – Examiner to ask:			
	'How would you treat this patient?' DC Cardioversion		**1**	**0**
	Total Score			

Global Rating	**1** Clear Fail	**2** Borderline	**3** Clear Pass	**4** Very Good	**5** Outstanding

Candidate Number:	University:
Date:	Year of Study:

STATION 4 – ARTERIAL BLOOD GAS INTERPRETATION

	Scenario 1 – Examiner to ask:			
	'What type of respiratory failure does she have?' Type II		1	0
	'What type of acid-base disturbance does she have?' Respiratory acidosis (1) with partial metabolic compensation (1)	2	1	0
	'How would you treat this patient?' Nebulisers, oxygen (high flow), steroids, intravenous antibiotics (2=any three suggestions, 1=any two suggestions, 0=one or none)	2	1	0
	Scenario 2 – Examiner to ask:			
	'What type of acid-base disturbance does he have?' Metabolic acidosis (1) with partial respiratory compensation (1)	2	1	0
	'Explain the measured pO2.' The patient is hyperventilating to bring down the CO2 to compensate for the acidosis, and this has the side-effect of increasing the O2		1	0
	'Which electrolyte is it most important to measure in this situation?' Potassium is likely to rise in renal failure (1) and can cause cardiac arrhythmias (1)	2	1	0
	'What are the 3 most common causes for chronic kidney disease?' Hypertension, diabetes, glomerulonephritis (2=three suggestions, 1=any two suggestions, 0=one or none)	2	1	0
	Scenario 3 – Examiner to ask:			
	'What is the likely diagnosis and what is the first-line investigation?' Acute pancreatitis (1), amylase or lipase (1)	2	1	0
	'What type of acid-base disturbance does he have?' Metabolic acidosis		1	0
	'Calculate the anion gap.' ($[Na - (Cl + HCO3)]=24$)		1	0
	'Give 3 other common causes for raised anion gap.' Lactic acidosis, ketoacidosis, toxins (such as ethylene glycol, methanol, aspirin, cyanide), renal failure (2=any three suggestions, 1=any two suggestions, 0=one or none)	2	1	0
	Total Score			

Global Rating	**1** Clear Fail	**2** Borderline	**3** Clear Pass	**4** Very Good	**5** Outstanding

Candidate Number:		University:
Date:		Year of Study:

STATION 5 – INTERPRETATION OF BLOOD RESULTS

	Scenario 1 – Examiner to ask:			
	'Give 3 possible causes for his electrolyte abnormalities.' Not absorbing potassium through the gut; vomiting; inadequate oral intake (2=all three suggestions, 1=two suggestions, 0=one or none)	**2**	**1**	**0**
	'Explain his renal function tests.' Hypovolaemic renal failure (1) due to vomiting and inadequate fluid absorption from the gut (1)	**2**	**1**	**0**
	'Which of his blood tests may be exacerbating his condition?' Low potassium decreases gut motility		**1**	**0**
	'What would you prescribe to help this condition?' The patient requires IV potassium		**1**	**0**
	Scenario 2 – Examiner to ask:			
	'Describe 3 of the most likely causes for this lady's electrolyte disorder.' Syndrome of Inappropriate ADH (SIADH); dehydration due to infection; medications (especially diuretics), renal disease (2=any three suggestions, 1=any two suggestions, 0=one or none)	**2**	**1**	**0**
	'What is the most severe complication of this disorder?' Neurologic complications due to brain oedema (this is caused by intracerebral osmotic fluid shifts)		**1**	**0**
	'What is the most likely diagnosis now?' SIADH		**1**	**0**
	'What would you expect the urine osmolality to be?' It is likely to be high (>100 mOsm)		**1**	**0**
	'Why does this condition cause hyponatraemia?' There is an excess (and inappropriate) level of ADH (1), which acts on the cortical and medullary collecting tubules in the kidneys to increase absorption causing a dilutional hyponatraemia (1)	**2**	**1**	**0**
	'What are the treatment options for this patient?' Fluid restriction, furosemide, hypertonic saline (2=three suggestions, 1=two suggestions, 0=one or none)	**2**	**1**	**0**
	'What complication is she experiencing?' Over rapid correction of the hyponatraemia is causing rapid shifts in osmolality in the brain (1) and this may lead to central pontine myelinosis (1)	**2**	**1**	**0**
	'What is the first thing that should be done to prevent this developing?' Stop the hypertonic saline		**1**	**0**
	Total Score			

Global Rating	**1** Clear Fail	**2** Borderline	**3** Clear Pass	**4** Very Good	**5** Outstanding

Candidate Number:	University:
Date:	Year of Study:

STATION 8 – INTERPRETATION OF URINE DIPSTICK

Scenario 1 – Examiner to ask:			
'What is the most likely diagnosis?' Urinary tract infection		1	0
'Give 3 predisposing risk factors.' Female gender, age, increased sexual activity, presence of long term urinary catheters, anatomical abnormalities (i.e. vesicoureteric reflux) immunosuppression (e.g. steroid usage, diabetes) (2=any three suggestions, 1=any two suggestions)	2	1	0
'What is the mechanism by which the urine dip is positive for nitrites?' Some bacteria have the enzyme nitrate reductase which convert nitrates in to nitrites		1	0
'What common organisms are responsible?' Escherichia coli, proteus mirabilis, staphylococcus saprophyticus (2=all three suggestions, 1=any two suggestions, 0=one or none)	2	1	0
'Suggest a suitable first-line antibiotic for treatment.' Trimethoprim, nitrofurantoin, amoxicillin and in later stages or with a history of known antibiotic resistance, co-amoxiclav (2=any two suggestions, 1=any one suggestions, 0=none)	2	1	0
'If the patient became agitated to the extent that you are worried they may be a danger to themselves or others, what medication might you consider prescribing?' Haloperidol or lorazepam		1	0
Scenario 2 – Examiner to ask:			
'What is the most likely diagnosis?' Renal colic/renal stone/ureteric colic		1	0
'What important differential should be excluded, and how is this done?' Abdominal aortic aneurysm needs excluding (1) Investigations for determining this differential include either ultrasound or CT (1)	2	1	0
'What investigation would you perform to confirm your diagnosis?' KUB radiograph with intravenous urogram (IVU) or a CT KUB		1	0
'Give 2 risk factors for this condition.' Anatomical abnormalities (e.g. horseshoe kidney), gout, hyperparathyroidism, dehydration, metabolic abnormalities increasing solute in the urine (e.g. hypercalciuria), cystinuria, drugs (e.g. thiazides), deficiency of citrate in the urine (2=any two suggestions, 1=any one suggestions, 0=none)	2	1	0
'What medical management would you institute?' Analgesia (i.e. paracetamol, rectal diclofenac), alpha-adrenergic blocker (e.g. tamsulosin), hydration (2=any three suggestions, 1=any two suggestions, 0=any one or none)	2	1	0
'What could explain this clinical picture and results?' Obstructed, infected renal system		1	0
'What is the acute treatment for this?' To relieve the obstructed system and allow drainage/treatment of infection by insertion of a nephrostomy (1) or surgical stone retrieval (either antegrade or retrograde ureteroscopy) (1) under antibiotic cover	2	1	0
Total Score			

Global Rating	1 Clear Fail	2 Borderline	3 Clear Pass	4 Very Good	5 Outstanding